Internal Medicine and the Structures of Modern Medical Science

THE UNIVERSITY OF IOWA, 1870–1990

Internal Medicine
and the Structures of
Modern Medical Science

THE UNIVERSITY OF IOWA, 1870–1990

Lee Anderson

WITH A PROLOGUE BY
François M. Abboud

IOWA STATE UNIVERSITY PRESS / AMES

To Kathy, my friend and my wife,
without whom nothing ever seems to get done.

LEE ANDERSON, an Iowa native, received his bachelor's degree in pharmacy and his Ph.D. in history from the University of Iowa. He practiced pharmacy in Virginia and taught history at Nebraska Wesleyan University and the University of Iowa before founding a public history firm, A&P Historical Resources, in Iowa City with his wife, Kathy Penningroth. Anderson's books, articles, and current research span the history of medicine, pharmacy, and nursing.

© 1996 Iowa State University Press, Ames, Iowa 50014

∞ Printed on acid-free paper in the United States of America

First edition, 1996

Parts of chapters 1 and 2 first appeared in *The Pharos* 55 (1992); *The Annals of Iowa* 51 (1992); and in the *Journal of the History of Medicine and Allied Sciences* 46 (1991). They appear here by kind permission of the publishers.

Library of Congress Cataloging-in-Publication Data

Anderson, Lee
 Internal medicine and the structures of modern medical science: the University of Iowa, 1870–1990 / Lee Anderson. — 1st ed.
  p.   cm.
 Includes bibliographical references and index.
 ISBN 0-8138-2332-3 (alk. paper)
 1. University of Iowa. Dept. of Internal Medicine—History. I. Title.
 [DNLM: 1. University of Iowa. Dept. of Internal Medicine. 2. Internal Medicine—history—Iowa.
3. Education, Medical—history—Iowa. WZ 70 AI8 A5i 1996]
 R747.I683375A53 1996
 616'.009777'655—dc20
 DNLM/DLC
 for Library of Congress   95-26592

CONTENTS

Photos appear after pages 84, 152, 246.

PROLOGUE

The Challenge of Professionalism

O
N Wednesday, March 27, 1996, the main headline on the front page of the *Iowa City Press Citizen* read, "UI Cuts to Affect 121 Jobs," and *The Daily Iowan* announced, "UIHC Cutbacks Start This Week." This is a landmark event, perhaps not in magnitude, considering the fact that University of Iowa Hospitals employ more than 7,600 individuals, but in what it actually represents: an unprecedented urgency to control expenses in the face of shrinking revenues for our university-owned teaching hospital. Business and government are no longer willing to support the national health care expense budget that has risen from $500 billion to almost $1 trillion within the last ten years. Health care costs are estimated to have reached approximately 14 percent of the gross national product. A major fiscal reform of our health care system is taking place.

I have been in academic medicine for forty-one years, at Iowa for the last thirty-six years, and am now in my twentieth year as chairman of the Department of Internal Medicine. We all have enormous pride in the extraordinary accomplishments of our department, our College of Medicine, and our Hospitals and Clinics. I hold a sense of deep gratitude for the privilege of being part of and serving a magnificent patient care, education, and research complex, which has been recognized as the best academic environment for medical education in the country.

The story of our department began in 1870. Looking back, I can discern three distinct cycles of progress in Iowa medicine that parallel American medicine. The first began in the latter part of the nineteenth century and the first half of the twentieth century. That period saw our medical school transformed from a "trade school" to a "medical science center." The second cycle, which covers the golden age of biomedical research, and the third cycle—the explosion of tertiary care and medical technology, fueled by the federal dollar and the insurance industry—bring us to the last decade of this century. We are now entering a fourth cycle. The events unfolding in the 1990s are viewed with disillusionment, anxiety, and even shock. Yet they are not at all unique to the University of Iowa. In fact, Iowa has been relatively sheltered from a corporate seizure of the health care system which has been raging through most academic medical centers. Tremors of economic uncertainties are shaking the roots of our values and the branches of our mission.

CORPORATE INVASION OF MEDICAL SCIENCE CENTERS

This assault began just as Lee Anderson, the author of this extremely well researched history of our Department of Internal Medicine, laid down his pen. Anderson presents an informative and erudite analysis of the evolution of internal medicine and the structures of modern medical science from 1870 to 1990. His treatise should help us understand how we came to this point and, hopefully, give us insight into the future. In his Epilogue, Anderson refers prophetically to the "risk [of] losing control of the practice of medicine to government agencies, the health insurance industry, and the growing roster of other economic and political interests." He ends his Epilogue with the following sentence: "Now, however, thanks to the extraordinary exertions of the past three decades, the department looks toward its future from an acknowledged position of national leadership, and perhaps the chief question for the future is whether it can combine that newfound prominence in scientific research with its traditional strengths in the human dimensions in medicine."

Anderson was concerned about the preservation of the human dimensions of medicine in the face of a growing scientific focus. I believe we are confronted now with the added challenge of preserving our professionalism despite a tightening corporate clutch on our medical centers. Health Maintenance Organizations (HMO's), driven by profit, promise comprehensive health services at reduced premiums but are accused of restricting expensive care of patients who need it.[1] Physicians employed by HMO's are faced with a dilemma. On one side, the cost-cutting mentality of their employers restricts expensive but necessary diagnostic and therapeutic interventions. On the other, their solemn covenant requires that their patients' needs come first. Academic medical centers are viewed as expensive providers of tertiary care. Their

---

[1] *The New York Times,* Vol. CXLV, no. 50:378, March 26, 1996, "H.M.O.'s in Tucson May Offer a Model for Medicare's Future."

subspecialties are often excluded from participating in the care of patients enrolled in HMO's without a significant reduction in their costs. A major part of those costs is for the support of the educational and research missions which have been subsidized incrementally by revenues from services to patients since the 1970s. Many universities have divested themselves of their teaching hospitals, transferring them to health management corporations to avoid bankruptcy, with the pious but unrealistic hope that the new corporate magnates will altruistically see the great societal good in supporting their academic medical centers.

In Iowa City we have been fortunate, thus far, that the new cycle manifests itself not in a corporate takeover, but in the adoption of corporate principles in the management of the health science enterprise. Some view this phase as a fundamental change in our "academic culture." I want us to preserve the ideals and professional values of our culture, but acquire a business sense and a management style that will allow us to survive. As a department and a College of Medicine, we have ended 120 years of our history with the glorious success described in the last chapter as "The Challenge of Excellence." We have attained prominence in scientific research and have been listed among the top ten departments in federal funding. Right in the middle of the cornfields of Iowa, we have gained national recognition as the largest university-owned hospital in the nation. We have an excellent record in medical education and postgraduate training. Where will the corporate invasion and the challenge to our professionalism take us?

Our new leaders, R. Edward Howell, Hospital Director, and Robert P. Kelch, M.D., Dean of the College of Medicine, have been at Iowa now for about a year and a half. They have joined hands in the utilization of resources, in the control of expenses, and in planning for our future patient care initiatives. They have established a "Corporate Leadership Group" to manage the business of our College of Medicine and University Hospitals and Clinics as a joint "Clinical Enterprise." Their challenge, our challenge, and the challenge of every academic medical center is to preserve our basic mission as we adopt management styles necessary for fiscal solvency. Embracing corporate principles is sound, though the real crisis may not be one of financial survival, but rather one of the survival of professionalism. Some wonder whether we can serve two masters.

This issue has been the subject of numerous editorials. The most recent one was on March 15 in *Annals of Internal Medicine* entitled, "The Patient-Physician Covenant: An Affirmation of Asklepios." The authors find it necessary to proclaim once again (as Hippocrates did more than 2,000 years ago) that "Medicine is, at its center, a moral enterprise grounded in a covenant of trust. ... Our first obligation must be to serve the good of those persons who seek our help and trust us to provide it. Physicians, as physicians, are not, and must never be, commercial entrepreneurs, gateclosers or agents of fiscal policy that runs counter to our trust."[2]

We certainly need to accept a business approach that emphasizes institutional priorities, efficiency, and austerity. To this end, we have reduced our UIHC bed capacity by 25 percent to cut inpatient costs and expanded and restructured our ambulatory services. We have established a non-tenure clinician-educator track for our faculty, and revised our practice plan to include "clinical incentives." We have participated in managed care. We now hold equity in an integrated health care delivery system in the state, have established a limited HMO, and are contracting for the development of a network of "providers." Our goal is to maintain the flow of patients essential for our educational mission. We wonder, what impact will these evolutions have on our institutional character and mission? As we support our deans, hospital directors, and executive officers in these academic-business ventures, we the faculty should keep the bush of our traditional academic-professional values burning brightly to light the road. We must survive despite corporate greed.

How will this fourth cycle unfold? We may have to wait another ten or twenty years for a historical update to find an answer to those questions. For the sake of our patients, our covenant, and our mission, I hope this fourth cycle will unfold into as glorious an outcome as the previous three.

In this history you will read how three different cycles evolved and overlapped since 1870, bringing us to the beginning of this last decade of the millennium.

FROM TRADE SCHOOLS TO MEDICAL SCIENCE CENTERS

The first cycle was one of transition from a trade school to a medical science center. At Iowa, it took forty years from 1870 to 1910 before the transition could even begin. It spanned the terms of four chairs, beginning with William S. Robertson, the first chair (1870–87) of the Department of Internal Medicine (then referred to as the Department of Theory and Practice of Medicine); followed by the chairmanship of William D. Middleton (1887–91); Lawrence Littig (1891–1903); and finally, Walter Bierring (1903–10). Lee Anderson addresses that period in the first chapter entitled "The Emergence of Internal Medicine." He describes the contributions of these individuals as they struggled to establish a credible educational program in the College of Medicine. Despite a genuine commitment to education, their efforts seemed to come to naught and

---

[2]Cassel, C. K.: The Patient-Physician Covenant: An Affirmation of Asklepios. *Annals of Internal Medicine,* 124(6):604, 1996.

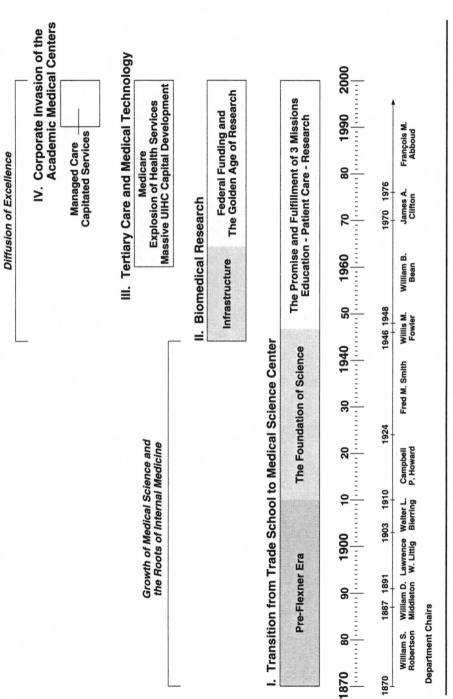

Cycles of evolution of academic internal medicine at the University of Iowa.

culminated disastrously in the Flexner indictment. In an entertaining account, Anderson reflects on the Abraham Flexner visit to Iowa City in April of 1909 that took eight hours and fifteen minutes:

> Flexner arrived in Iowa City at 4:00 P.M. and departed at 12:15 A.M. the following morning. When challenged about the brevity of his inspection tours, Flexner was fond of quoting a favorite anecdote: "You don't need to eat a whole sheep to know it's tainted." ... He did not like what he saw ... contending that "the hospital is, in its teaching aspects, headless" ... furthermore, "the present clinical department is on a high school basis." ... All in all, in Flexner's view, it was arguable whether or not the school was worth salvaging. (p. 20)

Flexner's prediction that "this small inland residential community" may not be worth salvaging was wrong. The transition from a trade school to one of the most prominent academic medical centers has occurred, and eighty-six years after Flexner left Iowa City our success story continues.

THE GOLDEN AGE OF MEDICAL RESEARCH

Although the seed of this golden age of medical research may have been planted by the fifth and sixth chairmen of medicine [Campbell Palmer Howard (1910–24) and Fred M. Smith (1924–46)], it took almost fifty years through the Depression and World War II for that seed to germinate. Howard and Smith were committed to scientific excellence. Both were physician-scientists pledged not only to patient care and education but also to research. The three-legged stool was conceived, but it needed the convergence of science, medical technology, and private and federal support to build it. Campbell Palmer Howard was a protégé of Sir William Osler and he was Osler's godson. He came from McGill University upon the advice of Osler and charted a scientific direction for both the Department of Internal Medicine and the College of Medicine. He returned to Montréal in 1924 and was elected member of the American Society for Clinical Investigation (ASCI) and president of the Association of American Physicians (AAP) in 1930. Fred M. Smith's tenure as department chair was the longest since the school's beginning. He served for twenty-two years, was a member of both the ASCI and the AAP, and was considered an inspiring leader in scientific medicine.

Under the leadership of Howard, research became part of the departmental mission. The Central Interurban Club for the exchange of research among academic physicians in the Midwest was established and would later become the current Central Society for Clinical Research. A milestone of that period was the

Rockefeller Foundation matching gift of $1,125,000 made on December 7, 1922, for a new University Hospital.

Anderson reflects on the period from 1929–1945 as one of hardship, Depression, and war. Yet, this was also the time of early development of the scientific base of the clinical subspecialties of internal medicine, and the establishment of residency training programs and the specialty boards in internal medicine. He relates the exploits and recognitions of some faculty members during the war years. Notable among those were the contributions of Elmer DeGowin and Robert Hardin to storage and preservation of blood and to blood banking. Hardin's efforts had a significant impact on the decision to airlift large quantities of preserved blood from the United States to Europe. During that same period Anderson laments a decline in facilities and programs in academic medicine. The Depression and war years took their toll. The hope of a new academic dawn was soon to be fulfilled, however.

In the 1950s and 1960s, the research programs in several research-oriented medical schools progressed at an unbelievable pace. It became apparent that the medical education enterprise would benefit enormously not just from the scientific advances and concepts that permeated the educational system but also from the financial support that was provided by the federal government through the National Institutes of Health (NIH). For a couple of decades, it seemed as though the NIH coffers would expand endlessly. Our medical education systems and the financial stability of our medical schools depended on the federal research dollar. Some schools, including Iowa, worried that federal "soft money" might too rapidly become a major source of funding of education and would in time put the educational enterprise in jeopardy. Others more visionary and entrepreneurial viewed the federal support of research and education as an opportunity for strengthening both the scholarly and fiscal bases of the medical centers. They recruited faculty driven by scientific curiosity and a desire for the academic rewards and recognition that came with NIH grants.

The period from 1945–1960 was one of opportunity and growth. The momentum for the creation of a major research complex took much longer to build at Iowa than at many other centers. Although the infrastructure for research was being developed, our department and medical school did not emerge as a potential powerhouse for research until the latter part of the tenure of William B. Bean. In the meantime, several state schools (such as the University of California in San Francisco, the University of Washington in Seattle, and Southwestern Medical School in Dallas) gained enormous academic prestige and recognition rivaling the private eastern schools. In each of these universities, the faculty of the departments of internal medicine were leading a research effort which encompassed not only clinical and patient-oriented research but also basic scientific research. The "indirect cost" of the federal grants represented a major financial resource for the entire university.

William B. Bean was appointed in 1948 as the eighth chairman following the brief appointment of Willis S. Fowler as acting chair for two years. It quickly became evident that Bean was facing major political, organizational, and recruitment challenges that would delay the "Golden Age of Medical Research" from reaching Iowa until the 1970s. Upon his arrival, Bean had to implement the newly established faculty practice plan, which was slandered by some as "socialized medicine." In addition, a graduating class of only fifty-seven students in 1948 alarmed the state legislature and the state medical society. Anderson notes that there was a common opinion among private practitioners of that era that those who did research, i.e., academic physicians at the university, were just a degree above "the moron" while many academic physicians thought that "only doctors of poor mentality . . . were practicing on the outside." Clearly, the political climate was, to say the least, not ripe for a focus on research and federal funding. Bean's priorities had to be increased enrollment, the creation of a general practice residency training program that would keep physicians practicing in Iowa, and the mending of fences between the university and private practice. Anderson gives great credit to Virgil Hancher, then President of the University of Iowa, who argued that federal aid to medical education was directly proportionate to expansion in enrollments:

> Hancher was critical of the medical profession's vocal opposition to federal aid in medical education. It was hypocritical ... for physicians to cry "socialized medicine" at the mention of federal aid to medical education while simultaneously castigating medical schools for failing to educate more physicians. (p. 136)

William B. Bean headed the department until 1970. By the middle of his term (1958–59), the department counted among its faculty seven professors, six associate professors, and eight assistant professors. Within this small nucleus was an intellectual force that would rapidly expand into our modern Department of Internal Medicine over the subsequent three decades. It included the names of Elmer DeGowin, Lewis January, Robert Hardin, and Margaret Ohlson as professors; Henry Hamilton, Paul Seebohm, Raymond Sheets, Walter Kirkendall, James Clifton, and Ernest Theilen as associate professors; and George Bedell, John Eckstein, Ian Smith, William Connor, and Roberta Bleiler as assistant professors. I joined the department in 1960 and became assistant professor in 1961. This team provided the blueprint. Several who are now emeritus professors provided leadership and deserve to be proud of their accomplishments. It was through their efforts in the 1960s that NIH-funded research at Iowa slowly but surely reached the threshold that would rise eventually to its steepest slope: a 1000 percent increase in our department between 1976 and 1996, from $2.5 million to approximately $30 million. Only a few other departments in the university could boast such an increase in NIH funding. The basic science departments were soon to achieve an equally impressive record.

Two important elements contributed to this success. The first was the emergence of leaders within the department who would take on major responsibilities for the development of interdisciplinary and interdepartmental research programs. The *research center* concept was essential in galvanizing scientific talents from various disciplines and various departments to converge on specific research initiatives and to respond to NIH programmatic developments. A second element was the erection of a major state-of-the-art biomedical research building later to be named after Dean John W. Eckstein. There, the best scientists and eventually Howard Hughes Investigators from our Department of Internal Medicine (Michael Welsh, M.D.), the Department of Physiology (Kevin Campbell, Ph.D.) and the Department of Biochemistry (John Donelson, Ph.D.) were housed. They would develop their laboratories and benefit from an interactive environment and splendidly equipped core research facilities to maximize research productivity.

THE EXPLOSION OF TERTIARY CARE AND MEDICAL TECHNOLOGY

We are now living this fabulous third cycle which began in the early 1970s while our research enterprise was growing at an impressive rate. It is characterized by a mushrooming of specialized and comprehensive clinical services provided by excellent clinical faculty, experts in every subspecialty of medicine and surgery. A very strong statewide and regional referral system has provided the essential network of patients. One of the boldest plans for modernization of the UIHC was initiated and over the course of twenty-five years, at a cost of approximately $400 million, four pavilions were erected to form one of the most attractive medical centers in the country. Miraculously, this was without any state appropriation. Reimbursement from patient care services supported by private insurance and the federal Medicare program provided the financial undergirding of this mammoth project. Anderson writes about the "Growth and Change in the Technological Age," an age deplored by some as expensive "half-way technology" and hailed by others as life-extending. The capital development was to take us into the twenty-first century with more than 1,000 beds, replacing an outdated turn-of-the-century hospital. Subspecialization was rampant.

With science and medical technology, the American medical education and health care systems were second to none in the world. At Iowa, the success of our scientific and patient care enterprises seemed unparalleled. Our Department of Internal Medicine was the envy of most. James A. Clifton became the ninth department head, serving between 1970 to 1976. He formalized the administrative structure of the department into subspecialty divisions, developed the template, and recruited the key individuals who would take us to the next phase of accomplishment. Thanks to him we were superbly poised to engage in the enormous expansion in patient care and research that was to come.

In 1976 I became the tenth department head, 106 years after William S. Robertson (who was born 100 years before me) had occupied the first chair. By the 1980s, with the legacies of William Bean and James Clifton as heads of medicine; the leadership of John Eckstein as dean; and the administrative skill of John Colloton as director of the UIHC, our department had become the flagship of the college. It rocketed into an orbit of unprecedented scientific and clinical accomplishments fueled by the recruitment of outstanding faculty from renowned medical schools. Iowa City was dubbed as the "best kept secret in academic medicine."

The success story of our department had to be told. A *Brief History of the Department of Internal Medicine at Iowa* had been written by Walter L. Bierring in 1958, based on the biographies of the first eight department chairs. Since the 1960s the evolution of internal medicine and the parallel changes in our department had progressed at such a pace that it seemed essential to create a new and comprehensive historical record. A history of the department, particularly in the last thirty years, had to be commissioned. Either Lewis January or Robert Hardin, who were emeritus professors of the department, could have done the job and the history would have contained a treasure of insights and personal views of the characters and personalities of the people who made the department what it is now. Their national leadership positions would also have provided a perspective on the evolution of academic internal medicine. We opted, however, for a historian from the cadre of faculty in the illustrious Department of History in our College of Liberal Arts. Lewis E. January recommended Lee Anderson and his choice proved ideal. My charge to the author was made in a letter to Lewis January dated November 25, 1987 which reads as follows:

Dear Lew,

You asked me for the goals and scope of our planned departmental history. Here is what I think.

The Department of Medicine at Iowa is 117 years old, founded in 1870. A history of the department between 1870 and 1958 was written by Walter L. Bierring, M.D., (the fourth department head) and published in 1958 by the State University of Iowa. This period covered terms of the first eight heads of Medicine including almost half of Dr. Bean's term in office. During that time, American medicine defined for itself a more rigorous, scientific basis following the Flexner report on medical education and began to emerge as the world's leader with the explosion of medical science and the enormous support of the federal government through the NIH. The earlier history was narrated more or less through biographical accounts of the department heads and the programs they developed and individuals they recruited. During the last thirty years, several major developments have occurred in academic internal medicine and our department, and its leaders have been the major participants.

I would like the history of the last 30 years to reflect the changes in the discipline of internal medicine and the parallel changes in our department. For example, the following factors have greatly influenced medical education and internal medicine throughout the country.

1) The increasing dependence of medical education on NIH funds and research support defined the quality and character of our system of education and our faculty in the 60's and 70's. More recent restrictions of federal research support pushed some faculty away from academic medicine into practice and others into clinical research sponsored by pharmaceutical companies.

2) Pharmaceutical companies are now creating major research enterprises which compete for academic basic researchers.

3) The increasing subspecialization and the role of ABIM and its sub-specialties making internal medicine the leading specialty with more than 30% of the graduates going into internal medicine. In Iowa, however, relatively more graduates have elected family practice and the surgical specialties.

4) The "privatization" of University Hospitals and the shift from "indigent" care to "private" care creates greater dependence of medical education now on private practice income.

   We find that in the 80's we have a different source of subsidy of medical education. The support of patient care through Medicare and Medicaid programs and through third party payors is beginning to redefine the quality and character of our system of medical education and of our faculty and academic specialists.

   Just as academic medicine is becoming more dependent on income from practice, most teaching hospitals are operating as independent corporations for financial reasons, and decisions on programmatic practices may not be in the academic interest.

5) The differing priorities of teaching hospitals and medical schools have created new tensions in many academic centers.

6) The technological advances increased cost of care enormously and attracted many graduates to specialties where manual dexterity and "invasive" procedures were recompensed at higher rates reducing the attractiveness of cognitive disciplines.

7) The exorbitant cost of care brought restrictive regulations on utilization of beds and services by the feds and private insurers which required that greater efforts of our faculty be channeled into documentation of services and away from teaching, research, and academic pursuits.

8) Competition between academic clinicians and private clinicians became almost vicious in many centers and threatened the stability and the very fabric of academic internal medicine.

9) VA hospitals have assumed a major role in the support of medical centers providing research funds and space and educational opportunities for students and fellows in exchange for high quality patient care by expert professors-specialists.

I would like the history of our department to be reflected against this background. The leadership provided by the heads of the department and, just as importantly, by the senior faculty who were national leaders of their organizations during those years should be highlighted in the context of the changes that have taken place.

Examples of changes in the department:

1) Multiple subspecialties were born.

2) Enormous growth in research (basic research) in Internal Medicine.

3) Exodus of some faculty to industry.

4) Enormous expansion of clinical activities leading to an ambitious and successful faculty recruitment effort helped immeasurably by the physical expansion of the hospital.

5) Expansion of residency training programs with research opportunities. Excessive training of clinical subspecialists.

6) Erosion of academic time by regulatory agencies and their requirements.

7) The role of the academic physician as *private* doctor had been reduced in the 60's and 70's and is now returning in the 80's and requires reeducation.

8) Greater dependence on referring physicians requires new and better ways of communication.

9) Competition from emerging tertiary care centers in Iowa—our response?

10) New emphasis on ambulatory care, on geriatrics, nutrition, clinical epidemiology, genetics, etc.

   • Expansion of University Hospitals without state appropriation; stability of referrals and increased subspecialty in-patients units.

   • Expansion of VA—new clinical building and research facilities. Expanding VA research budget.

11) Medicare and third party payors restricting funding of postgraduate education to residents and excluding fellows—new sources of funding for fellows.

12) New Human Biology Building.

13) Major interdisciplinary centers crossing divisional and departmental barriers—leading role of the Department of Medicine.

14) Establishment of tenure track and adjunct appointment for Ph.D.s in medicine.

15) Presidencies of the major organization led by members of our department: American Heart Association, American Diabetes Association, American College of Physicians, American Federation for Clinical Research, American Academy of Allergy, American Board of Internal Medicine, etc. Their impact.

16) Impact of deans and university presidents on the institution and department.

17) How our faculty meet these challenges.

Lew, is this what you wanted?

Sincerely,

Frank

In retrospect, the charge was encompassing. Lee Anderson's account has captured the evolution in internal medicine as an academic discipline and the parallel changes in our department, viewing the accomplishments of its faculty through the objective eyes of an "outsider." The account took three and a half years to research and write. It is replete with detail, factual and analytical, yet it retains the warmth, the intensity, the creativity, the curiosity, the compassion of the actors and the intellectual genius, the competitive spirit, the ambitions, and even the political machinations of many stars of this production. If history repeats itself, we can expect a future as vibrant, as dramatic, as changing, and as promising as Anderson portrayed the past. The young academic internists will fulfill their dreams and hopes through their mission against significant odds. We shall see them as teachers, as administrators, and as researchers. Some of them will be visionary planners and entrepreneurs. Others will hunger for recognition, nurture their pride, and sometimes unfortunately their greed, but our devout hope is that, above all, their covenant with their patients will never be betrayed.

FRANÇOIS M. ABBOUD, M.D.
Edith King Pearson Professor
Head, Department of Internal Medicine
The University of Iowa College of Medicine

ACKNOWLEDGMENTS

WHEN I began work on this project in the fall of 1988, I was, as historian and outsider, quite uncertain of my place in a busy department of medicine in one of America's largest academic medical centers. However, the patience and kindness of department faculty and staff helped to make the ensuing three-year collaboration an extraordinarily enriching experience for me. No doubt it was less so for my hosts, who were gracious enough to hide that fact. Many people shared their wisdom with me during the course of my research; to them I am grateful. Because of my ignorance or because of the press of time and circumstance, there were surely many voices I did not hear; to those I extend a sincere apology.

My thanks go especially to Dr. François Abboud, a very busy man who was nonetheless generous of his time in attending to my requests and occasional complaints; to Dr. Lewis January, a kind and gentle man, truly a man for all seasons, committed to excellence in the department of medicine, in the arts, in Hawkeye athletics, and in his friends and colleagues; and to Randy Jordison, Ruth Dawson, Bill Radl, and all the administrative staff who helped at various points along the way. Special thanks are due also to university archivist Earl Rogers and his staff, whose willingness to aid and accommodate never ceases to amaze, and to the staff of the University Hospitals Dietary Service, who kindly made available their collection of materials on Kate Daum. Inevitably, this work is inadequate witness to the faith of all those who, in whatever way, gave their encouragement and support. It is surely inadequate as well as tribute to those whose careers enliven its pages.

Three journals have kindly consented to the use of portions of my previously published articles: "'A Great Victory': Abraham Flexner and the New Medical Campus at the University of Iowa," *The Annals of Iowa* 51 (Winter 1992); "'Headlights Upon Sanitary Medicine': Public Health and Medical

Reform in Late Nineteenth-Century Iowa," *Journal of the History of Medicine and Allied Sciences* 46 (April 1991); and [with Lewis E. January], "Walter Bierring and the Flexner Revolution at the University of Iowa College of Medicine," *The Pharos* 55 (Winter 1992).

We are grateful for the financial support for this project generously provided by the Iowa Medical Society; Marion Merrell Dow, Inc.; Bristol Myers Squibb; and Pfizer, Inc.

INTRODUCTION

Internal Medicine and the Uses
of Medical History

THIS is a study of a single department of internal medicine, that of the University of Iowa College of Medicine. Internal medicine at the University of Iowa began inauspiciously in the late nineteenth century, survived a serious early twentieth-century crisis to achieve a position of modest national prominence by the late 1920s, then slipped into a quiet provincialism during the lean years of the Depression and World War II. After 1945, however, the University of Iowa Department of Internal Medicine blossomed into a dynamic and imposing educational and scientific enterprise, sprung improbably from the cornfields of Iowa. In its way, then, the history of internal medicine at the University of Iowa is a quintessentially American rags-to-riches story. Just as important, it is a story that in many ways parallels the rise of modern American medicine.

The name "internal medicine," taken from the German *innere Medizin,* was in common use in the United States by 1900.[1] Internal medicine was a product of nineteenth-century advances in physiology, biochemistry, bacteriology, and pathology as well as of new diagnostic techniques, such as auscultation, and of new technologies, such as the thermometer and the stethoscope.[2] In the language of the late nineteenth century, internal medicine promised to be simultaneously conservative, because it employed nonobtrusive modes of diagnosis and therapy, and radical, because it would relieve underlying causes of disease.

Yet the history of internal medicine is more than a history of science and technology. The professionalization and institutionalization of American medicine—processes begun in the late nineteenth century—were also significant factors in creating internal medicine. For example, internists initially defined their specialty in opposition to surgery and the self-importance of surgeons; somewhat later, many—like William Osler—defined their specialty in opposition to the movement of medical science from clinic to laboratory; and in the twentieth century, internists have continually redefined internal medicine in response to newly emergent knowledge, technologies, and specialties.

In addition, political, economic, and social factors have helped to define the nature and scope of internal medicine. Among the more obvious of those are the authority wielded by state and federal governments over medical practice and medical education, the institutional controls implicit in university and medical college settings, the constraints on medical practice and on medical research imposed by public, philanthropic, and corporate funding agencies, and the ill-defined and often contradictory desires and expectations of the consuming public.

In light of such complexities, as well as the central place of internal medicine in modern American medicine and especially academic medicine, the historiography of internal medicine is surprisingly sparse, even as historians have generally broadened and enriched our perspective on medical history in general.[3] That fact alone would seem to justify a study such as this. At the same time, there are admitted disadvantages and limitations to the case study approach, as historians will only too willingly testify. How "typical," after all, is any single case? And admittedly, the University of Iowa Department of Internal Medicine, past and present, might be either typical or unique, depending upon the kinds of questions asked and comparisons made. For example, the history of internal medicine at Iowa of course differs in many particulars—some of them important ones indeed—from the history of internal medicine at Johns Hopkins University, but does that make the Iowa case exceptional or typical? Furthermore, as Hopkins' own boosters attest, the world of medical science and education has come to look more and more homogeneous in recent decades.[4]

Throughout most of their history, both internal medicine and medical education in general at the University of Iowa have shared many characteristics of their counterparts elsewhere in America. From 1870 to 1910, medicine at Iowa was undistinguished by modern standards. Clinical faculty held part-time posts and generally commuted long distances to attend to their teaching duties; facilities, especially clinical facilities, were marginal; and the overall quality of medical education was low, at least by today's standards. Still, during those four decades, medical education at Iowa made significant strides, in no small part because of the contributions of internal medicine, and by the advent of the twentieth century, the University of Iowa College of Medicine had become a respectable institution.

Nonetheless, Abraham Flexner, in his 1909 survey of medical schools for the Carnegie Foundation for the Advancement of Teaching, argued that the college in Iowa City was not worth the investment needed to salvage it—this after a hurried assessment of faculty, facilities, curriculum, and pedagogical methods. Moreover, Flexner aimed his harshest criticisms at the clinical facilities that were chiefly the province of internal medicine, then under the direction of Walter L. Bierring.[5] The result was a crisis—for Bierring, for internal medicine, for the college, and for the university.

The College of Medicine survived that crisis, due chiefly to the concerted efforts of University of Iowa president George E. MacLean and William R. Boyd, president of the finance committee of the state board of education. After a nationwide search, internal medicine at Iowa gained new credibility with the hiring of Campbell Palmer Howard, a product of McGill University, a protégé of William Osler, and a promising young scholar of impeccable credentials. In addition, in August 1911, John G. Bowman, ex-secretary of the Carnegie Foundation, took office as University of Iowa president, seeming to guarantee continued administration support for medical education. It should be noted that Walter Bierring, too, survived the crisis of 1910, his long and distinguished career in American medicine including service as president of the American Medical Association, as regent of the American College of Physicians, and, at different times, as head of both the American Board of Internal Medicine and the American Board of Preventive Medicine.[6]

In the second decade of the twentieth century, internal medicine at the University of Iowa entered a new era, marked by a new scientific orientation and by an unprecedented expansion of physical facilities. The construction of the new medical campus west of the Iowa River, financed in part through Rockefeller moneys secured through the influence of Abraham Flexner and completed in the late 1920s, was the capstone to that remarkable era of expansion and a symbol, too, of the maturation of American medical science and education. However, despite the excitement and promise of those years, the subsequent fifteen-year period of depression and war was one of hardship for the University of Iowa College of Medicine in general and the Department of Internal Medicine in particular. The draining combination of fiscal stringency and wartime emergency measures left the department to begin the postwar era with a depleted faculty, a seriously diminished reputation, and an uncertain future.

Yet World War II marked a second major turning point in the history of medicine at the University of Iowa, as it did throughout the United States.[7] Spurred in part by the successful wartime marriage between the federal government and scientific research, in part by the developing Cold War, in part by wartime evidence of serious health deficiencies in American society, and in part by the contributions of medical science to the war effort, unimagined sums of federal money flowed into medical research, and to a lesser extent into medical education, in the postwar years. "Biomedical research," it seemed, "could solve the problems of disease if only [Congress] would provide adequate funding."[8] And the University of Iowa Department of Internal Medicine experienced explosive growth in size and stature, as federal funds fueled both the rise of "big medicine" and the diffusion of excellence in medical science.

In the midst of prosperity, many problems remained, some holdovers from an earlier era, some products of prosperity itself, and some reflecting complex changes in postwar American society. Major controversies over the delivery of health care and its cost and the relationship of academic medicine to the medical profession and to the university, were, in varying degrees, holdovers from an earlier era. In contrast, the exclusion of women and minorities from medicine became a major issue only in the postwar era, and while women and minorities made sharp enrollment gains in the late 1960s and 1970s,[9] their recruitment to faculty positions lagged, especially in the oldest and most prestigious internal medicine subspecialties. At the same time, the increasing specialization in research, training, and practice in the postwar years accelerated the fragmentation of internal medicine into a diverse cluster of subspecialties.

In those and in many other ways, the history of internal medicine at the University of Iowa reiterates much of modern American medical history, from the institutionalization of scientific medicine and the reform of medical education in the late nineteenth and early twentieth centuries to today's technology-driven science and practice. But despite the immediacy of that history and its implications for both present and future in American medicine, the status of medical history has long been problematic in the academic institutions where much of that history is made.

Physicians, like most other Americans and certainly like most professionals, are ambivalent about their history. On the one hand, they entertain an active mythology, consisting chiefly of tales of heroic individuals and events. On the other hand, physicians seem often to disparage, or at least to have little time for, history proper. Surely physicians' ambivalence toward their professional history reflects the intensely scientific and technological nature of modern medicine, a condition in which the past seems at best a curiosity and at worst an irrelevancy. After all, in a technological world, as Henry Ford is supposed to have said, "history is bunk."

That was not always so. At the turn of the century, major figures in American medicine were firmly convinced of the importance of history in medical education and practice. For William Osler, for example, history had didactic value. Following on that tradition, physicians, most of them academics or retired academics, dominated the field of American medical history well into this century. Although their generally uncritical celebrations of medical progress lent a whiggish cast to medical historiography, celebrating great men, great moments, and the march of progress, those enthusiastic amateurs performed valuable services in historical research, preservation, and bibliography.[10]

In the second and third decades of this century, a small band of professional medical historians, for whom William Lloyd Garrison was pioneer and exemplar, augmented and to some extent challenged the amateur strain in

American medical historiography. Later, in the 1930s and 1940s, Henry Sigerist's social history approach carried medical history farther beyond its early great-doctors and great-moments focus. Ironically, though, as medical history was successfully institutionalized in America, the triumphs of scientific medicine and the demands of scientific education crowded medical history from the medical curriculum and, to a large extent, from professional consciousness as well. Moreover, the kinds of critical interpretations of American values and institutions inspired by Henry Sigerist's socialist leanings were not kindly received during the Cold War years of the late 1940s and 1950s.

Throughout that half-century of development in American medical history, one thing remained more or less understood: only a physician could legitimately claim to be a medical historian. For example, Richard H. Shryock, who was not a physician but who possessed an impressive list of publications in medical history, declined to label himself a medical historian. At the same time, faculty in departments of history—typically preoccupied with political, diplomatic, and intellectual history—remained unconvinced of the legitimacy of medical history, in much the same way that they questioned other non-traditional areas such as labor history or women's history.[11]

It was not until the late 1960s and 1970s that American medical history became the multifaceted and often contentious enterprise it is today.[12] And it is no coincidence that the resurgence of medical history has paralleled the rise of social history, labor history, and women's history, with their questioning attitudes toward traditional approaches and interpretations of the past. Likewise, it is no coincidence that the resurgence of medical history has occurred during a time when the status of medicine has been as uncertain and its future as clouded as at any time since the late nineteenth century.

A striking element in the recent flowering of medical historiography, and also a principal source of contentiousness, has been the growing numbers and influence of non-physician historians. That trend was obvious already in the early 1960s; the 1962 publication of Charles Rosenberg's *The Cholera Years: The United States in 1832, 1849, and 1866* is cited often as a watershed in the professional makeup of medical history. By the 1970s and 1980s, the increasing importance of health care issues in American political discourse further enhanced the status of medical history and further accelerated the demographic shift within the community of medical historians.

At times, tensions between physician- and non-physician historians have broken out into open warfare. Physician-historians have often complained that non-physicians tend to write medical history without a feel for medical science and practice. Meanwhile, non-physician historians have complained that physicians tend to write medical history without a feel for the political, social, and economic contexts of scientific and professional developments. In short, one group complained about the writing of medical history without medicine, and the other complained about the writing of medical history without history.

That was not an entirely new debate but echoed a long-standing discussion over the relative importance of internal versus external factors in medical history.[13] Nonetheless, it is true that the changing demographics of the community of medical historians, reinforced by the contentious political atmosphere of the late 1960s and early 1970s, sharpened the argument. Moreover, at its extremes, the historiographical debate threatened, it seemed, to reduce physicians to historical caricatures, posed as other-worldly idealists on the one hand and as shameless political manipulators on the other.[14]

To a considerable extent, as the historiography of medicine has become richer and more sophisticated in recent years, the conflict among physician and non-physician historians has been muted.[15] For their part, physicians have shown a broader and deeper interest in medical history as their domain has been pressured by the activism of disgruntled consumers, the intervention of increasingly skeptical state and federal governments, the aggressive expansion of corporate business in the health care marketplace, and jurisdictional competition from other health care professionals. Simultaneously, non-physician medical historians have come increasingly to appreciate that collaboration with physicians can enrich their understanding of medical history, giving a far more complete picture of physicians in their multiple roles as scientists, teachers, healers, and members of a large and influential profession.

Recent efforts to inject "humanism" into medical education and practice have also underscored the relevance of medical history. The place of humanism in medical education is yet another old thread in American medicine. In the mid-nineteenth century, for example, Daniel Drake argued that history, French, Greek, and Latin were essentials of the physician's education. Many medical educators of the early twentieth century would have agreed at least in principle with Drake's program. As medicine had become more professionalized, it also became—in some ways and with respect to white males at least—more democratic in recruitment,[16] and one of the supposed virtues of a humanist emphasis in medical education was to insure that the new physician-scientist was also a physician-gentleman.[17]

The humanism of the post–World War II period, however, was quite different both in origin and in emphasis. It followed in large part from criticism—scattered in the 1950s but more widespread and sustained by the 1970s and 1980s—of the narrowly scientific, biomedical model of disease, a model focused on disease entities rather than patients and one that interposed more and more technology between physician and patient.[18] Ironically, most of the celebrated triumphs of scientific medicine—from insulin therapy to heart transplants—hinged upon that disease model, but critics pointed out that the model pushed the patient's experience of illness into the background, elevated objective signs elicited by technological aids above the patient's subjective symptoms,[19] and fostered the false assumption that "to know the disease and its treatment" was "to know the illness and the treatment of the ill person."[20] In the modern world of technological medicine, as Edmund Pellegrino has observed, "The physician became our Merlin, at once beneficent and threatening."[21] Moreover, physician and patient became strangers.

William Bennett Bean, who headed the University of Iowa Department of Internal Medicine from 1948 to 1970, was an example of the early postwar voices calling for a compromise between technology and humanism in medicine and lamenting the "false dichotomy" between the sciences and humanities in medical education and in medical practice.[22] What William Bean and others proposed was the resurrection in medicine of the healing metaphor—one of the most powerful and persistent forces in western culture and the ultimate source of the physician's cultural authority. Modern medical science has shifted the emphasis in medicine from healing toward techniques of disease management, supposing that the art of healing and the science of medicine are the same thing, but critics maintain that patients seek healers, not scientists or experts in disease management.[23] In this light, one of the uses of medical history is to rediscover the physician as healer and to provide a different perspective on age-old problems of health and illness as well as on the physicians' broader role in society.

Internal medicine, because of its central place in the past and present of American medicine, provides a fertile and still largely untapped resource in which to trace many of the changes and challenges in American medicine over the past century, to address many major historiographical issues, and to reflect upon the uses of medical history. In particular, the history of the University of Iowa Department of Internal Medicine is neither a story of the inexorable march of progress nor one of the self-interested pursuit of power. Rather, it is a very human story of individuals who sought, albeit sometimes mistakenly and sometimes with unintended consequences, to change the world in ways they understood to be for the better.

I

The Growth of Medical Science
and the Roots of
Internal Medicine

1870–1945

1

The Emergence of Internal Medicine

1870–1910

THE development of internal medicine at the University of Iowa was part of the late nineteenth- and early twentieth-century "transformation" of American medicine. In those few decades, the changing locus of medical practice and the shifting relationship between physician and patient altered long-standing patterns of behavior among American health care consumers and vested unprecedented authority—cultural as well as scientific—in physicians. A concomitant restructuring of American medical science and medical education ushered in the era of scientific medicine and transformed traditional chairs of theory and practice of medicine, like that at the University of Iowa, into modern departments of internal medicine.[1] Thus, the early history of internal medicine at the University of Iowa reflected much of the complexity and ambiguity—and irony as well—of a critical era of American medical reform.

The late nineteenth-century reform of American medicine was in large part a local phenomenon, defined and initiated by local elites in the several states, and was at the outset largely undifferentiated—that is, small circles of physician-activists pursued a broad variety of goals. William S. Robertson, Professor of Theory and Practice of Medicine at the University of Iowa from 1870 to 1887, was typical of such reformers. Robertson's energies touched every aspect of Iowa medicine; indeed, one could argue that his chief contributions came not in internal medicine but in the building of Iowa medical organizations and institutions, ranging from the College of Medicine to the Iowa State Board of Health.

Thanks in part to the work of William Robertson and his colleagues, Iowa medicine was substantially changed by the 1890s, and medical reform had gained momentum and had also become more specialized. Robertson's successors in internal medicine at the University of Iowa became, to an increasing extent, participants in a growing national, and even international, community of medical science, and their interests centered more and more on the improvement of medical education and medical science. Their exertions helped to build the University of Iowa College of Medicine into a recognizably modern institution by the early 1900s, its laboratory facilities, hospital, faculty, and curriculum considerably improved from what William Robertson had known in the 1870s and 1880s.

By the early twentieth century, the reform of medical education had likewise gained a significant national dimension, as organizations such as the Association of American Medical Colleges and the Council on Medical Education and Hospitals of the American Medical Association sought to order American medical education in much the same way that the trusts sought to order the chaotic American economy. The result was a collision between the uneven pace of local reform, such as at the University of Iowa, and an increasingly powerful vision of national standardization. Abraham Flexner's 1910 report, *Medical Education in the United States and Canada,* symbolized that collision, and Flexner's devastating assessment of the University of Iowa College of Medicine, and especially the Department of Internal Medicine, cast the future of the college in doubt and sparked a desperate scramble to salvage the school.

At the outset, then, this chapter casts a wide net, describing the nature of late nineteenth-century Iowa medicine and the strategies and goals of medical reformers like William Robertson. Reiterating the tendency toward specialization in medical reform in the 1890s and early 1900s, the text then turns more specifically to the development of the University of Iowa College of Medicine and ultimately to the Department of Internal Medicine itself, culminating in the changes consequent to Abraham Flexner's visits in 1909.

HEADLIGHTS UPON SANITARY MEDICINE

To a modern observer, Iowa might have seemed infertile ground for medical reform at any time in the last century. The nineteenth-century health care market was chaotic and oddly democratic, with drug suppliers, especially druggists and patent medicine manufacturers, playing major roles, while the physician's role was far more limited than today.[2] Indeed, prior to the mid-1880s anyone could profess to be a physician in Iowa, and civil suits for malpractice were the only real limitation on practitioners' claims to competence. In nineteenth-century

Iowa, as in most of America, the family was the chief primary care provider, and the principle of self-medication that lay at the heart of domestic medicine was based in an eclectic pharmacopoeia drawn from regular and sectarian medicine, family "recipes," and native American traditions and products.

Throughout the century, disease was a constant threat to all ages and social classes, although the young and women of child-bearing age were especially at risk. The disease environment was not static,[3] and by the 1870s its characteristics were typical of developed societies before the era of scientific medicine: childhood diseases—notably diphtheria, scarlet fever, and measles—were the dominant features, but smallpox and typhoid fever were of sporadic significance and the incidence of tuberculosis was on the rise. Low population densities, the comparative cost of professional care, cultural biases against elitist professional monopolies and "big government," and the dismal state of both transportation and medical science all accounted for the apparently paradoxical combination of low demand for physicians' services and a burdensome, if ever-changing, disease environment.

Organized medicine scarcely existed in nineteenth-century Iowa but was one of the twentieth-century symptoms of medicine's professional maturity. The earliest Iowa physicians were, of necessity, jacks of all trades, combining the skills of general practitioner, surgeon, and apothecary; and many were farmers, bankers, or businessmen as well.[4] The limited demand for professional health care pushed physicians, regular and sectarian alike, into intense competition with one another for the relative few available patients.[5] The fiercely competitive health care market strained professional relations to the breaking point and stunted the growth of medical institutions—e.g., medical schools, medical societies, and medical journals. Where such institutions survived, they did so only through the determined efforts of a handful of physicians.

Prior to the passage of Iowa's first physician licensure statute in 1886, the would-be physician could expect little return from an investment in formal medical education. Preceptorship was the dominant mode of medical training, as young men, and occasionally young women, "read" medicine with an established practitioner, supposedly absorbing both the science and art of medical practice from the study of a few standard texts, from observation, and from hands-on experience. While this could be adequate, and perhaps even exemplary, training, it was not always so. At the same time, the education afforded by medical schools was none too good, in Iowa or anywhere in America, before the 1890s. In part that was because nineteenth-century medical science generally offered neither useful insight into disease processes nor effective therapies; in short, there was little recognizable medical science to be taught in the schools. In the early 1880s, an Iowa physician exclaimed, "Never before did a human life stand so good a chance in the hands of a good physician,"[6] but medical practice was still—and would remain for nearly a generation—more art, or "bedside manner," than science. Although it is true that surgeons rapidly broadened their array of invasive procedures in the last half of the century, it often seemed that the ordinary physician could do little more than soothe pain and diarrhea with opiates and induce sleep with chloral hydrate, making the superiority of regular medicine over sectarian alternatives or self-medication a matter of speculation. Thus, too, general practitioners looked upon surgeons with envy and a fair degree of resentment.

The inadequacy of nineteenth-century medical education also reflected the generally low level of public education. A high school education was uncommon in the nineteenth century; requirements for medical school admission were correspondingly low; and in any event, prevailing norms of decorum among nineteenth-century university students left much to be desired. Another of the limits on medical education was the lack of public and private financial support for medical research and education. Nineteenth-century medical schools were chiefly entrepreneurial ventures, so-called proprietary schools where, as Daniel Drake observed in the 1830s, faculties were too small and too often deficient in learning, school sessions were too short, laboratory facilities were too few, clinical training was nearly nonexistent, and medical pedagogy was uninspired.[7] Students seeking medical degrees endured two-year courses of lectures and demonstrations delivered over a sixteen- to twenty-week academic year, with the second-year course duplicating the first.

Enterprising Iowa physicians contributed to the proprietary medical school boom. The College of Physicians and Surgeons of the Upper Mississippi opened in Davenport in the fall of 1849, offering the first course of medical lectures in Iowa. The following summer proprietors moved the school to Keokuk where it became the Keokuk College of Physicians and Surgeons. The school continued operations for some sixty years, and from 1851 to 1869 it served as the Medical Department of the University of Iowa. Similar schools, although with lesser credentials, appeared in Des Moines, Sioux City, and other communities at different times,[8] and the more ambitious graduates of such schools might complement their rudimentary training with a year or more of clinical work at one of the older teaching hospitals in New York or Philadelphia.

Given the primitive state of medicine in Iowa and in America at large, nineteenth-century medical reform was dependent on the labors of scattered, ill-defined groups of physician elites. It was they who built the new institutions and promoted the new medical science of the late nineteenth-century. The leadership of eastern elites—men like William Welch and John Shaw Billings—was important, and historians have given such figures their due. However, in medicine or in any other occupation, professionalism was, and largely still is, mediated at the state level. State legislatures, for example, enacted physician licensure statutes, established educational standards for physicians, set the boundaries of professional jurisdiction, and financed medical education.

Through their work at the state level, then, William Robertson, his Iowa colleagues, and their counterparts in other states laid much of the groundwork for modern American medicine.

The son of a Columbus City, Iowa, physician of some note, William Robertson was gifted with a dynamic personality, tireless energies, and professional ambitions to match. Organizer of a broad-ranging medical reform campaign, Robertson's achievements included a principal role in the early development of the College of Medicine at the University of Iowa, creation of the Iowa State Board of Health in 1880, and passage of Iowa's first physician licensing statute in 1886, all critical steps in the advent of modern scientific medicine in the state. In addition, Robertson was an influential figure in the Iowa State Medical Society and member of the American Medical Association and American Public Health Association. Above all, William Robertson, like many other medical educators of his time, was an institution-builder whose many other interests often overshadowed his role in medical education.[9]

William Robertson was part of a new physician elite that crystallized in Iowa after the Civil War as the states of the Midwest joined the mainstream of American economic and political life. Iowa's population, for example, rose from 192,000 in 1850 to more than a million in 1870. Thanks in no small part to the advancing railroads, urbanization and economic development followed apace, while physician numbers rose proportionately as well. In turn, revolutions in demography and transportation significantly altered the Iowa State Medical Society, which had been since its founding in 1850 largely the instrument of medical school proprietors. After the Civil War, local medical societies grew in number, spurred often by the arrival of graduates from medical schools in Chicago and the east. For example, of the ten physicians who organized the Upper Cedar Valley Medical Association in 1871, two were graduates from Rush Medical College in Chicago, two from the University of Michigan, two from New York City schools, and one from Yale University.[10] In the 1870s delegates from local societies far outnumbered representatives from the proprietary medical schools in the membership list of the state medical society, and those new members slowly opened the door to new leadership with a new and ambitious professional agenda.

The professional ambitions of Iowa's new physician-reformers coalesced around a handful of closely related goals: a greater political role for physicians, beginning with public health administration; state regulation of medical practice; and gradual reform of medical education around the newly emergent principles of scientific medicine. And in an age when American society was increasingly commanded by public and private corporations, reformers offered a new definition of medical professionalism grounded in the principle of corporate organization, using an organized medicine to bolster the physician's claim to professional authority.[11] Moreover, reformers argued, that claim should be tied to rigid standards of occupational entry and performance enforced by the state.

From the first, Iowa's physician-reformers promoted a wide-ranging agenda for professional medicine. In the 1870s and 1880s, at a time of growing concern over public health issues, the promise—as yet largely unrealized—of scientific medicine along with the mysterious but unmistakable decline in mortality rates spawned plans for an ambitious system of "medical police" that would mobilize the state's police power in defense of the public health, safety, and morals.[12] The building of the University of Iowa College of Medicine, founded in 1870, was only a small part of that agenda; indeed, the reform of medical education must have seemed pedestrian in comparison to the excitement generated by men like Pasteur and Koch and the obvious implications of their work in the realm of public health.

William Watson, president of the Iowa State Medical Society, outlined the medical police principle in 1868, contending that "the state should use every means in her power to promote the most healthy and efficient condition of her people."[13] During the 1870s, the terms "medical police," "sanitary police," and "state medicine" became part of the lexicon of Iowa's medical reformers. At the same time, there was a growing middle-class audience for schemes of social regeneration couched in the language of science and offering scientifically trained professionals to minister to the manifold evils of gilded age society, including the weakening of traditional communities, values, and hierarchies and the massive influx of immigrants.[14] In courting that public health constituency, reformers' arguments for "a wholesome regard for medical police," took on a starkly utilitarian cast. In 1883, William Robertson, for example, noted that "as you increase the number of healthy persons, or diminish the days of sickness, you add so much to the national wealth." Furthermore, he contended, just as governments collected statistics on cotton and other crops, so, too, should they collect statistics on the "human crop." "A man's health," Robertson intoned, "is [his] property."[15]

Reforming physicians argued that "sanitary science is but an expression of the higher development of the medical sciences."[16] Thus, one Iowa physician claimed, with more enthusiasm than accuracy, that physicians should administer "the science of public health" because of their "proficiency in that kind of knowledge."[17] Another volunteered Iowa's physicians to perform such "sanitary work without fee or reward," asking only "to be recognized, to be organized into boards to become more efficient."[18] Still another concluded that it was the duty of physicians to stand "as headlights upon sanitary medicine."[19] Reformers also forecast a vast expansion of physicians' authority; "the duties of the sanitary physician," they assured their listeners, would "in places interlace with those of the moralist and priest."[20] Carried away with the excitement of the moment, one Iowa physician exclaimed, "Questions that are moral to-day will be medical tomorrow."[21]

State licensing of physicians was an extension of the medical police concept. Physician licensure would assure higher standards of medical education and reserve the practice of medicine to "those who are properly qualified physicians,"[22] while it eliminated the "knavish quacks [who] protract sickness and increase the death rate."[23] Also, the policing of physician competence would insure the accuracy of vital statistics reported to state agencies by local practitioners. In short, reforming physicians promised nothing less than the dawn of a new era in which medicine would claim "its rightful influence over those who gracefully yield it homage and pay tribute to the full measure of its gravity."[24]

Despite such reassurances, the plans of William Robertson and other reformers encountered considerable resistance from Iowa physicians. As Charles Rosenberg has pointed out, nineteenth-century American medicine was characterized by "democratic assumptions that allowed every would-be practitioner to call himself 'doctor,'" and a good many Iowa physicians were sensitive to any suggestions, especially medical licensing and educational reform, threatening to unbalance that "linguistic fiction of medical equality."[25] Nonetheless, in June 1879, after a decade of exhortation and often bitter debate, the Iowa State Medical Society authorized a committee on state medicine, with William Robertson as chair, "to secure legislation relative to the practice of medicine and to the establishment of a State Board of Health."[26]

After securing a pledge from the Hahnemann Medical Society of Iowa "to work side by side in any movement which would give us an efficient sanitation and an operative medical practice act,"[27] Robertson carried his campaign to the state legislature. In the nineteenth century, the Republican Party—the party of mainline Protestant denominations, main street business, and mainstream culture—dominated Iowa politics, and by the 1870s Iowa Republicans were accustomed to using the power of government to uphold the existing social order. Moreover, Robertson himself held a seat in the Iowa Senate in 1880, while John C. Schrader, Professor of Obstetrics and Gynecology at the University of Iowa, chaired the senate committee on medicine, hygiene, and surgery.

The Eighteenth General Assembly of 1880 was typically receptive to public policy innovations. In addition to a prohibition amendment to the state constitution and a law to regulate the practice of pharmacy, state legislators approved Robertson's plan for a state board of health empowered to act "for the preservation or improvement of the public health." However, the House of Representatives balked at the companion proposal to regulate the practice of medicine. One opponent of physician licensing, reflecting common sentiment, charged that the plan was "not only absurd, but an infringement upon personal rights."[28] And although the Iowa State Medical Society subsequently approved a resolution urging "every member to use his influence with the members of the General

Assembly" to secure physician licensing, Robertson did not have his physician licensing statute until 1886—until, that is, both physicians and the wider public had grown accustomed to state intervention in matters of health.[29]

The new board of health, under William Robertson's vigorous leadership, made the most of its statutory mandate, investigating outbreaks of infectious disease, marshalling state and local resources to control their spread, compiling vital statistics, and sharing information about infectious disease with public health authorities in other states. At a time when scientific medicine was in its infancy and disease etiology was still largely a mystery, the board's actions were sometimes wrong-headed and occasionally colored by ethnic and class prejudices; nonetheless, the board was a valuable forum bringing public-spirited, politically involved physicians and at least the fundamentals of modern medical science to public attention.

The board of health, although it was the greatest triumph of Robertson's first generation of medical reformers, was in some respects a disappointing tool for the propagation of scientific medicine. First, while the board's disease containment actions, particularly its rigid quarantine guidelines, did indeed bring the emerging precepts of scientific medicine to bear upon the most intimate details of Iowans' private lives, the board's actions often met fierce resistance both from practicing physicians and the public. Many physicians resented the intrusion of the state into the physician-patient relationship, while the stigma of infectious disease brought embarrassment and inconvenience to individuals and significant commercial harm to local communities. Second, there was widespread resistance, especially among physicians, to the expansion of "state medicine" beyond its original, narrow mandate to control infectious disease. Practicing physicians zealously guarded their free enterprise ideal against intrusions from public institutions like the state board of health.

There were, then, strict limits—perhaps unexpected ones—to what the board of health could accomplish in the way of medical reform. That lesson was one factor in the shifting of many reformers' attentions to medical education; more general acceptance of a new scientific professionalism in medicine, they thought, would come only through the education of a new generation of physicians. That realization focused renewed attention on the University of Iowa College of Medicine, an institution that was ill-equipped for such an important mission during William Robertson's tenure.

THE MOST COMPLETE MEDICAL COLLEGE

Medical education at the University of Iowa developed at a snail's pace in the 1870s and 1880s. That was so in part because there was no overriding sense of crisis in medical education. After all, physicians were not even agreed on the need of formal professional education, and in any event few could have guessed what the future held for American medical education. Besides, it was plain that the training offered at the university in the 1880s, whatever its shortcomings, was far better than anything available in Iowa in, say, the 1850s. Reformers like William Robertson, wrapped in the excitement of public health reform, took for granted that medical education would continue its gradual course of improvement.

At its founding in 1870, the University of Iowa College of Medicine was part of a national trend that would eventually make higher education more democratic and make the American university into a center for the discovery of new and useful knowledge.[30] More immediately, the College of Medicine was the product of a mixture of university boosterism and professional ambition. Its most visible and influential supporters were John P. Irish, an Iowa City newspaper editor, state legislator, and university trustee; John F. Dillon, a Davenport physician-cum-lawyer, federal judge, and later chief justice of the Iowa Supreme Court and professor of law at Columbia University in New York; and Washington F. Peck, a young Davenport physician-protégé of Dillon's, an 1863 Bellevue Hospital Medical College graduate, Civil War veteran, and subsequent professor of surgery and dean of the new college.[31]

The proposal to establish a publicly supported school of medicine on the state university campus roused a wave of resistance from the proprietors of existing medical schools. Since the 1850s, those proprietors had beaten back several proposals to organize a school in Iowa City, and they could still count on considerable support from their alumni. In 1870, for example, graduates of the Keokuk College of Physicians and Surgeons made up nearly 25 percent of the membership of the Iowa State Medical Society. In addition, a good many physicians were, as a matter of principle, wary of state intrusion into the free market for medical education; just as many opposed state regulation of medical practice. In an 1870 resolution, a majority of the Iowa State Medical Society labeled the proposed college in Iowa City "a useless expenditure of public money" entailing the "unnecessary multiplication of medical colleges." In addition, they condemned college organizers as "injudicious and injurious to the interests of the medical profession."[32] However, despite loud opposition, the university's board of trustees approved the new medical college, and the trustees' decision survived a subsequent challenge in the state legislature as well before the school opened in October 1870.[33]

The Iowa City community gave the new college a mixed reception, an ambivalence heightened by a sensational grave-robbing incident. Scarcely two months after the college opened, the body of an Iowa City woman disappeared from a fresh grave in the city cemetery, and according to the Iowa City *Republican,* "Suspicions at once fell upon the Medical Department of the

University." The connection between medical schools and grave-robbing was common currency at the time, and in this case it was true: the cadaver was indeed in the school's dissecting room. Before the sheriff could obtain a search warrant, however, the conspirators slipped the corpse out a window, took it away on horseback, and hid it in a haystack. Facing a public relations disaster, Dean Washington Peck issued a statement assuring one and all that "faculty are in no way concerned in the drama."[34] Nonetheless, James H. Boucher, Professor of Anatomy, resigned in the wake of the scandal and was eventually arrested along with three students. To make matters worse, newspapers across the state picked up the story, triggering a firestorm of outrage that the struggling school barely survived.

The school overcame public embarrassment and political opposition due largely to the leadership of a determined group of faculty members bonded by circumstance, by experience, and by professional ambition: William Robertson (professor of theory and practice of medicine), Washington F. Peck (professor of surgery and dean), William Drummond Middleton (professor of physiology), and John C. Schrader (professor of obstetrics and gynecology). All were young; Robertson, at age thirty-nine, was the oldest, while Schrader was barely in his thirties and Middleton and Peck were just twenty-six and twenty-eight respectively. Also, Middleton had studied under Washington Peck and, like Peck, had journeyed to New York to attain a degree from Bellevue Medical College. Likewise, William Robertson, who had taken a degree from Jefferson Medical College in 1856, attended Bellevue in the winter of 1868–69. In addition, Peck, Robertson, and Schrader had served as army surgeons during the Civil War; Middleton, meanwhile, was an infantryman from 1861 to 1865. Despite Peck's position as dean, William Robertson, as elder statesman, was the dominant figure, much as he was in the larger medical reform movement in Iowa.

At its opening, the University of Iowa College of Medicine differed little from competing proprietary schools. While the lecture room was "tolerably filled with students" on the opening day of classes,[35] one newspaper commented that, "on account of lack of facilities," the school could "scarcely turn out anything but quacks as graduates."[36] Installed in cramped quarters consisting of little more than a dissecting room and large lecture room and with just $3,000 appropriated for equipment, the college struggled for some years on income from student fees and faculty members' private practices. In 1873, the board of regents turned over the "Mechanics Academy"—the university's first classroom building and most recently a student dormitory—to serve as a hospital, but neither the board nor the legislature provided funds for renovation or for equipment.

Given the limited economic return from formal education and the competition from proprietary schools, it was not easy to attract students. Nor was it easy to keep them; few students in the school's first decade fulfilled graduation requirements of two courses of lectures and two years' work with a physician-preceptor. In 1879, for example, the school conferred just fourteen diplomas. Among those graduates there was one woman; however, although much remarked at the time and since, the enrollment of women was as much testament to the school's weakness in recruiting male students as to its commitment to the principle of coeducation. It was a truism of the time that medical school faculty almost universally preferred "a white skin and a male apparel" in their student body.[37] Indeed, as enrollments mushroomed at the University of Iowa College of Medicine from the initial class of thirty-seven in 1870 to 202 in 1895, female enrollments in fact dropped from eight to four, or from just under 22 percent to less than 2 percent.

William Robertson and his colleagues were well-intentioned, but their other interests, coupled with the lack of financial support and their relative isolation, hindered the development of medical education at Iowa. Reflecting universal practice, Robertson and other clinical faculty were only part-time instructors; their educational roles were adjuncts to private practice and other professional activities. They were also usually non-resident, and by the 1870s expanding railroad networks made it possible for Washington Peck and William Middleton, for example, to commute from Davenport, some 60 miles away. Teaching schedules reflected the needs of non-resident faculty, and William Robertson's schedule was typical: one-hour lectures on Monday and Thursday mornings followed by afternoon clinics. The bulk of instruction was didactic, consisting of repetitive lectures and readings, and Robertson's lectures reflected the undifferentiated nature of internal medicine: general pathology and descriptions of specific disease conditions, etiology, clinical history, diagnosis, and therapy.

In light of his obvious leadership skills, it is ironic that Robertson was universally remembered for his trying habit of reading his lectures very rapidly from prepared notes, and on at least one occasion he stormed from the hall when challenged by students to speak without his well-worn notes. It should be noted, however, that medical students of that era were barely housebroken; brawls in and out of the classroom are part of the early lore of the medical college, including battles pitting older medical students against younger, medical students against dental students, and medical students against law students.

Despite an Iowa physician's counsel to "draw the chalk line from pathology to therapeutics and hew to it,"[38] the unfolding scientific revolution had, at the outset, a marginal impact on internal medicine at Iowa, and much of what passed for medical science in William Robertson's time was of the parochial, seat-of-the-pants variety. However, that did not necessarily mark medicine at Iowa as backward. Internists throughout America held to a tradition of sometimes haphazard clinical observation—drawing mostly upon private, paying patients—rather than embracing laboratory research. In part that reflected the lack of public support for research facilities. In part it reflected the fact that the germ theory, as an example, although an enormously fruitful concept, was of limited practical utility to the clinician whose job was to treat ill patients. And in part, too, resistance to laboratory science was one legacy of early nineteenth-century French influence in American medicine,[39] an influence that eschewed system and causation.

Besides, being up-to-date with the latest literature had its perils as well. Physicians who saw the new scientific medicine as a tool to distance medicine from "quackery" often dressed ill-informed speculation in the new methodology and language. There was, as one critic noted, a powerful temptation toward publication "of half-knowledge, of doubtful fact, and of loose inquiry," all of it proclaimed as scientific medicine.[40] Moreover, to many internists it seemed that modern science, especially the germ theory and the associated "German method," would reduce diagnosis and therapy to rote, making "the detection of disease ... a mechanical process with no place for history, physical diagnosis or logical reasoning"—in short, no place for the clinician and perhaps not even the patient.[41] Internists, then, might concede that "the greatest advance of our time is the ardent study of the causation of disease,"[42] but they did not rush to the laboratory. Clinicians and laboratory scientists early in the history of scientific medicine were deeply divided over the choice of bedside or bench as the proper locus of medical science.[43]

Nonetheless, in the 1880s and especially in the 1890s, an accelerating rate of investment in medical education accompanied the state's expanded role in public health, and that, combined with advances in science and technology, brought significant improvements in facilities and curriculum at the University of Iowa College of Medicine—improvements that, by the early twentieth century, set the college apart from competing proprietary schools. The college entered the 1880s with an elective three-year graded course in addition to the traditional two-year ungraded format. In 1882, after a concerted lobbying campaign spearheaded by Washington Peck, the medical faculty occupied new quarters constructed with a $35,000 appropriation from the previously tight-fisted state legislature.[44] The facility was, its boosters claimed, "the most complete medical college building in the West." In addition, the privately financed Mercy Hospital that opened in Iowa City in 1886 provided additional opportunities for clinical instruction. In 1882, William Robertson instituted a course of lectures on sanitary science and public hygiene,[45] and also in the 1880s, William Middleton introduced the microscope, first in physiology and subsequently in medicine as well, and also championed the use of the thermometer in diagnosis.[46]

Middleton succeeded Robertson in the chair of theory and practice of medicine upon Robertson's death in early 1887; however, Middleton's tenure was short, interrupted by his elevation to professor of surgery in 1891.

Middleton's successor, Lawrence W. Littig, marked an important passage in the history of internal medicine at Iowa. An 1883 graduate of the college, Littig was the first of many alumni to hold positions in internal medicine at Iowa. More importantly, Littig had worked under William Osler in Philadelphia, and from 1886 to 1888, reflecting the growing influence of European medical science on American medicine, had studied abroad, first in London and Paris and then joining the growing numbers of American medical students drawn to German and Austrian universities. The German experimental approach to medical science was a major attraction to American students like Littig.[47] However, critics noted, likely with some justification, that a continental tour often overshadowed the lure of science for many students. At the same time, given the rapidly changing nature of German higher education, not all American students shared the same experience in their German studies.[48]

Whatever the case, the more serious students, and Lawrence Littig appears to have been one of those, returned home inspired by the promise of experimental science and sometimes, too, by the model of the full-time teacher-investigator, but they returned to institutions where laboratory facilities were largely unknown and where the laboratory method was little appreciated.[49] Certainly Littig, who had studied bacteriology with Koch, encountered both strictures at Iowa, but he was a determined innovator—sometimes an irascible one by all accounts—and unlike William Robertson, Littig's energies were focused chiefly on medical education. He introduced the stomach tube, centrifuge, and oil immersion lens to internal medicine at Iowa and took a leading role in the creation of a separate chair of Pathology and Bacteriology in the college. Littig's tenure also saw the lengthening of the college's program of study to four years of 26 weeks in 1895 and the opening of a new university hospital in 1898. Despite his credentials, however, Lawrence Littig, like his predecessors Robertson and Middleton, made little mark as a researcher. Burdened with lectures, demonstrations, and clinical duties as well as his private practice, Littig had little time for independent research, even if facilities had been available.

In part because internal medicine lacked a well-defined scientific tradition, internists in Littig's time struggled to establish an identity. They still lagged well behind surgeons in status, both within the profession and without. Washington Peck's early position as professor of surgery and dean of the College of Medicine and William Middleton's progression from internal medicine to surgery and then to dean suggest the existing hierarchy. Ironically, Lawrence Littig, who later lamented the prevalent notion "that the surgeon has the larger brain with deeper convolutions,"[50] resigned the chair of theory and practice of medicine in a huff in 1903 when, after William Middleton's death, he was passed over for promotion to the chair of surgery, and possibly the position of dean as well.

Walter Bierring, a protégé of Littig and his successor as professor of theory and practice of medicine in 1903, was another important transitional figure in internal medicine at the University of Iowa. In addition, Bierring was at the center of the crisis provoked by Abraham Flexner's visits in 1909. A figure of wide acquaintance and considerable notice both in his own time and since, Walter Bierring was, to a far greater extent than his predecessors, a participant in the global medical scientific community. During an extraordinarily long and varied career as medical educator, scientist, and general booster of professional medicine, Bierring wrote scores of articles on a variety of topics and held dozens of professional society memberships and offices. He was, for example, a regent of the American College of Physicians throughout the 1930s, president of the American Medical Association in 1934–35, and a principal in the creation of the American Board of Internal Medicine in the mid-1930s, serving subsequently as the board's first chair. He was also president of Alpha Omega Alpha, the national medical honor society, for over thirty years. At his death in 1961, one writer eulogized him as "Iowa's Osler," and William Bean, then chair of internal medicine at Iowa, referred to him as "the grand old man of American med-icine."[51]

With Washington Peck and William Middleton as preceptors, Walter Bierring enrolled at the University of Iowa College of Medicine in 1889 and received his degree in March 1892. Bierring was an especially promising student at a time when the quality of medical students was yet decidedly mixed, and upon graduation he accepted the new chair of Pathology and Bacteriology that Lawrence Littig had engineered.[52] Before taking up that position in 1895, however, Bierring followed Littig's example and embarked on a graduate tour of some of continental Europe's prestigious centers of medical science. At the University of Heidelberg, the University of Vienna, and the Pasteur Institute, he rubbed shoulders with the likes of Ernst, Billroth, Roux, and Pasteur and returned to Iowa City well prepared, it seemed, to contribute substantially to the development of internal medicine, serving as a model of the emerging clinical scientist, "equally at home in the laboratory and at the bedside."[53]

In 1895, five years after Behring and Kitasato's initial work on diphtheria antitoxin and just a year after the first published trials on human subjects, Bierring set out to prepare his own serum in Iowa City—with the aid of his colleague John C. Schrader, "who kindly provided the horse for the experi-ment." Because diphtheria was the most feared of childhood diseases in the late nineteenth century, the discovery of the antitoxin had caused a sensation in America. One of Bierring's contemporaries noted that "everyone started making diphtheria serum" in the mid-1890s, most with more enthusiasm than skill, and the result, he remarked cryptically, was "many [patients] killed."[54] However, Bierring's skill, or luck, was better than most; in addition, he pledged to try his product first "in very large doses on [himself]." At any rate, Bierring claimed to have used his serum successfully in "over 300 cases of diphtheria,"[55] and his was reputedly the first successful production of the antitoxin west of New York City. Buoyed by success, Bierring envisioned state-supported production in order to make his serum affordable and readily available, but his youthful ambition was derailed by the Iowa State Medical Society, whose members, like physicians in other states, let him know that the state had no business engaging in competition with private enterprise.

That early episode aptly displayed both Bierring's talent and his ambition. Undaunted, Bierring went on to build a career as teacher and clinical investigator that was, in the context of turn-of-the-century American medical science and education, respectable and perhaps exemplary. Reflecting the unspecialized nature of internal medicine, Bierring published a variety of clinical observations during his career at the university from 1895 to 1910. Most of those appeared in the *Transactions of the Iowa State Medical Society* and the *Iowa Medical Journal,* the latter established in 1895, but a few of his works reached a national audience through the *Journal of the American Medical Association.* In view of Bierring's training and accomplishments and given the standards of the time, he presented impeccable credentials when the chair of theory and practice came vacant in 1903, and there seems little reason to question his selection for the position.

During his seven years as head of the Department of Theory and Practice, Bierring supervised the continued expansion and improvement of medical education at Iowa. Unlike his predecessors, Bierring enjoyed the luxury of a part-time clinical assistant, Clarence Van Epps, who supervised the expansion of the modest clinical laboratory at the University Hospital and who also taught courses in clinical microscopy. For his part, Bierring was particularly proud of his emphasis on the teaching of diagnostic techniques, from simple history-taking to more complex diagnostic procedures and tests. As part of that regime, he instituted a regular system of ward rounds for senior students. Along with changes in curriculum and pedagogy, the expansion of facilities continued. The college occupied new quarters after a disastrous fire in 1901, and in 1905 a new wing was added to the University Hospital, pushing total capacity to near 200 beds.

When Walter Bierring assumed the post of hospital director in 1908, the University of Iowa hospital was in a state of transition mixing modern and nineteenth-century features. At a time when few medical colleges enjoyed the unrestricted use of hospital facilities, the University of Iowa Hospital was unusual, a clear illustration of the benefits of state university affiliation, and it was fast becoming a sizable business venture, accounting for more than 10 percent of the university's total revenues by 1910. Controlled by the university's board of regents, with medical college department heads comprising its staff, the hospital's chief purpose was clinical instruction. However, like its nineteenth-century predecessors, the university hospital welcomed only patients suffering from "acute, curable, and non-contagious diseases," and it likewise retained a good deal of the nineteenth-century hospital's moral baggage in its strict rules for patient behavior.[56] As a facility for clinical instruction, the hospital's major weakness, as had been true since the 1870s, was the small population base of the Iowa City area, and although Bierring and others had suggested that the hospital serve as a referral center for indigent patients from across Iowa, several years passed before the legislature approved such a plan.

At the end of the first decade of the twentieth century, then, medical education at the University of Iowa blended the old and the new. Walter Bierring and others were well aware of needed improvements; still, the University of Iowa College of Medicine had become a recognizably modern institution. The school offered a four-year graded course; two years' college work, including twenty-two semester hours of physics, chemistry, and biology, was required for admission; laboratory science was a prominent part of the non-clinical curriculum, notably in physiology, anatomy, and chemistry; Walter Bierring, as head of internal medicine, had a respectable record as educator and scientist; the hospital had been significantly upgraded since its opening in 1898; and total capital investment in the expanding medical school complex stood in excess of $500,000.[57]

In 1909, however, the two-decades long experiment in educational reform at the College of Medicine ran afoul of a plan for the sweeping reformation of American medical education, and in 1910, with the University of Iowa College of Medicine facing a crisis of survival, Walter Bierring was none too gently discharged as head of internal medicine.

ANTIQUATED METHODS OF TEACHING

By the early 1900s, thanks to medical licensing statutes that conferred automatic licensure upon degree-holders, the gap between the best and worst among American medical colleges had widened enormously. At the bottom were operations that were little more than fly-by-night diploma mills, while at the top were schools that approached the best in Europe. The University of Iowa and similar schools made up a second rank where the pace of reform in medical education trailed that at the best-endowed schools, mostly in the east, but where reformers nonetheless held similar aims. On the whole, however, leaders of the national movement for reform in medical education did not make such distinctions, but tended to see only a wasteland beyond Johns Hopkins, Harvard, Pennsylvania, and a handful of other schools, and the reformers' aim was to make up the difference between the best and worst medical schools at a single stroke through the imposition of nationwide standards.

The Progressive era of the early twentieth-century provided a nurturing environment for such a campaign. With its faith in science and professional prowess and its often deep-seated distrust of democracy and democratic institutions, Progressivism was a cultural and political response to the many alarming changes in a rapidly industrializing society, and it was marked by a determined and sometimes desperate public faith in material progress fostered by science and by science-inspired technologies. For example, Thomas Edison was a cultural hero to his generation, as was Henry Ford. In that context, the prestige of scientific medicine received an enormous boost from turn-of-the-century technological innovations, of which x-ray machines were the most dazzling. Such new technologies made it seem plausible to suppose "that solutions to disease and death were as close as the nearest patent office," while "new and better machines seemed only a step away."[58]

Under the circumstances, wholesale changes designed to make medical education more scientific would, according to reform proponents, put medicine in the vanguard of twentieth-century American society.[59] Accordingly, the reformers' program emphasized the teaching of science, both in pre-clinical and clinical subjects. Reformers also demanded a new emphasis on scientific research among medical faculty, under the assumption that good researchers were the best teachers.[60] "Medicine to-day is applied science," wrote Frank Billings in 1903, and "it must also be an experimental science."[61] Moreover, Victor Vaughan argued, "The university professor who does not devote a considerable portion of his time to honest and earnest endeavor to extend the bounds of knowledge is unworthy of his position and should be replaced."[62] Finally, reformers were generally agreed on the ideal of full-time teaching by resident faculty in clinical subjects, an ideal well beyond the reach of all of America's medical schools at the time.[63]

The package of reform proposals blended altruistic and economic motives. The investment in new laboratory and hospital facilities as well as faculty salaries required to implement the sweeping package of reforms would be far greater than the weakest schools, chiefly proprietary operations, could bear; thus, they would be forced to close or to consolidate with other institutions. The elimination of a vast majority of the proprietary schools would, at one fell swoop, boost the average level of medical education and improve the public image of American medicine. At the same time, such a drastic restructuring of American medical education would bring a precipitate fall in the numbers of physician graduates, easing the widely perceived problem of overcrowding in the profession.[64]

In all, then, Abraham Flexner's survey of American and Canadian medical education, begun in December 1908 with the results published in June 1910, was symptomatic of an era. Flexner, although not a physician, held a degree in classics from Johns Hopkins University, and his older brother Simon had gone to Hopkins to study medicine in 1895 and stayed for ten years as an assistant to William Welch. Not surprisingly, then, Abraham Flexner began his research into medical education with the premise that in Johns Hopkins he had seen a "small but ideal medical school."[65] Nor is it surprising, in light of the forces behind Flexner's work as well as his personal background, that his report was—with the exception of a handful of elite schools—a devastating indictment of medical education that supported a draconian proposal to reduce the number of medical schools in the U.S. and Canada from 155 to 31.[66]

Flexner first visited the University of Iowa College of Medicine in April 1909.[67] This, like all his visits to medical campuses, was a whirlwind affair; Flexner arrived in Iowa City at 4:00 P.M. and departed at 12:15 A.M. the following morning.[68] When challenged about the brevity of his inspection tours, Flexner was fond of quoting a favorite anecdote: "You don't need to eat a whole sheep to know it's tainted." And in many cases at least that was no doubt true. Yet Flexner was also a prickly man whom his critics, and there were many of those, labeled "erratic" and "hasty in judgment."[69] Abraham Flexner's judgment, hasty or not, was that he did not like what he saw during what he admitted was an "all too brief visit to Iowa City."[70]

Ten years later the Iowa State Board of Education recalled Flexner's observations in 1909 as "frank and to the point";[71] certainly Flexner's conclusions set off shock waves on the University of Iowa campus. While the basic science instruction offered in the College of Medicine, he reported, was "generally good and in some points excellent," "the clinical situation is of a different order altogether." In a stinging blow to Walter Bierring and the Department of Internal Medicine, Flexner contended that "the hospital is, in its teaching aspects, headless" with "no hospital records worthy the name" and no obvious pattern "on which the bedside teaching was conducted"; furthermore, "the present clinical department is on a high school basis." More generally, he cited a lack of contact between preclinical instructors and non-resident clinical faculty, particularly when the dean, James Guthrie, and professor of surgery, William Jepson, commuted long distances from their private practices. Furthermore, there was disorganization in the hospital administration suggesting "antiquated methods of teaching"; and there was a lack of clinical material for adequate instruction. All in all, in Flexner's view, it was arguable whether or not the school was worth salvaging; surely Iowa medical students would do better in Chicago or Minneapolis than in such a "small inland residential community."[72]

At the time, clinical instruction was the weakest point in American medical education, while, as Kenneth Ludmerer argues, "the strength of the country's medical schools had clearly come to lie in the basic science instruction of the first two years."[73] Nonetheless, Flexner's dismal portrayal of medical education at Iowa and at many other schools was overblown. There was, as German visitors of the time attested, much to be admired about American medical education in the early twentieth century.[74] Not only were American medical schools "attracting the most capable undergraduates" and, like Iowa, raising their admission standards as they improved their facilities and curricula; it was also the case that the best graduate opportunities in America were comparable to those available in Europe.[75]

Also, although the development of the modern hospital was "one of the prerequisites to any major change in the clinical curriculum,"[76] the weaknesses in clinical instruction were on the whole neither so bad as Flexner portrayed them nor, as the future would prove, so difficult to remedy. In fact, Flexner's survey provided a snapshot of American medical education in transition from a nineteenth-century regime that divided education between the "book-learning" of the medical schools and the practical training of the preceptor relationship to one in which both components were encompassed by the medical school and associated hospital facilities. At the University of Iowa that transition was well underway in 1909; the hospital facilities fulfilled Flexner's basic criteria which dealt with size and relationship to the medical school—that is, university-owned and run by the medical college.

Flexner's preliminary report, although harsh, was also curiously inconsistent, suggesting that his assessment was clouded by the assumption that the most cost-efficient way to improve American medical education would be to close vast numbers of medical schools. For example, even as he questioned the wisdom of maintaining a medical school in Iowa City, or anywhere in Iowa, Flexner admitted that a first-rate care facility would "probably draw to Iowa City all the clinical material that is needed." Moreover, he noted, "the clinical teaching can be improved without any greater expenditure than is involved in securing a permanent resident dean, a permanent resident surgeon, and a hospital head."

Ironically, President George MacLean had come to the University of Iowa in 1899 with his own credentials as an educational reformer and with great hopes for the university, and enrollments had doubled in MacLean's decade-long tenure. MacLean was not disposed to take Flexner's challenge lightly in as much as the Carnegie Foundation stood behind Flexner, and the American Medical Association's Council on Medical Education and Hospitals, too, approved of his mission. MacLean also very much needed Carnegie Foundation money, not only for teacher pensions but for university expansion as well. Yet neither was he willing to see the college of medicine, fast becoming a hallmark of the modern university, go down the drain without a fight or, just as bad, see it transferred to the capital city of Des Moines. MacLean, then, did not protest Flexner's findings directly but sought a compromise solution that would save the medical school.

President MacLean immediately circulated Flexner's preliminary report to all medical faculty with a charge to "read it ... and send me the points that could be made in answer to it."[77] Instructors in non-clinical areas were reluctant to comment on Flexner's criticisms of clinical faculty. Charles S. Chase, professor of materia medica, noted simply, "It seems to me they [i.e., clinical faculty] can best speak for themselves."[78] And Elbert W. Rockwood, professor of chemistry, suggested that Flexner's opinion "may not be worth more than that of an Iowa farmer."[79] Walter Bierring and other clinical faculty, meanwhile, were adamant that Flexner's charges were ill-informed. Bierring's response was tempered, but William Jepson, professor of surgery, was livid, charging that "the facts intended to be set forth [in Flexner's report] are so far from the truth that a relationship cannot even be recognized." Indeed, Jepson sputtered, it appeared that Flexner was "drumming up trade ... for Minneapolis and Chicago."[80]

Perhaps because of President MacLean's reputation in educational reform circles, Carnegie Foundation president Henry S. Pritchett asked Flexner to make a second visit to the Iowa campus. With Dean R. H. Whitehead of the University of Virginia College of Medicine in tow, Flexner returned to Iowa City in early November 1909, but his opinion was little changed from April. "There has been a certain degree of activity," he noted, combined with "a genuine desire to improve conditions." Still, he doubted that anyone really understood what needed to be done, and the crux of the problem, he speculated, might be "that the clinical teachers are not themselves in all respects modern men."[81] Whitehead, like Flexner, praised the pre-clinical instruction at the college but noted a "marked contrast with the condition of affairs in the clinical branches"; the "lack of material," he noted, was a serious handicap and "seemed greatest in internal medicine."[82]

However, Whitehead, whose own school was located in a community similar to Iowa City, did not say that the University of Iowa College of Medicine should be abandoned. And although Flexner was still highly critical, he had softened his position after a lengthy discussion in Iowa City with William R. Boyd, a Cedar Rapids journalist and president of the finance committee of the state board of education, who assured Flexner that the board was prepared to meet his demands.[83] Both Whitehead and Flexner were agreed, though, that if the school were to survive, it desperately needed "a leader well versed in the methods of modern medical pedagogy" and capable of attracting other top-notch faculty.

The combined medical faculty responded to Flexner's and Whitehead's reports with a resolution—offered by William Jepson—defending Dean James Guthrie and excoriating the "report[s] of Dr. Whitehead and Dr. Flexner" that "by implication charge our Dean with the responsibility for the discreditable condition in which he [sic] claims to find the department."[84] Clearly the medical faculty understood that Dean James Guthrie was the "leader" to whom Whitehead and Flexner referred and that Guthrie's position was therefore in jeopardy.

Clearly, too, university officials and the board of education were under pressure to demonstrate their commitment to reform, most likely through dismissal of one or more of the clinical faculty implicated in Flexner's report. But it was not Dean Guthrie or even William Jepson who was sacrificed. Prodded by Boyd and MacLean, the state board of education, at a December 1909 meeting, charged its faculty committee with finding "means of improving the college."[85] Recent "radical departures in medical education," the board concluded, mandated larger state appropriations, expansion of the hospital as already planned, and the attraction of more clinical material to the hospital through provision of free beds to be apportioned among Iowa's counties. However, the most important step, in keeping with Flexner's and Whitehead's criticisms, was recruitment of a "thoroughly equipped internist." This should be, it was decided, "a man of wide reputation" and an outsider who would end what Whitehead had described as "the vice of inbreeding" in faculty recruitment.[86]

Whether the implicit reference to Walter Bierring reflected Flexner's November chat with William Boyd is unknown, but Walter Bierring's removal, although no one said as much, had become the price of saving the college. Admittedly, as hospital director and vice-dean of the college as well, Bierring shared responsibility for whatever deficiencies may have existed at the college; however, that responsibility was Bierring's largely by default. Bierring was, after all, an Iowa City resident, while Dean Guthrie commuted twice weekly from his Dubuque obstetrical practice, and William Jepson made improbable 600-mile weekly round trips from his Sioux City surgical practice. Neither Guthrie not Jepson was in a position to contribute much to administration, to teaching, or to collegiality at the college.

Taking into account the often bewildering intricacies of institutional politics, Bierring was perhaps the most vulnerable of the clinical faculty. To some extent the fate of each of the principals hinged on the strength of their personal relationships with President George MacLean and the members of the state board of education, and both Guthrie and Jepson had many well-placed friends. Beyond that, Bierring was formally out-ranked by Dean Guthrie, and in any event the firing of the dean would only have heightened already rampant speculation about the shaky future of the college. Guthrie in fact played a central role in recruiting Bierring's successor and remained as dean until 1914. On the other hand, William Jepson, as professor of surgery, also outranked Walter Bierring, and Bierring's position may have been weakened by the resignation of his mentor, Lawrence Littig, in 1903 when Jepson had received the chair of surgery.

Whatever the rationale, the rapid-fire developments of late 1909 and early

1910 left Walter Bierring in an unenviable spot. President MacLean seems to have hoped to allow Bierring a graceful exit by delaying the search for a new head of internal medicine. There is no evidence that MacLean made any move to initiate a search, and it was not MacLean but James Trewin, president of the state board of education, who finally wrote Abraham Flexner in April 1910 seeking advice on Bierring's successor.[87] Tellingly, Bierring's name did not appear in the board of education's May 26, 1910, listing of medical faculty salaries, even though it was not until early June that Bierring and the faculty committee of the board of education reached a convenient impasse—apparently over Bierring's refusal to give up his large private practice—that led to his dismissal.

At any rate, by June 24, 1910, when MacLean formally notified Bierring of the board of education's action, the search for a successor was well under way, a search that was without precedent in the medical college's previous experience. President MacLean and William Boyd understood that it was essential to answer Flexner's charge of provincialism "among the weak schools of the west" and to assert the university's adherence to reform ideals. The search for Walter Bierring's successor, then, had as much to do with the increasingly complicated politics of medical education as it did the specific qualifications of the candidates. Just as certainly it was neither Walter Bierring's abilities nor his private practice that was the proximate cause of his dismissal. Johns Hopkins, after all, did not have a full-time head of internal medicine until 1915. MacLean and Boyd realized that they were, for the first time, playing to a constituency beyond the borders of Iowa, and under the circumstances it was important that they secure not just the best and brightest candidate to head the department of internal medicine, but the best and brightest candidate from the east.

Henry Pritchett had responded to Trewin's April letter to Flexner suggesting Joseph Pratt of Harvard and three others as likely candidates for the Iowa position, all of them Johns Hopkins graduates.[88] With Bierring's fate settled, President MacLean, too, entered the search, seeking advice from Dean F. F. Westbrook of the University of Minnesota College of Medicine and Frank Billings of Rush Medical College. MacLean also dispatched Dean James Guthrie to the Carnegie Foundation offices in New York City and to Harvard in search of recommendations. Guthrie also attended a March meeting in Baltimore on medical education where he had access to Johns Hopkins faculty, and he visited Dean Whitehead in Charlottesville on his return.

In early June 1910, President MacLean invited Joseph Pratt to visit the Iowa campus. Pratt was a Harvard physician who had worked under William Osler at Johns Hopkins and had been a founding member of Osler's Interurban Clinical Club. However, Pratt gave Iowa only brief consideration, noting that "the opportunities for me are better in Boston than in Iowa City." Chief among those opportunities was his remunerative private practice.[89] Attention then shifted to John Phillips of Western Reserve in Cleveland, and Phillips visited Iowa City in mid-June, a trip that "was a revelation to him" according to Dean Guthrie. But Phillips, like Pratt, withdrew from consideration, apparently before receiving any firm offer. Like Pratt, Phillips' reason for withdrawing—also ironic in light of the supposed grounds for Walter Bierring's dismissal—was his reluctance to leave "his very large clinic."[90]

As the search progressed amid considerable statewide publicity as well as speculation about the fate of the medical college, there was some pressure from Iowa medical and political circles to choose an Iowa physician for the post. The most likely of those was W. E. Sanders, an Alta, Iowa, physician with connections to Johns Hopkins and a man who was recommended to MacLean by both James Trewin and another board of education member.[91] MacLean treated Sanders and other Iowa candidates gently, even inviting Sanders for a brief campus visit; but the president tactfully explained that the local candidates had "come into competition with one or two men who have had great advantage in education and in proving out in teaching positions."[92]

Chief among those "one or two men" was Campbell Palmer Howard of McGill University in Montreal, a name suggested by Abraham Flexner.[93] Campbell Howard was not only superbly qualified but also carried the Hopkins mystique and enjoyed a close family connection with William Osler. Campbell Howard's father, R. Palmer Howard, was a prominent late nineteenth-century internist, head of internal medicine at McGill, one of Osler's teachers, and a founding member (1886) of the Association of American Physicians—an elite organization of mostly east coast physicians devoted to "the advancement of scientific and practical medicine." William Osler was, in fact, Campbell Howard's godfather, and Howard's name appeared among the contributors in the 1905 edition of Osler's *Principles and Practice of Medicine*.

For Campbell Howard, the Iowa job beckoned as a stepping stone. Howard was stymied at Montreal General Hospital, where he was assigned to the outpatient service, his prospects for advancement blocked by the tenure of senior men. The move to Iowa, as William Osler advised him, would be a good career move under the circumstances, one that would surely lead to "a chair in one of the big universities."[94]

Dean Guthrie testified that Campbell Howard was "the man highly endorsed by all of the Baltimore [i.e., Johns Hopkins] people."[95] And, by early July, Campbell Howard had become the consensus choice to succeed Walter Bierring. Howard visited the Iowa City campus on July 12, 1910. Later the same day the medical faculty "unanimously recommended" him to President MacLean and the board of education. A week later, Howard telegraphed his conditions for acceptance, including a salary of $4,500, two assistants at $2,000 each, and

$1,500 for equipment.[96] Bierring, in comparison, had earned $1,100 for his part-time services. MacLean immediately urged the board of education to offer Howard a salary of $4,000, to be increased to $4,500 in the second year, two assistants with first-year salaries considerably below the $2,000 requested, and $500 "for apparatus and supplies." Moreover, this was, MacLean argued, "a critical moment in the history of the College of Medicine," and either William Boyd or Dean Guthrie, he said, should go to Montreal to negotiate directly with Howard.[97] Just two days later, the Faculty Committee of the board of education concurred, authorizing university officials "to make all practical efforts to secure Dr. Campbell P. Howard."[98]

On Tuesday, July 26, with William Boyd in Montreal, President MacLean waited anxiously for word of Howard's acceptance and agonized over "leaks" to the press about Boyd's mission.[99] On Wednesday morning MacLean received Boyd's message: "Howard will come."[100] MacLean promptly sent two letters to Campbell Howard, one welcoming him to the faculty and a second reiterating the terms that Boyd had offered.[101] But the deal was not yet sealed. Howard wrote to MacLean on August 3 to clear up some ambiguities regarding laboratory equipment and expenses. He also noted that he would "have a chat with Dr. Osler" about Iowa's offer, and "if he approves of my going to Iowa City, as I feel certain he will, I will write you my official letter."[102] A few days later the board of education confirmed Campbell Howard's appointment, and internal medicine at Iowa had survived its most serious crisis.

CONCLUSION

In one sense at least, Campbell Howard's appointment opened a new era at the University of Iowa College of Medicine; the recruitment of an internist of "wide reputation" marked the unmistakable integration of the University of Iowa College of Medicine into a larger world of medical science and education. Moreover, both George MacLean and William Boyd appreciated that a new political context had fundamentally changed the guidelines for faculty selection. If that loss of autonomy was one of the costs of saving the College of Medicine, they were willing to pay it.

Yet for all the excitement surrounding it, the extent of the "Flexner revolution" at the University of Iowa should not be overstated. The response to Flexner's report did not profoundly alter the course of development established well before his visits. The reforms associated with Flexner's name were built upon foundations laid by a generation of reformers like William Robertson and his successors in internal medicine at Iowa. It was they who first introduced scientific medicine to a skeptical public and fought for improvements in public health and for passage of a physician licensure statute, while building the College of Medicine at the University of Iowa and shepherding it into the modern era. In like manner, the immediate future of internal medicine at the University of Iowa rested upon the skills and reputation of Campbell Howard.

2

The Making of the Modern
Department of Medicine

1910–1928

WHEN Campbell Howard came to Iowa as an ambitious young man of thirty-two to head the Department of Internal Medicine, his immediate task was to help rebuild an institution in turmoil in the wake of Abraham Flexner's disastrous report. Indeed, for both the Department of Internal Medicine and the College of Medicine, Campbell Howard's solid credentials and reputation were essential ingredients in nearly two decades of rapid expansion that constituted a now forgotten golden age, a formative era that in many important respects laid the foundations for the remarkable developments of more recent decades.

In those years, the Department of Internal Medicine shared with American academic medicine in general the excitement of scientific advance along with continuous institutional construction and reconstruction, marking the maturity of American medical education and the emergence of the teaching hospital as the centerpiece of the hierarchical regionalism that has remained the guiding principle in the organization of American health care.[1] At the University of Iowa, the new medical campus that grew on the west bank of the Iowa River between 1918 and 1928—boosted, ironically enough, by Abraham Flexner—symbolized the newfound dynamism and authority of academic medicine and the rising public confidence in, and expectations of, the new medical science and technology.

For the University of Iowa Department of Internal Medicine, the years from 1910 to 1928 brought significant growth in faculty numbers and a more rigorous approach to clinical education, including the institutionalization of the fifth year, or graduate hospital internship. Just as important for the long term, those critical years saw the introduction of systematic scientific research to the department and the fuller integration of department faculty into the rapidly developing network of regional and national scientific organizations.

Rapid growth appeared at times to exact a high price. In both the College of Medicine and in the Department of Internal Medicine, for example, there were sometimes bitter conflicts over policies, personalities, and the distribution of power. Meanwhile, many Iowa doctors resented the fact that the University of Iowa's new medical elites were, to an increasing extent, not Iowans at all but outsiders bent upon reshaping the college in their own image. Campbell Howard was a lightning rod for such complaints, in part because of his pugnacious nature but chiefly because his hiring had set the precedent for a new and unsettling policy of faculty recruitment. In short, then, there was more to this golden age than triumph and celebration.

THE NEW MEDICAL EDUCATION AT THE UNIVERSITY OF IOWA

The incorporation of the medical school into the university complex was one of the striking features of America's new medical education that emerged in the late nineteenth century. Given its increasing emphasis on the teaching of practical knowledge, the university seemed the logical home for the medical school; after all, as one enthusiastic university booster claimed, "The university idea involves the cooperative intellectual and moral effort to collect, disseminate and apply knowledge for man's needs."[2] Thus, when controversy erupted in 1920 over whether to locate the University of Virginia's new medical school complex in Charlottesville or Richmond, Theodore Hough argued that "the clear trend ... is toward bringing the medical school into the closest possible contact with the rest of the university." Both the interdependence of medicine and the basic sciences and the need of curricular flexibility in medical education, Hough argued, demanded placement of the medical school with the university in Charlottesville. And to buttress his argument, Hough pointed to the University of Iowa as a model.[3]

In Iowa, the consequences of the movement of medical education toward the university were profound. In 1900, there had been four medical schools in the state, located in Sioux City, Des Moines, Keokuk, and Iowa City, but by the autumn of 1913 the Sioux City school had closed, the Keokuk school had merged with the Drake University School of Medicine in Des Moines, and the latter had in turn merged with the College of Medicine at the University of Iowa.

The concentration of medical education at the University of Iowa, coupled with the university's formal adoption in 1910 of standards of admission prescribed by the Association of American Medical Colleges,[4] drastically altered the demographics of medical education in Iowa. While Iowa medical schools had enrolled 660 students and granted 130 degrees in 1903–04, enrollment dropped to 109 and graduates to 13—all at the University of Iowa—in 1913–14.[5] Meanwhile, a decline in female graduates—just four in 1907—had begun even before the shrinkage in enrollments.[6]

At the University of Iowa and elsewhere, much was expected of the marriage of medical education and the university, and to some extent those hopes were fulfilled. Certainly the association meant a measure of financial stability for medical schools, and medical schools in turn added to the prestige of universities and swelled the ranks of politically influential alumni. Moreover, because of the university association, medical schools became home to medical scientific research and were the birthplaces of a new academic medicine,[7] which, in the following decades, exerted significant influence on the professional development of American medicine.[8]

Yet, while the university medical school became the focus of medical reform in Iowa and in much of America, the marriage of medical education and the modern university was, and still remains, at times an uneasy one. The close interaction of medical faculty and students with the rest of the university community envisioned by early twentieth-century reformers seldom materialized, and as medical school complexes grew in size through the 1920s and 1930s, their degree of isolation, often physical as well as psychological, grew as well. That isolation was evident at the University of Iowa with the movement of the medical campus "across the river"—i.e., from the east to the west side of the Iowa River that now divides the campus.

When Campbell Howard arrived at the University of Iowa, however, his concerns were far less philosophical and far more practical. His paramount aim was to introduce to internal medicine at Iowa the fundamentals of scientific medicine as he had observed them at McGill and Johns Hopkins, and to do that he needed money, personnel, and equipment, all of which had been major concerns in his negotiations with President MacLean. From Montreal, Howard brought Louis Baumann, a graduate of the College of Physicians and Surgeons of New York, to conduct the research laboratory of the medical clinic, a facility that Howard hoped to model on the Medical Chemistry Laboratory at McGill.[9] Campbell Howard was not disappointed; in 1916, he praised Baumann's work in blood chemistry and metabolism, noting that Baumann was "well known in the physiological-chemical fields." In fact, Howard testified, Baumann was "doing more for the recognition of the medical school in the scientific world than any two of us clinicians."[10]

By 1915, other major figures of Campbell Howard's team were also in place. Clarence Van Epps, whom Walter Bierring had recruited to the faculty, had become full professor, and when Howard recommended the differentiation of neurology from internal medicine in the mid-1920s, Van Epps became professor and head of the new department, where he remained into the 1950s. By 1915, the department also included Clifford W. McClure, clinical microscopist, and Frank J. Rohner, clinical assistant, the latter a 1911 Iowa graduate who had subsequently served a year as Howard's intern. In addition, the department employed a lecturer in pediatrics until, with Campbell Howard's concurrence, pediatrics became a full-fledged department in the fall of 1915.[11] Finally, the still new field of radiography fell within the purview of internal medicine, and Howard in fact took some personal interest in it, incorporating x-ray films in a 1914 article.[12]

Faculty salaries grew rapidly as Campbell Howard built his department. Total salaries for internal medicine faculty rose from $4,250 in 1909–10, Walter Bierring's final year as department head, to $14,000 in 1914–15 and to $25,000 in 1921–22, an increase reflecting both growing faculty numbers and a substantial rise in salary rates. While Walter Bierring had received $1,100 for his part-time services in 1909–10, for example, Campbell Howard's salary was more than three times that, and his successor, Fred Smith, joined the faculty in 1924 at $7,000, both of them on a part-time basis and both augmenting their salaries substantially by returns from private practice.

Higher faculty salaries accompanied an increased teaching load under a significantly revamped curriculum. Clinical instruction, in particular, demanded much more faculty time in the 1920s than had been the case prior to 1910. There were also important changes in teaching style and cognitive emphasis in medical education. Keys to the new medical education were the active participation of the student in the learning process and the development of critical thinking skills under close faculty supervision. Expanded clinical instruction for junior and senior students, like laboratory experience in the basic sciences, exemplified the heightened emphasis on what Kenneth Ludmerer calls "learning by doing."

Through the 1920s, the pre-clinical curriculum of anatomy, histology, embryology, physiology, pathology, bacteriology, and chemistry remained substantially the same in organization, if not in content, as in Walter Bierring's time, but the clinical subjects expanded significantly, as the curriculum was broadened and innovations were formalized. By 1921–22, for example, Campbell Howard was teaching theory and practice of medicine to both junior and senior classes; in addition, he shared responsibility for the course in clinical medicine in which senior clerks demonstrated clinical cases for their junior and senior colleagues. Howard also taught ward classes—the formal program of clinical clerkship for seniors—and participated in the twice-weekly internal medicine clinic designed to meet both patient service and instructional needs.

Campbell Howard idolized William Osler, who was both his godfather and an exemplar of the new scientific medicine, and many years later, Walter Bierring credited Campbell Howard for having "brought the spirit of Osler to the State University of Iowa."[13] Osler's *The Practice of Medicine* was Howard's classroom bible, and he could, his students claimed, recite line by line from it. Howard's intellectual accomplishments in the clinic and the classroom made an impression on colleagues and students alike. One of his students remembered Howard's classroom demeanor as "pretty tough." He did not mince words in discussion of general academic standards or in dealing with individual students. Campbell Howard, "a big man physically and mentally," was perhaps not well liked by all his students, but "everybody respected him."[14]

Curricular innovation imposed additional burdens not just on faculty but on the college's physical plant as well, requiring ever larger facilities and more expensive equipment. Overcrowded classes were a common worry and brought a faculty recommendation to limit enrollment to "legal residents of Iowa" or to students who had completed at least the last year of pre-medical studies at an Iowa college.[15] Although the state board of education turned down that proposal, informal mechanisms accomplished much the same reduction in enrollments. Rising expectations for student performance, for example, resulted in a very high attrition rate; in 1922, the total medical student enrollment of 325 was made up of 137 freshmen, 81 sophomores, 55 juniors, and just 38 seniors. Similarly, the jump in tuition from $50 in 1912–13 to $175 for Iowa residents and $350 for non-residents by the early 1920s worked both to hold down enrollments and to "practically eliminate students from outside the state."[16]

In the decade from 1910 to 1920, medical education in America also expanded beyond the four-year program as the hospital internship became increasingly common.[17] The question of whether or not to make the so-called "fifth year" mandatory was much debated at the University of Iowa and elsewhere. The issues were two: first, whether or not the internship was needed at all, and, second, whether the internship would be a part of the undergraduate program—thus, supervised by the medical schools—or become a graduate requirement for licensure. Responding to a query from the Council on Medical Education and Hospitals of the American Medical Association in May 1916, the University of Iowa medical faculty passed a resolution against instituting a mandatory fifth-year requirement.[18]

Prior to the 1920s, there was little standardization in internship programs, and for several years the Department of Internal Medicine at the University of Iowa operated what would be known a half century later as a "straight internship," with interns assigned exclusively to internal medicine. The more familiar "rotating internship" came later. The number of interns—all of them Iowa graduates—assigned to the department expanded rapidly. In 1910–11, Campbell Howard supervised a single intern, but the number rose to two in 1915–16, three in 1918–19, four in 1920–21, five in 1922–23, and reached six in 1925–26.

Moreover, even though the number of female students in the College of Medicine had fallen to minuscule proportions, Campbell Howard often included one woman among his intern selections. The expansion of the ranks of interns highlighted new problems for the College of Medicine ranging from lack of housing to disciplinary concerns. Already in 1912, the hospital staff recommended that "for the sake of discipline" the interns should "be prohibited from visiting the nurses' home."[19]

In many respects, the teens and twenties of this century were an important period in the development of academic medicine and medical education at the University of Iowa, just as was the case across America. For Campbell Howard and his colleagues in the Department of Internal Medicine, the new era meant more time devoted to the teaching of undergraduates, and it brought the additional burden of instruction of interns as well. For students, meanwhile, the changes in medical education meant a more diverse and more demanding curriculum and more time spent in learning situations, whether classroom, laboratory, or clinic.

THE DEPARTMENT AND COMMUNITIES OF MEDICAL SCIENCE

The new medical schools of the early twentieth century were to be centers of scientific research as well as of medical education. In an era when internal medicine in America earned considerable prestige from an impressive list of advances in immunology, endocrinology, nutrition, and metabolism built on a combination of clinical insight and laboratory work,[20] scientific research for the first time achieved significance as a standard by which individuals and departments were measured.

In 1915, Lee W. Dean, dean of the College of Medicine, worried that the college "had gained a wide reputation for the excellent character of its equipment and instruction" but that the same was not true of its "interest and attainments in research." Newspapers, too, criticized the university more generally for not having "reached out after men and women who are pre-eminent as scholars."[21] In response, the medical faculty recommended to the state board of education a requirement that all instructors "engage in some definite form of research work,"[22] and in January 1916, university president Thomas H. Macbride issued a letter to all medical faculty stating research expectations.[23] Thus, at Iowa as elsewhere, the reward system for medical faculty began a long and subtle shift from teaching toward research.[24]

The new emphasis on scientific research in academic medicine sparked an exponential growth in scientific associations and in professional journals, and

Campbell Howard participated in both developments. He circulated the results of his research—on subjects reflecting both his broad interests and the still largely unspecialized nature of internal medicine—in professional journals such as *Archives of Internal Medicine* and the *American Journal of the Medical Sciences*.[25] At the same time, he was prominent in the closer integration of midwestern internist-researchers into the larger American community of medical science. In 1911, Howard was chosen an associate member of the Association of American Physicians, and in 1914 was elevated to full membership.[26] In December 1919, Campbell Howard joined major figures in midwestern medicine—including George Canby Robinson, George Dock, James B. Herrick, and Frank Billings—in creating the Central Interurban Club, an organization modeled on the Interurban Clinical Club founded by William Osler in 1905 and one dedicated to furthering research, teaching, and fraternity among academic physicians in the Midwest.

Members of the Central Interurban Club in turn created the Central Clinical Research Club, meant specifically to engage junior faculty in scientific work. Campbell Howard saw to it that his colleagues, Wesley E. Gatewood and Frank J. Rohner, were early members.[27] Howard was also involved with the American Society for Clinical Investigation, an organization founded in 1908 by aggressive young researchers promoting the new concept of clinical investigation, and he served on the first editorial committee of the *Journal of Clinical Investigation*.

The benefits of such connections with the larger world of internal medicine were evident also at the University of Iowa. Just a few months after the successful isolation of insulin in 1922,[28] Howard conferred in Atlantic City, New Jersey, with Simon Flexner of the Rockefeller Institute about a new insulin project then in the planning stage. The project, using Rockefeller funds, was meant to publicize the insulin discovery by subsidizing insulin therapy for diabetics at selected sites around the country and educating practicing physicians in diabetic management with insulin. Through subsequent negotiations with Flexner, Howard secured a $10,000 grant in 1923, and in the next twelve months 144 patients at the University Hospitals received insulin therapy, thirty physicians received training in its use, and the college established a "diabetic home" with its own dietitian to accommodate the influx of diabetic patients.[29]

In all, the emergence of scientific research and the elaboration of networks of communication among academic physicians may well have been the most striking and most important single change in academic medicine in the early decades of the twentieth century. Not only did the promulgation of faculty research requirements, as at the University of Iowa, add a new element to the academic physician's job description; it also solidified academic physicians' larger sense of community and shared purpose and in doing so set them further apart from the private practitioners whom they trained.

THE UNIVERSITY HOSPITALS AND PRIVATE PRACTICE

The modern hospital was another defining characteristic of the new scientific medicine. The number of beds in American hospitals exploded from just 42,000 in 1909 to over one million in 1932.[30] The University of Iowa Hospital that Walter Bierring had known in the first decade of the century sprouted new wings of six and seven stories in 1912 and 1914; in addition, an isolation hospital opened in 1918 at the corner of Jefferson and Gilbert Streets. Meanwhile, completion of the Children's Hospital in 1919, marked the opening of the new 58-acre medical campus west of the Iowa River. In addition, the Munger Bill passed by the state legislature in 1910 empowered local governments to levy taxes for the construction of community hospitals across Iowa, the first of those opening in Washington, Iowa, in July 1912.[31]

The University of Iowa hospitals were, first, sources of clinical material for instruction and for research for the College of Medicine. In the early twentieth century, indigent patients received care on an ad hoc basis, admitted to the hospitals on the basis of a letter "from a physician, a clergyman, or a county officer."[32] However, in October 1914, the medical faculty submitted to the state board of education a draft of legislation to bring "crippled and afflicted" children to the University Hospitals at public expense,[33] and in the following year the General Assembly approved the Perkins Bill—named for its sponsor Senator Eli C. Perkins—that opened the university hospital to children from all ninety-nine Iowa counties and to adult patients confined in other state institutions.

Already in November 1916, University Hospitals admissions included fifty-three "Perkins" cases out of the total of 287 patients admitted that month.[34] Perkins cases, many of them involving complicated orthopaedic procedures, generated considerable revenue, enough, staff physicians feared, to "occasion very critical comment by the State Executive Council."[35] To be sure, as indigent admissions spiraled rapidly upward, from some 400 in 1915–16 to more than 2,200 in 1919, hospital income from state patients rose dramatically, totaling over $95,000 in the 1917–18 fiscal year, some 40 percent of all hospital revenues. Furthermore, in 1919, the Thirty-eighth General Assembly of Iowa passed the Haskell-Klaus Law, which provided care at university hospitals for Iowa's indigent adult population. As a result, the university hospitals admitted nearly 3,000 adult patients at state expense in 1920, and in fiscal year 1920–21, state payments for patient care surpassed a half million dollars.[36]

The hospital also served as a supplementary source of income for clinical faculty, in direct conflict with the full-time system espoused by Abraham Flexner. In 1913, during the search for a new head of surgery to replace William Jepson, Abraham Flexner volunteered to secure "a first rate surgeon, willing and eager to devote his entire attention to the subject and not to practice."[37]

Supporters of full-time contended that it would "raise clinical departments up to the status of true university departments" and integrate clinical faculty more fully into the university structure.[38] Furthermore, they argued, time spent with private patients detracted from time clinicians could spend in research, as well as tainting scientific medicine with the unsavory odor of commercialism. The private practice issue even commanded attention from the popular press in Iowa, as the *Des Moines Register and Leader* ran a major story on the $1.5 million gift—with the full-time plan as *quid pro quo*—from the General Education Board to Johns Hopkins University in 1914.[39]

Whatever the supposed virtues of the full-time system, income from private patients was a critical element in recruiting figures of Campbell Howard's stature to the University of Iowa College of Medicine, and internists and surgeons, as the oldest and most powerful groups of clinical faculty, guarded their hospital prerogatives jealously. Campbell Howard's mentor William Osler was the full-time plan's most influential and perhaps most bitter opponent. Backed by the promise of "big Rockefeller cheques," Osler charged in 1915, the full-time plan "has been forced on the profession by men who know nothing of clinical medicine." "To have a group of cloistered clinicians," he continued, "would be bad for teacher and worse for student."[40] The full-time system, another critic argued, was the product of the false notion that medicine can be made a strict science, removed from the idiosyncrasies of individual patients.[41]

Ironically, in the wake of Abraham Flexner's 1909 visits, the system of private practice had become more institutionalized at the University of Iowa. In 1915, the medical faculty voted to set aside the third floor of a new hospital wing for private cases,[42] and by the early 1920s private practice privileges, in the dean's estimation, boosted Campbell Howard's annual income to nearly $20,000, more than four times his academic salary.[43] In 1922, a faculty committee, of which Campbell Howard was a member, offered several arguments in favor of private practice. Private patients, the committee claimed, added variety to the clinical material available for teaching purposes, and barring private practice would also close the "best equipped, most efficient hospital in the state" to private patients. Finally, without the added income from private practice, the committee noted, it would be impossible to keep top-notch faculty.[44] Campbell Howard was as outspoken as his mentor Osler on the subject of the full-time plan. "Even before I saw Osler's letter to the trustees of the Johns Hopkins," Howard claimed on one occasion, "I was against the scheme." "Wherever it has been tried," he charged, "it has proved a distinct failure." Not only did clinical teaching suffer as a result, but also, in Howard's view, "the much-talked-of 'research' has not yet materialized."[45]

Still, the medical faculty was aware of the potential for abuse of the privilege of private practice, and in fact the faculty itself was divided on the issue. Some favored an "open hospital," with outside physicians admitted to practice, while others favored a strictly "clinical hospital," with no private patients at all. In 1915, faculty members compromised on new rules to regulate private practice. The new rules mandated, first, that clinical teachers confine private practice to the area of their specialties; second, clinical teachers must, the faculty ruled, be willing "to make private practice wholly secondary to teaching"; third, the rules required clinical faculty to spend a minimum of three hours in the hospital each day; finally, the university hospitals were effectively closed to outside physicians.[46] Subsequently, Campbell Howard threatened to resign if those new rules were changed.[47] Moreover, when Dean Lee W. Dean recommended to President Jessup in 1920 that private practice be limited to two hours per day and eliminated altogether when sufficient funds became available to raise salaries to a competitive level, he added the cautionary note, "I would recommend that Dr. Howard be always exempt from this provision."[48]

The question of private practice at the University Hospitals was a divisive issue in Iowa medicine, sparking biting criticism from the Iowa State Medical Society and especially Lawrence W. Littig, the former head of internal medicine who had gone from the university to private practice in Davenport, Iowa. In a 1912 article in the *Journal of the American Medical Association,* Littig made scarcely veiled allusions to the private practice controversy in commenting on the adverse affects of "commercialism" in medicine, a subject, he said, that "will not down until the medical profession mends its ways."[49] More importantly, though, Littig chaired the Iowa State Medical Society Committee on Medical Education in 1914 that compiled a scathing report on the College of Medicine in general and the conduct of the University Hospitals in particular. "The hospital," Littig wrote, "is being liberally patronized by private patients," and the faculty were "neglecting their work to attend to private practice." Perhaps still smarting from Walter Bierring's dismissal in favor of Campbell Howard, Littig professed astonishment that the head of internal medicine "has a free office ... where he receives his private patients." "The University Hospital," he concluded, "should be used only for teaching purposes."[50]

Perhaps more ominously, the private practice controversy sparked an anonymous charge of fee-splitting by physicians at the University Hospitals, a charge that reached the American Medical Association in 1914. In response to the allegation, Arthur Dean Bevan, chairman of the AMA's Council on Medical Education and Hospitals, dispatched a stern letter of inquiry to President Macbride, reminding him that such practices were sufficient cause for withdrawal of the college's accreditation.[51] While publicly denying the charge, Macbride and many others privately conceded that the practice was commonplace.

What made the private practice issue especially sensitive was the fact that it was outsiders, like Campbell Howard, who were the chief beneficiaries of practice privileges in the University Hospitals. Lawrence Littig's 1914 report for the Iowa State Medical Society, for example, included alumni complaints about the hiring of "Eastern Graduates as teachers in the University." Even James Trewin, president of the state board of education, harbored reservations on that score and in 1914 opposed the promotion of professor of surgery Charles J. Rowan, an 1898 Rush Medical College graduate, to the post of dean of the college. Trewin warned darkly of a "clique in the Medical College which ... has sought to obtain control" and recommended Lee Wallace Dean for the post. Dean was a native of Muscatine, Iowa, an 1896 University of Iowa graduate, an early student of Walter Bierring, and had been a College of Medicine faculty member since 1898.[52]

In 1914, a Fort Dodge physician summed up the situation by noting that "the medical department of the university is in bad odor with the medical profession of the state,"[53] a situation that was neither new nor easily resolved but one that had become increasingly troublesome. In the face of that, the university administration and the faculty of the College of Medicine sought to mend professional fences. President Macbride invited the Iowa State Medical Society to hold its 1916 meeting at the university, promising to make laboratories and other facilities available.[54] Also, beginning in 1920, Campbell Howard energetically promoted outreach programs of summer graduate work for practicing physicians.[55] Similarly, the college invited all practitioners in the state to its annual Alumni Clinic, later called simply the Annual Clinic, an occasion for technical demonstrations, talks by nationally known figures in medicine, and fraternal activities of various kinds that attracted as many as 150 Iowa physicians by the late 1920s.[56]

Despite such well-intentioned efforts, a degree of animosity remained a constant feature in the relations of the college and the medical profession at large. To a considerable extent that animosity was symptomatic of the closer integration of the College of Medicine into the rapidly evolving world of medical science and education. As we have already seen in the case of Campbell Howard, that process of integration entailed a significant shift in faculty recruitment practices, and it also meant a subtle reorientation of academic physicians toward a larger scientific community, all of which contributed to the troubled relationship between College of Medicine faculty and Iowa's practicing physicians.

A GREAT VICTORY: THE CAMPAIGN FOR THE NEW HOSPITAL

The future of medical science and medical education at the University of Iowa hinged upon continued growth of the physical plant, but facilities on the old medical campus, repeatedly enlarged and improved since the 1890s, were pushing the limits of available space by the mid-teens. In 1917, Campbell Howard was part of a faculty committee charged with preparing a plan "for an entire group of medical and hospital buildings" to be located on a tract of land west of the Iowa River.[57] The plan encompassed a spacious 1,000-bed general hospital supported by a medical laboratory building, a nurses' dormitory, a psychiatric hospital, and the children's hospital—the last already under construction. The combined total of patient beds in the new facilities would be some five times that of the old, part of an ambitious plan of "state hospital service" designed to make the University Hospitals more accessible to Iowans, in effect to make the university hospitals the equivalent of today's tertiary care facility.

The Department of Internal Medicine was directly linked to hospital expansion in two ways. First, the reputation of the department under the leadership of Campbell Howard was a key to the growing reputation of the college as a whole. Looking back on Campbell Howard's years at Iowa, the Iowa City Press Citizen in 1936 noted that it was "largely Dr. Howard's influence and work which raised this medical staff and this hospital to a class A institution."[58] Second, without the new laboratory and hospital facilities, the potential for continued growth in the department was limited. In the original plan for the hospital, the department was allotted 105 beds, eighty-five for clinical cases and 20 for private patients; subsequently, the medical faculty increased that allotment to 100 clinical and thirty private beds,[59] although an agreement with the state medical society sharply limited actual private admissions.

Construction plans were not appreciably delayed by the war effort of 1917–18, but with total costs for buildings and equipment estimated as high as five million dollars, original plans called for a piecemeal approach, beginning with the Children's Hospital, completed in 1919 at a cost of some $250,000. However, by the early 1920s, hope centered on attaining philanthropic funding for a concerted building effort. That idea appears to have originated with William Boyd, president of the state board of education's finance committee,[60] but the fact that the college had become, by the early 1920s, a regular stop for Rockefeller-sponsored dignitaries, foreign and domestic, was surely a factor in the scheme. By May 1921, the state board of education had composed a formal declaration of purpose for the college, a document designed expressly for use in soliciting aid.

Quite improbably, Abraham Flexner's personal interest in the building project was a decisive factor in its success.[61] Since 1912, Flexner had been an assistant to General Education Board Secretary Wallace Buttrick, and the GEB, thanks to a generous endowment from the Rockefeller Foundation, had taken an active role in the reform of medical education, with Abraham Flexner a central figure in its activities. By 1920, in the wake of what Steven Wheatley has called an eight-year "organizational whirlwind" that bestowed substantial gifts on several private medical colleges,[62] both the General Education Board and Rockefeller Foundation stood at a crossroads, their trustees uncertain over the best way to apply the Rockefeller millions earmarked for support of medical education.

Abraham Flexner visited the University of Iowa campus on December 8 and 9, 1920, shortly after a meeting in New York with university president Walter A. Jessup, and at that point was drawn into the planning process for the new hospitals complex. A few days after his visit, Flexner wrote Dean Lee Wallace Dean asking for details of the building plan,[63] the first in a long series of communications between Flexner and university officials. In Flexner's recollection, William Boyd subsequently appeared in New York to describe the plan in person. While Flexner was generally enthusiastic about the project Boyd outlined, he objected to the piecemeal approach that would, he complained, stretch construction into the unforeseeable future. "By the time the plant and reorganization were completed," he later noted, "we should all be dead and gone." After a hasty consultation with President George E. Vincent of the Rockefeller Foundation and Secretary Buttrick of the General Education Board, Flexner claimed to have proposed to Boyd a plan "to put the entire reorganization through at once," with the Foundation and the GEB together providing half the estimated cost of $4.5 million.[64]

Flexner's memory of events was at the very least somewhat streamlined. He appears, first, to have telescoped two or more meetings with William Boyd, and perhaps with other university representatives as well, into a single account. In any event, it is impossible to say which of several meetings Flexner was describing. More importantly, Flexner's influence over the selection of projects to receive support was not so immediate as he later remembered, and frustrating delays repeatedly stalled his plan for the University of Iowa and threatened at times to undermine it altogether. In addition, Flexner neglected to mention in his account that he initially envisioned the Carnegie Corporation, with his old Carnegie Foundation boss Henry S. Pritchett at the helm, as an equal partner with the Rockefeller philanthropies in the Iowa project.

Likewise, Flexner was less than clear on his motivation. His developing relationship with William Boyd was no doubt an important factor in the outcome, but that relationship, by Flexner's own recollection, was an effect not a cause of his meetings with Boyd in the early 1920s. It seems likely in fact that Flexner was by 1920 entertaining doubts about the hierarchical system of medical education he had fostered since 1910 and that he sought to promote a first-rate facility at the University of Iowa in order to weaken the influence of elite eastern schools and perhaps also to bolster his own position of leadership in American medical education. The Iowa project, he noted to President Jessup in 1922, would counter the fact that "leadership in medical education in this country has lain with endowed institutions."[65] Certainly, Flexner was straightforward in his hope that an infusion of Rockefeller money at the University of Iowa would spur similar projects at other midwestern institutions.[66]

Based on Flexner's reassurances, William Boyd was optimistic after his trip to New York in early 1921. "I believe these people [i.e., the Rockefeller philanthropies] are going to do something worthwhile for us," Boyd wrote President Jessup from New York.[67] But events proceeded much more slowly than Flexner had led Boyd to expect. Dean Lee Wallace Dean met with the "Rockefeller people" in New York in May 1921, and on May 25, Flexner assured Jessup that he would "bring the matter to Dr. Buttrick's attention just as soon as I have opportunity enough to go into it thoroughly with him."[68] Three days later, the Iowa State Board of Education presented its formal report to the GEB, and Jessup wrote Flexner, "We are awaiting the final decision of your board with the keenest expectancy."[69] In early June, however, the word from Flexner was discouraging; it had been "impossible to take up your application with Dr. Buttrick at this time," he wrote. However, Flexner continued, "I hope in the fall to go over the matter with him."[70]

Six months later, in December 1921, William Boyd met again with Flexner, but still no firm commitment materialized from any of the promised sources. Finally, in May 1922, after yet another meeting with Abraham Flexner, Boyd assured President Jessup that the details were "all arranged." The General Education Board, the Rockefeller Foundation, and the Carnegie Corporation, Boyd reported, were each agreed to provide one-sixth of the total cost of $4.5 million, contingent upon the Iowa legislature's pledging matching funds.[71]

On May 24, 1922, the executive committee of the Rockefeller Foundation made a formal pledge of $750,000, conditioned on a similar commitment from the General Education Board, but Abraham Flexner notified President Jessup two days later that because of a crowded agenda the GEB had not made a final decision at its May meeting. However, Flexner promised, much as he had the previous year, that the trustees would discuss the Iowa proposal at a special meeting in the autumn.[72] The GEB's agenda for that May meeting may indeed have been as crowded as Flexner claimed, but the real obstacle to the Iowa proposal was the vehement opposition of Frederick T. Gates, who was John D. Rockefeller's longtime adviser and GEB chairman from 1907 to 1917. Gates argued for a strict division between public and private spheres of endeavor; he saw no future in investing money in the University of Iowa in particular and argued in general that if a public university needed money, the taxpayers should provide it.

Between the late spring and early fall of 1922, once bright prospects had grown dim indeed. The Rockefeller Foundation was on board, and Foundation President George Vincent visited the Iowa campus in August. However, a matching commitment from the General Education Board no longer seemed a sure thing, Abraham Flexner's assurance and support notwithstanding. Moreover, after a long silence, Henry S. Pritchett of the Carnegie Corporation reminded President Jessup in a late October letter that Carnegie's policy was "not to make grants to tax-supported institutions." A few days later, Pritchett wrote again, this time warning darkly, "I think it unlikely ... that the Carnegie Corporation will be able to make this appropriation."[73] Indeed Pritchett's prediction was right, and likely the most immediate reason was, as Pritchett explained, the Corporation's heavy commitments elsewhere.[74]

Abraham Flexner appears not to have been surprised by the Carnegie Corporation's withdrawal; indeed, two days before Pritchett's first letter, Flexner had inquired of President Jessup, "What plan would you expect to pursue" in the event "that the Carnegie Corporation does not make the appropriation requested?"[75] Jessup could only respond weakly, "We have not even considered any other outcome." If the Carnegie people did not come through, Jessup said in despair, it "would probably make our whole program impossible."[76]

In the meantime, however, Flexner had, as promised, carried the Iowa case before the trustees of the General Education Board at a special October meeting. As expected, Frederick Gates made a lengthy and impassioned plea in which, in Flexner's words, he "tore the whole proposition to pieces."[77] Gates reiterated his philosophical objections to the joining of private philanthropy and public institutions; he also remained skeptical that the University of Iowa College of Medicine could become a school of national prominence. To invest the GEB's money in the Iowa scheme, Gates maintained, "is to take a gambler's chance with our money."[78] But Flexner argued in response that the proposed gift to the University of Iowa would not only make Iowa a first-rank school, but would, out of "friendly rivalry," spark similar improvements at other midwestern schools at no expense to the General Education Board.[79]

Gates and Flexner were the dominant personalities on the board, each accustomed to having his way. Although they had worked more or less in concert in the previous decade, this issue split them apart. The trustees' subsequent endorsement of Abraham Flexner's position was a resounding victory for Flexner, a shattering defeat for Gates, and a pivotal moment in the history of the GEB.

Buoyed by his success with the GEB and undaunted by the Carnegie setback, Flexner was as determined as ever in early November, assuring Iowa officials that "we shall sink or swim together."[80] In fact, Flexner had already hatched an alternative scheme calling for the Rockefeller Foundation and General Education Board to shoulder the full $2,250,000 by themselves. At Flexner's behest and with his advice, the Iowa State Board of Education in late October and early November prepared several drafts of another detailed request for assistance, reiterating both the need for and benefits of the new hospitals complex. On November 9, the board submitted its final draft, along with a personal note from Iowa Governor Nathan Kendall, to both the GEB and the Foundation.

From that point, all the pieces fell into place just as Flexner hoped. In a telegram dated November 23, 1922, he notified President Jessup confidentially that the GEB trustees were prepared to raise their contribution to one fourth of the $4,500,000. The next day, Flexner mailed formal notification of the gift to the secretary of the state board of education.[81] Still, the Rockefeller Foundation trustees had not yet decided whether to commit an additional $375,000, and Jessup—obviously and understandably on pins and needles—pestered Flexner for news on that front. Finally, on December 7, the Rockefeller Foundation trustees approved a matching gift of $1,125,000.[82]

The gifts from the Rockefeller philanthropies were the largest ever bestowed on a public institution, and unlike the previous gifts to private schools such as Johns Hopkins, Harvard, and Washington University, there was no full-time quid pro quo. Officials in the College of Medicine and the university administration were justly elated at their success; however, their job was only half finished. Now they faced the sobering task of convincing state legislators to match the contributions from the GEB and Rockefeller Foundation.

William R. Boyd, Walter Jessup, and the other principals had conducted their negotiations with the Rockefeller interests well out of the public eye. They preferred not to have their plan become the subject of public debate until the Rockefeller commitments were sealed. After all, despite an extensive public relations effort, including film clips of John D. Rockefeller handing out dimes to children, the Rockefeller name was still closely identified with monopoly capitalism. That connection by itself might be expected to spark controversy in Iowa; moreover, university officials worried that the appearance of eastern interests, Rockefeller or otherwise, commanding the development of medical education in Iowa might also be a potentially explosive political issue, especially among Iowa physicians.

The depressed agricultural economy of the postwar years also clouded prospects for winning matching funds in the amount of $450,000 per year for five years from the Iowa legislature. As William Boyd at one point commented to Abraham Flexner, even in the best of circumstances, Iowa farmers were not "accustomed to think in terms of seven figures."[83] When state aid to elementary and secondary education amounted to just $500,000 annually, an annual appropriation of $450,000 for construction of a medical campus at the university was a staggering sum.

In addition, Iowans had long displayed a considerable ambivalence toward the university itself. Because of its liberal arts emphasis, it was often labeled an elitist institution. The university's location in Johnson County, a notoriously "wet" and largely Democratic county in a "dry" and largely Republican state, was another source of irritation and suspicion, adding a taint of iniquity to the school's elitist reputation. In any event, mothers and fathers in far-flung rural districts of the state had traditionally been reluctant to entrust their children to the university's care.

Taking all that into account, university officials devised a carefully orchestrated publicity campaign. Concerned first with timing, officials delayed formal announcement of the grants until December 27 in order to avoid having it lost in the pre-Christmas bustle while still capitalizing on the good will of the holiday season. Desiring also to publicize the story as widely and positively as possible, the university sent nearly nine hundred letters to major figures in Iowa politics, business, and education, as well as to a variety of organizations, ranging from the Iowa Bankers Association to the Iowa Federation of Women's Clubs. The university also distributed a lengthy press release that many Iowa newspapers printed either verbatim or in excerpted form.

University officials emphasized the need for expanded hospital facilities to serve the needs of patient care and medical education. They also celebrated the extraordinary opportunity the grants presented, noting proudly that this was the first time the Rockefeller agencies had bestowed such a gift on a public medical school. "If ever a godsend came to an institution," William Boyd noted for the record, "it is this proffer to the university." Officials were careful also to mention Abraham Flexner only in passing, while effusively praising the initiative of Iowans William Boyd, Walter Jessup, and Governor Nathan Kendall, though Kendall had played only a tangential role in the drama.[84]

The university's public relations effort also included a glossy brochure titled "Facts Relative to the $2,250,000 Gift to Iowa" targeted specifically at members of the Iowa legislature. The "Facts" reiterated the service of the University Hospitals to the state and especially the hospitals' services to indigent children, but it relied more on an emotional appeal than on reasoned argument and the recitation of statistics. Heart-rending before-and-after photos of patients, mostly children whose deformed limbs had been reconstructed in the orthopaedic clinics, were meant to soften even the hardest critic.

In the first days of January 1923, university offices received congratulatory letters and telegrams from individuals and organizations as diverse as the Iowa Pharmaceutical Association, the American Farm Bureau Federation, and the American Legion.[85] Former university president George E. MacLean wrote, "Oh, that Middleton [i.e., William Drummond Middleton] might have lived to see the day."[86] Public officials, too, added their voices. U.S. Representative Cyrenus Cole, for example, pointed to "the 5,000 crippled children who have been made whole and happy" by university physicians. "Which of us," Cole went on, "is so poor, not in purse, but in mind and heart" as to oppose acceptance of the Rockefeller gifts?[87]

Favorable editorial comment appeared in dozens of newspapers in many Iowa towns, from Waterloo, Clinton, and Davenport to Council Bluffs and Atlantic.[88] The coverage of the *Evening Gazette* of Cedar Rapids was perhaps typical. Seldom a friend to the university, the Gazette nonetheless gave the story front-page treatment on December 27 and called the Rockefeller funds "a Christmas gift." A follow-up story the next day offered laudatory comments from community leaders, including a declaration from Cedar Rapids Mayor C. D. Huston that the project "should have the interest, sympathy and support of every man and woman in the state."[89]

But there were rumblings of discontent as well. The *Des Moines Register*, a politically important—and Republican—newspaper often among the university's most vocal critics, ignored the story altogether in its year-end editions, a silence that spoke loudly indeed in Iowa City. In addition, the Farmers Union of Emmet County declared, "We are unalterably opposed to the accepting the Rockefeller Foundation or any similar donations,"[90] and an agricultural publication, *Iowa Homestead*, shared similar sentiments. Here were examples of the tight-fisted farmers, fearful of a boost in property tax rates and resentful of what they perceived as an "elitist" university, who had prompted William Boyd's remark to Abraham Flexner, and farmers would hold 64 of the 108 seats in the Iowa House in the Fortieth General Assembly of 1923.

Troubling, too, was the silence of Iowa's physicians. This silence, like that of the *Register*, was disappointing but not surprising. Recognizing that the medical community's silence in January 1923 was a political embarrassment, President Walter Jessup inquired of Dean Lee Wallace Dean about the prospects of an endorsement from the *Journal of the Iowa State Medical Society*. Dean conceded the desirability of such an expression of support; however, he continued, his chief concern was to see "that an editorial which would not be favorable did not appear" in the organ of the state medical society.[91]

Nonetheless, Jessup had received a private message of support from *Journal* editor and longtime college supporter Dr. David S. Fairchild. Fairchild's support encouraged Jessup to pursue the matter further, even though Fairchild was then in Panama, and the *Journal* was in the hands of an acting editor. Jessup wrote medical society secretary Tom B. Throckmorton and asked if, on the basis of Fairchild's letter, Throckmorton would provide an editorial endorsement for the *Journal*'s February number. Unfortunately, Fairchild's letter, which Jessup had intended to forward, was not enclosed with Jessup's, and Secretary Throckmorton responded peevishly, "I have no material here from which an editorial could be written." Furthermore, he said, he had little time to write such a piece. Although Jessup provided the missing letter from Fairchild by return mail, the exchange with Throckmorton underlined Dean's warning about dealing with the medical society and apparently spurred Jessup to make a direct appeal to Fairchild. In any event, the February 1923 issue of the *Journal of the Iowa State*

Medical Society contained a plea from Fairchild that Iowa physicians forget past divisions "and concentrate on the one great question of developing our Medical University."[92] Clearly David Fairchild, a widely respected elder statesman in Iowa medicine and a fifty-year member of the medical society, was one of the heroes of the hour.

There was reason, then, for Jessup, Boyd, and their supporters to suppose that an appropriation of matching funds by the general assembly was far from a sure thing. In retrospect, however, the political situation was not so bleak as it appeared. The enthusiastic initial public response to news of the Rockefeller largesse reflected Iowans' rapidly rising support for the University of Iowa. In the four years prior to 1922, the student body in Iowa City had doubled, reaching some 7,000 and surpassing enrollment at the Iowa State College in Ames, an agricultural college that had long enjoyed far wider public acceptance. Rising enrollments helped the university shed its image of elitism, significantly broadening its constituency among Iowans, and justifying larger appropriations from the Iowa General Assembly.[93] Between 1915 and 1920, annual appropriations for the university had risen from $812,500 to over $2.7 million.[94]

Moreover, in the late nineteenth and early twentieth centuries, a variety of mechanisms had spread the wonders of medical science to a large audience in Iowa as in the rest of America. The combination of an expanding system of public education and mass circulation media had played an important part in that, but the public relations efforts of the medical profession were important as well. For example, since the 1880s the Iowa State Board of Health had actively publicized the application of the principles of scientific medicine to the control of infectious disease; likewise, in the twentieth century the seeming miracles performed at the University Hospitals had bolstered public appreciation of medical science. Thus, in the late nineteenth and early twentieth centuries, medical advances such as the isolation of disease-causing organisms, the discovery and application of x-rays, the identification of vitamins, and the elaboration of a variety of sophisticated surgical techniques rapidly became part of public culture.[95]

Finally, even William Boyd's tight-fisted farmers were unusually buoyant in that winter of 1922–23. After the disastrous slide in farm prices in the immediate postwar years, 1922 had brought a substantial recovery in the prospects of Iowa farmers. For example, spot prices for corn in Chicago markets had risen from a low of forty-eight cents per bushel in January 1922 to seventy-six cents per bushel in December. While part of that rebound was due to a fall in production in key crop-growing states, Iowa's farmers had in fact enjoyed bumper crops. Thus, at year's end, the future of Iowa agriculture appeared far brighter than anyone could have imagined just twelve months earlier.[96]

Those factors, combined with the mobilization of an extensive network of alumni and other university supporters, help to explain why, contrary to the fears and expectations of many, the course of matching funds legislation through Iowa's Fortieth General Assembly in the first months of 1923 was largely anticlimactic. In the Senate, passage proceeded without a hitch, attracting petitions of support from a variety of civic and professional groups—such as the Ottumwa Kiwanis, the Independence American Legion, and Daughters of the American Revolution chapters in Des Moines and Sioux City—representing a substantial cross section of Iowa society. Bolstered by such backing, the bill passed the full Senate by a vote of thirty-three to fifteen.[97] In the House, support was equally broad, although a small band of opponents sought to sidetrack the bill through a variety of parliamentary maneuvers and harassing amendments. In the end, however, a recall vote by the full House pried the bill from the hands of a stubborn appropriations committee chairman, Republican A. O. Hauge of Des Moines. The bill's supporters also defeated killing amendments to include the College of Dentistry in the language of the bill, to earmark auto registration and driver license fees for the necessary appropriation, and to prohibit university employees from accepting outside pay for work in the University Hospitals. The House then gave final approval by an overwhelming eighty-seven to seventeen margin.[98]

The House vote was, Walter Jessup wired Abraham Flexner, "a great victory,"[99] and this time the *Des Moines Register* conceded the story front-page coverage under the headline "Iowa Assured of $4,500,000 Medical Unit."[100] Even before Governor Nathan Kendall signed the bill into law on April 4,[101] a second flood of congratulations poured into university offices. Among those messages were two of special significance. The first was from Abraham Flexner, who had been in a real sense the architect of this "great victory." "We are all delighted" was Flexner's simple message to President Jessup.[102] And from Walter Bierring came a gracious note: "You have won a great victory ... We all rejoice with you."[103]

EXIT CAMPBELL HOWARD, ENTER FRED M. SMITH

In 1910, William Osler had seen the Iowa position as a necessary step in Campbell Howard's advancement toward a chair at a more prestigious school. At the same time, Osler had feared Howard's isolation in the Midwest and had written to Frank Billings and James Herrick in Chicago to apprise them of Howard's move to Iowa, and in turn he encouraged Howard to contact them.[104] In his letter to Herrick, Osler described Campbell Howard as "my special friend" and lauded him as "one of the best ward teachers I have ever known."[105] Osler's greatest hope was that Howard might one day return to his alma mater McGill, and in subsequent years Osler repeatedly pestered authorities at McGill on that score. Meanwhile, however, Campbell Howard developed a genuine attachment to the University of Iowa, and the university clearly needed Campbell Howard. World War I posed the most serious threat to that relationship, as Howard—a Canadian citizen—volunteered for service with a Canadian hospital unit in France in early 1915. Upon leaving the university, he offered his resignation in the event "such a procedure is desirable,"[106] but the university administration declined, not expecting a lengthy war and anxious not to lose Campbell Howard. Still, during the summer of 1915, it became clear that there would be no quick resolution to the war, and in August Dean Lee Wallace Dean notified President Macbride that "the best thing to do is to declare the position of Head of the Department [of Internal Medicine] vacant." Perhaps, Dean suggested, they had "made a mistake in not permanently filling this position last spring."[107] Dean then notified Campbell Howard of the university's intentions and began a search for his successor,[108] but Dean was soon relieved to receive word from Howard that he would return in February 1916, an occasion for a faculty dinner and reception for all medical college and nursing school personnel.[109]

Aside from his wartime service, Campbell Howard showed little inclination to leave the University of Iowa. In 1915, for example, he declined a position as head of the medical service at Mercy Hospital in Chicago, partly because of Osler's reservations,[110] and in 1920 he declined a position at the University of Michigan.[111] Nonetheless, during the Christmas season of 1923, Howard began negotiations that would take him to his father's old position as Professor of Medicine at McGill and Physician-in-Chief at Montreal General Hospital, and in late March 1924 he notified Dean that he would likely accept the "recent offer to return to Montreal." The only remaining stumbling block, Howard reported, was the "question of academic salary."[112] Two months later Dean received Campbell Howard's formal letter of resignation in which Howard noted that his decision was "solely due to the strong personal and family associations with McGill."[113]

The resignation of a figure of Campbell Howard's stature and importance was cause for concern, particularly since the college of medicine had become, in part by design, the object of considerable public interest across the state. Consequently, Dean Lee Wallace Dean advised President Walter Jessup to release the news immediately: "I do not like the idea of having it gradually leak out."[114] Even at that, some fallout was unavoidable. "The brilliant scholar and his lovely wife," the Iowa City Press Citizen reported, "will be missed mightily in Iowa City."[115] Indeed, upon learning of Howard's resignation, the new hospital chemist wrote to decline the position he had only recently accepted.[116] Moreover, the Department of Internal Medicine was left in limbo through the summer with assistant professor Frank J. Rohner serving informally as head per

Campbell Howard's suggestion, and tensions, as we shall see, mounted in the now headless department.

The search for Howard's successor began immediately. Walter Bierring wrote to recommend an associate professor at Western Reserve in Cleveland, Dr. A. M. Blankenhorn, who later became head of medicine at the University of Cincinnati and who, Bierring assured his readers, "is not Jewish."[117] University officials briefly courted George F. Dick of Rush Medical College and later the University of Chicago, noted for his work with scarlet fever, but Dick withdrew from consideration.[118] The most serious candidate, as it turned out, was Fred M. Smith, an Illinois native, a 1914 Rush Medical College graduate, and later a student and colleague of James B. Herrick. Conceding that Smith had been "reared on the farm and lacks some of the polish, refinement, and scholarliness" of other men, Herrick nonetheless contended that "he has the right stuff in him." Furthermore, Herrick noted, Smith "knows his failings" and "is not in the least conceited."[119]

Following an internship at Chicago's Presbyterian Hospital, Fred Smith had held a faculty position at Rush Medical College since 1916, with the exception of a stint in the U.S. Army Medical Corps in 1918–19. Following in Herrick's footsteps in cardiology, Smith had made his reputation early on in the study of myocardial infarction, using dogs to demonstrate the electrocardiographic results of myocardial lesions.[120] Impressed with Smith's qualifications and his personality during a campus visit on August 8, 1924, Lee Wallace Dean enthusiastically endorsed Smith, noting that "he has the makings of a wonderful clinician" who could do "good research work" and was also a "good mixer" with faculty and students.[121] The head of surgery, Charles J. Rowan, also enthusiastically supported Smith. For his part, Fred Smith was favorably impressed with the University of Iowa and was scheduled to return with his wife a week later for a final tour.

Enthusiasm, however, was not universal. On August 11, Frank Rohner complained to Dean that the uncertainty of the summer months had left the Department of Internal Medicine in a condition "almost one of chaos." Rohner asked that he be formally appointed acting head, with Campbell Howard's salary, and also that he be promoted from assistant to associate professor.[122] The next day the other junior members of the department threw their support behind Rohner in a letter to President Jessup.[123] In addition, in a personal letter to Jessup, assistant professor Wesley E. Gatewood said that he "would be dissatisfied" with Fred Smith's appointment and that such an outcome would be "a definite retrogression" for the department. Gatewood, like Rohner, went on to demand more money and promotion to associate professor.[124] Meanwhile, Robert B. Gibson, who had taken over as head of the chemical research laboratory when Louis Baumann left in 1919, likewise sent a personal letter to Jessup. Gibson—who held a Ph.D., not an M.D., and later headed the new

Biochemistry Department—was disappointed that the administration had turned down a raise in pay requested for him by Campbell Howard. After all, he claimed, "This laboratory has been responsible for nearly all of the research that has come from the department." In fact, he continued, work "planned and carried on quite independently by the laboratory staff" had "added largely to Dr. Howard's own standing."[125]

On August 13, pressured by what must have seemed an incipient rebellion among the junior faculty in internal medicine, Lee Wallace Dean recommended Fred Smith's appointment, effective immediately.[126] President Jessup and the state board of education concurred and offered Smith a salary of $7,000, which he accepted. Campbell Howard voiced his approval to Dean, albeit in a back-handed way. "I feel that you have made no mistake," Howard wrote.[127] However, William Boyd fretted over the generous salary offer, particularly the reaction from the Department of Surgery. "Did Doctor Rowan know about this salary, and did he approve it?" Boyd asked Jessup. If not, Boyd warned, "'the fat will be in the fire' again"[128]—a reference to ongoing jealousies between internal medicine and surgery. Clearly Smith's reception, both in the department of internal medicine and in the college, was for a time an open question, and while Fred Smith's personable demeanor no doubt smoothed a good many ruffled feathers, some of the issues raised at his appointment soon provoked a far more serious crisis.

DESPOTISM AND PRIVATE PRACTICE

The brief flare of discontent at the time of Fred Smith's hiring was symptomatic of deep resentments festering just below the surface in the Department of Internal Medicine and in the College of Medicine, and as the spring semester drew to a close in 1927, those resentments flared in an ugly dispute that brought the resignations of Drs. Rohner and Gatewood in internal medicine, Rowan in surgery, and Griswold in hygiene and preventive medicine, as well as the superintendent of the hospital, Jesse L. McElroy, the hospital's director of nursing, Mae J. MacArthur, and the dean of the college, Lee Wallace Dean. Most simply, questions of privilege and power in the college sparked the blowup, and Dean was the immediate target of complaint.

Lee Wallace Dean was in some respects a reluctant administrator; his requests that President Jessup relieve him of the deanship were an annual ritual. At the same time, Dean was a tough administrator who, with control over an ever-increasing budget and with the unquestioned backing of presidents Macbride and then Jessup, had built the deanship into a centralized administrative system, replacing the loose collegiality and haphazard lines of communication of the James Guthrie era and before.

Only a few months into his job in November 1914, Dean had complained to President Macbride of the "lack of system" in the workings of the college. Too much important business, he said, bypassed the dean's office. Dean had then proposed regulations designed to enhance the power of his office, and Macbride had incorporated Dean's recommendations in his "Rules governing the conduct of business in the College of Medicine."[129] By 1927, however, Dean's success in centralizing power in the college, including his own authority over the University Hospitals, combined with charges that he favored his own Department of Head Specialties over others in assigning space and resources, laid him open to charges of "despotism" and "mismanagement" from faculty, hospital administrators, and nurses.[130]

The private practice versus full-time issue was central to faculty complaints. In the 1920s, the college had taken limited steps toward a full-time system. In 1924, Philip C. Jeans was hired to head a reorganized full-time Department of Pediatrics, and the university received a grant of $49,000 from the General Education Board to finance the experiment for five years.[131] Psychiatry, too, was on a full-time basis in the 1920s. However, bringing internal medicine and the surgical specialties into the full-time fold would not only have been a much more expensive proposition but would also likely have sparked a destructive power struggle. Instead, the 1920s saw the formalization of a system in which private practice was limited to half-time department heads, while associate and assistant professors were full-time on salaries generally ranging from $2,500–$3,000 but in exceptional cases as high as $5,000–$6,000.

The system of full-time for junior faculty was predicated on the assumption, in Lee Wallace Dean's mind, that junior faculty were in effect adjuncts or assistants to department heads. As Rohner's and Gatewood's independent scholarship suggested,[132] and as Robert Gibson had been only too happy to point out in 1924, Dean's vision of affairs was becoming rapidly outdated, a problem that had grown increasingly worse as faculty numbers rose from twenty-one in 1910 to fifty-five in 1927. Nonetheless, under Dean's regime, junior faculty were without power or privilege in their departments or in the college. Dean was especially vulnerable to criticism because he had—as professor of otolaryngology and oral surgery—an extensive private practice himself, while he maintained a steadfast opposition to half-time clinical appointments with private practice privileges for junior faculty. Moreover, Dean was not much inclined to seek or accept the counsel of junior faculty on important issues, as was evident in his handling of the Fred Smith appointment in 1924.

Long-festering issues of personality and administrative style came to a head in early May 1927, when Frank Rohner's, Charles Rowan's, and Jesse McElroy's abrupt resignations sparked a front-page banner in the Iowa City

Press Citizen: "Three Resign Posts on Iowa 'Medic' Staff."[133] The following day, perhaps to Dean's surprise, the state board of education accepted what had become more or less his annual letter of resignation from the deanship. However, Dean retained his position as head of the Department of Head Specialties for the time being. Four days later, internal medicine's Wesley Gatewood turned in his resignation, as did Mae MacArthur, the director of nursing. Finally, on May 12, Dean resigned his faculty position as well, amid reports in the *Press Citizen* of anonymous complaints from medical faculty about Dean's "high-handed manner" of administration. The *Press Citizen* also printed Dean's letter to President Jessup in which Dean complained, ironically enough, of the evils of private practice among the medical faculty.[134]

In response to Dean's charges, the remaining medical faculty, led by Junior Dean John T. McClintock, attacked Dean in an open letter to President Jessup and the state board of education. Charging Dean with "insincerity and duplicity," the faculty asked assurance that Dean's resignations from the deanship and from his faculty position would not be reconsidered and demanded further that the faculty have a voice in the selection of his successor.[135] To the embarrassment of the college, Iowa newspapers kept the affair simmering well into the summer, including a two-page spread as late as July 24 in the *Des Moines Sunday Register* that noted the medical faculty's "lack of respect and confidence in Dr. Lee Wallace Dean."[136]

For faculty in general, the central issues in the confrontation were Lee Wallace Dean's authoritarian leadership style, his alleged favoritism toward his own department, and the distribution of privilege and income in the college, especially income from private practice. For Frank Rohner of internal medicine, those grievances carried a personal edge. Rohner, an associate professor in 1926–27, had asked Fred Smith for a salary increase from $3,000 to $4,000 in April 1927, saying that he would otherwise resign. However, Dean had intimated to Smith that Rohner would not receive the raise. Consequently, Fred Smith noted that he was "not counting on [Rohner's] services the coming year."[137] Wesley Gatewood, also an associate professor in 1926–27, likewise had a long-held grudge against Dean. Gatewood's hiring in 1920 had been an important test case of Dean's developing policy of confining private practice to department heads, as Dean had pointedly insisted to President Jessup that Gatewood be hired strictly on a full-time basis.[138]

Meanwhile, before the storm broke, Fred Smith had taken a leave of absence from the Department of Internal Medicine to go to Vienna for a summer of study. Smith learned of the fiasco on May 27 through a simple, if desperate, telegram from President Jessup: "Gatewood, Rohner resigned. Can you return immediately." With his department apparently reduced to a shambles, Smith had few options and wired Jessup that he could indeed return and would do so as quickly as possible, but it was nearly three weeks before Smith arrived in Iowa

City to begin the reconstruction of his department.[139]

In the face of what proved a broad-based faculty revolt, the university administration and the state board of education were chiefly concerned with the maintenance of discipline in the College of Medicine. Moreover, Abraham Flexner entered the picture once again, advising William Boyd and the state board of education to stand firm against faculty demands. In addition, Flexner took a personal interest in the selection of a new dean, strongly recommending Henry S. Houghton, head of Peking Union Medical College and subsequently acting as intermediary in communications between the university and Houghton.[140]

The university administration's concern to stifle dissent in the college was apparent in its single-minded pursuit of Houghton without serious consideration of other candidates. Indeed, in their haste to settle the affair, university officials appealed to Houghton to take the job sight unseen. In many respects, Henry Houghton was the perfect man for the job, offering impeccable credentials and, by all accounts, overpowering personal charm. However, the administration also made one important concession to faculty grievances, making the deanship a full-time administrative position. Thus, when Houghton took over as dean on February 1, 1928, he was, unlike his predecessor, neither a department head nor a beneficiary of private practice.

As the university administration aggressively pursued Houghton to fill the deanship, Fred Smith—displaying a heightened sensitivity to the issues swirling about the college—petitioned President Jessup for a $1,000 salary reduction, claiming that his private practice income far exceeded his expectations.[141] Jessup and Smith also began a frantic search to fill the staff vacancies in internal medicine. At Smith's suggestion, President Jessup wrote to G. Canby Robinson expressing a keen interest in Dr. John B. Youmans—who later made a name at Vanderbilt for his work in nutrition—to fill the position vacated by Frank Rohner. Jessup begged Robinson to release Youmans "in view of our dire necessity," but Robinson declined.[142] At the same time, Fred Smith pursued Horace M. Korns of Western Reserve, offering a full-time salary of $6,000— twice Rohner's pay. In mid-July, Korns formally accepted the offer.[143] Later, Earle P. Scarlett was hired as instructor to take Wesley Gatewood's place, at a full-time salary of $3,000.[144]

By the beginning of the fall term of 1927–28, then, the damage had been repaired, at least superficially. But while calm was restored to the college and particularly to the Department of Internal Medicine, many of the problems that had sparked the spring blowup remained unresolved, and, as we shall see in later chapters, those problems grew more serious in some respects with the passage of time.

CONCLUSION: A DISTINCTIVE LANDMARK

Whatever the problems along the way, the years from 1910 to 1928 contributed much to the modern foundations of internal medicine at the University of Iowa. Above all, for internal medicine as for other clinical departments, the opening of the general hospital in 1928 capped an improbable rags-to-riches story of symbolic as well as practical importance. On the one hand, the new facilities symbolized the explosive growth of the new medical science and of the new medical education built around a more rigorously scientific curriculum. On the other hand, the stately north tower of the general hospital—in the words of one proud observer, "a distinctive landmark for the city and surrounding country"—was also graphic evidence of American medicine's apparent emergence as a "sovereign profession."

Just as important, the new hospital and laboratory facilities reflected a new public confidence in the powers of medical science to address society's ills, confidence built upon the public health triumphs of William Robertson's generation and bolstered in the early twentieth century by findings in basic nutrition, metabolism, and blood chemistry, as well as by "healthy baby" contests and the health-related advice columns that proliferated in the popular press. So powerful was the appeal of medical science that major political and economic currents of the era failed to slow expansion at the University of Iowa College of Medicine. For example, Campbell Howard's twelve-month absence in 1915–16 was arguably the major event of World War I for the College of Medicine, and ironically that came well before America's entry into the war. Similarly, the extended agricultural slump of the 1920s, although critically important to Iowa's economy, had little visible impact on the growth of the college.

The formal opening of the general hospital in November 1928 was occasion for elaborate celebration, and the guest list for the three-day dedication ceremonies represented much of the elite of American medical education, including James B. Herrick, Hugh Cabot, George Whipple, G. Canby Robinson, and Campbell Howard. William J. Mayo delivered a dedicatory address entitled "Looking Backward and Forward in Medical Education" as President George E. Vincent of the Rockefeller Foundation and a host of state and national dignitaries looked on. It was an occasion for expansive rhetoric and grand hopes, all of it consistent with the national mood in the waning days of the roaring twenties when anything and everything seemed possible.

3

Years of Hardship—
Depression and War

1929–1945

FOR the Department of Internal Medicine, the buoyant optimism of the 1920s scarcely survived into the 1930s, as the Depression brought severe budget reductions, staff cutbacks, and declining standards in both teaching and patient care. Those lowered expectations extended through the years of World War II, when wartime manpower demands and an accelerated schedule of instruction put further strains on faculty and facilities. By 1945, after a decade and a half of hardship, the department showed worrisome signs of deterioration.

However, the years from 1929 to 1945 did not constitute a lost era, either at the University of Iowa or elsewhere in American academic medicine. Medical science, for example, continued its development through depression and war, in part because medical research was not yet the capital-intensive enterprise we know today. The relatively meager internal funds allotted to sundry research projects at institutions like the University of Iowa produced significant dividends, and the 1930s also brought the first trickle of research grants from private foundations and industry. Moreover, World War II, despite the burdens it imposed on American medical colleges, provided an immediate boost to medical research and, just as important, laid the groundwork for a partnership between government and academic medicine that carried over into the postwar period.

The trend toward specialization in American medicine also continued through the 1930s and World War II. In academic medicine, specialized scientific organizations and publications proliferated, and scientific conferences and conventions became more numerous. By 1940, the aggressive medical researcher might well attend a half-dozen such gatherings each year. Meanwhile, the institutionalization of the graduate residency joined specialization in academic medicine to specialization in medical practice. Indeed, by the 1930s, the accelerating tendency toward scientific specialization in academic medicine had become a driving force behind the trend toward practice specialization. As a result, specialty definition and certification became a major issue in internal medicine in the 1930s as it did in other specialty areas.

While depression and war, then, posed serious challenges to the University of Iowa Department of Internal Medicine and to American academic medicine at large, they did not slow two of American medicine's fundamental tendencies: the growing sophistication of medical science, including the ongoing differentiation in its organizational structure, and the associated tendency toward specialization, both in medical research and in medical practice. Wartime experience, in fact, accelerated both the growth of medical science and the trend toward specialized practice.

THE DEPRESSION AND MEDICAL EDUCATION

From 1921 to 1933, over half of Iowa's banks disappeared through closure or consolidation, and behind the bank failures lay a disastrous, if irregular, downward spiral in the agricultural economy. By 1932, the prices paid for Iowa corn, hogs, eggs, and butter had fallen as much as 75 to 80 percent from World War I highs. With many farmers saddled with unmanageable debt burdens, eight of every one hundred Iowa farms were the object of foreclosure action in 1933 alone. Throughout those troubled years, property taxes, falling heavily on farmers, were the state government's chief source of revenue; sales and income taxes were reforms introduced only in the mid-1930s when farmers clamored for property tax relief.[1]

Given that backdrop, the surprise is not that the depression of the 1930s affected the University of Iowa College of Medicine; rather the surprise is, first, that the impact of the agricultural depression was so long delayed and, second, that the university's medical community, after nearly two decades of rising state support, seems not to have foreseen the approaching era of austerity. For example, the College of Medicine's operating budget for 1929–30 was $337,039, and college and university administrators projected increases of 8 and 10 percent in 1930–31 and 1931–32 respectively, a continuation of the pattern of expansion that had held during the 1920s.[2] Furthermore, salaries continued to rise well into the worst period of the depression: in 1930–31, for example,

Dean Houghton's salary rose from $12,000 to $15,000, while in internal medicine, Kate Daum went from $3,500 to $3,800 and Clarence Baldridge from $4,500 to $5,000. And as late as 1931–32, Willis M. Fowler received a raise from $2,500 to $3,000.[3]

From 1917 to 1929, state appropriations for all institutions of higher education in Iowa had nearly tripled, but, by 1931, state legislators had begun slicing the state board of education's budget for higher education. State legislators grumbled about unregulated growth "during our flush period,"[4] and charges of financial impropriety at the University of Iowa fueled further complaints as the depression deepened. During the great expansion of the 1920s, the proportion of University of Iowa revenues derived from state tax moneys had in fact fallen from 75 percent to just 54 percent. Nonetheless, for the 1931–33 biennium, state appropriations for the university fell 20 percent, from $2,500,000 to $2,000,000.[5] As a result, the per-student state appropriation for the university fell to $248 from a peak of $376 in 1924–25. Despite the frantic efforts of university administrators to defend their institution, legislators trimmed yet another $200,000 from the university's appropriation in the 1933–35 biennium.[6]

The budget of the College of Medicine reflected that retrenchment, falling to just under $300,000 in 1931–32 and to $265,000 in 1933–34, and the internal medicine budget fell in proportion, from $34,100 to $27,952. At the time, faculty salaries made up over 90 percent of departmental budgets; Fred Smith's entire administrative staff in internal medicine consisted of a single secretary at an annual salary of $900, while expenses for departmental supplies totaled less than $1,500 per year. Under the circumstances, declining budgets could only mean declining faculty salaries, and the state board of education instituted a 5 percent across-the-board salary cut for the 1931–32 academic year. In 1932, under increasing pressure from the governor's Interim Committee on the Reduction of the Costs of Government, the board decreed further salary reductions on a sliding scale of 15 to 30 percent for all faculty and staff.[7]

The burden fell hardest on junior faculty, whose salaries were often marginal in the best of times. In internal medicine, for example, Fred Smith and Horace Korns saw their $6,000 salaries cut 16.66 percent to $5,000, while James Greene—one of the younger and more promising additions to the department—took a 15.33 percent reduction from $3,000 to $2,540. College of Medicine Dean Henry Houghton, whose own salary was pared from $15,000 to $9,575, warned that such draconian fiscal measures "would necessitate return of all clinical chiefs to part time" and "would tend to lower scientific quality and prestige of the college of medicine."[8] President Walter Jessup, his salary cut by legislative mandate from $18,000 to $10,000, feared that deep salary reductions could well mean the loss of valued personnel, since there was "still sharp competition" from other institutions for faculty in highly technical fields such as medicine.[9] Ironically, those dire predictions about the effects of severe salary reductions were borne out when both Houghton and Jessup resigned, Houghton to become Director of Clinics at the University of Chicago and Jessup to head the Carnegie Foundation for the Advancement of Teaching.

Houghton's resignation left a temporary executive committee chaired by John T. McClintock in charge of the College of Medicine; however, the strict austerity program frustrated the search for a new dean. University officials could offer a salary of just $8,000, and medical faculty would not approve extension of private practice privileges to a new dean to make up the deficiency in salary. Finally, in 1935, President Eugene A. Gilmore recommended that the state board of education appoint Ewen Murchison MacEwen, head of the Department of Anatomy, to the post at a salary of $8,050.[10]

In the Department of Internal Medicine, a high rate of turnover in the bottom faculty ranks was one consequence of fiscal austerity. Most of the assistants and associates hired in the 1930s left the department after one or two years to enter private practice. Even James A. Greene, who was promoted to assistant professor in 1935 and subsequently carved out a solid career in academic medicine, was on the verge of resigning in 1936 to enter private practice in Sioux City.[11] Greene's retention was accomplished in part through a $250 raise drawn from off-budget sources. Other faculty, including Willis Fowler, Fred Smith, and Kate Daum, were also beneficiaries of a bookkeeping legerdemain that boosted some salaries beyond the institutional guidelines.[12] Still, the salary picture remained bleak through the 1930s, a far cry from the promise of the previous decade.

Austerity strained the facilities of the University Hospitals as well. A long waiting list of patients in all hospital departments had been one of the nagging problems of the 1920s; by 1929, over 1,000 patients awaited admission in the various hospital services.[13] Meanwhile, even before the depression, disgruntled legislators had fixed the hospital's annual appropriation for indigent patient care at $1,000,000, forcing the hospitals to operate at only two-thirds capacity. With the coming of the depression, the dilemma facing faculty and other hospital staff worsened, with deep budget cuts on the one hand and increased demands for service on the other. To a surprising extent, the hospitals managed to reconcile the conflict; as the number of indigent patients treated rose from 8,166 in 1928 to 11,324 in 1931, the cost per patient declined from $116.50 to $88.30.[14] However, the patient waiting list swelled to over 2,500.[15] Further complicating matters, dwindling numbers of paying patients dropped the average patient population per day from 672 in May 1930 to 597 in May 1931, and in the same year-to-year comparison total receipts for the month fell from $112,500 to $95,000.[16]

The situation on the three internal medicine wards reflected the general service bottleneck. In 1929, the department had, on paper, a capacity of ninety-seven indigent patient beds, plus five private beds, but budgetary restrictions had already reduced the effective indigent capacity to sixty-five. Meanwhile, the patient waiting list for internal medicine services stood at more than 250.[17] As the demand for service grew, the ceiling of sixty-five beds remained. For example, the department reported 1,953 indigent patient-days for the month of May 1930, an average of sixty-three patients per day, and 1,967 indigent patient-days, an average of just over sixty-three per day, in May 1931.[18] Meanwhile, the department's waiting list continued to grow. Finally, in order to introduce a measure of equity into the distribution of indigent beds and to answer rising criticism of the indigent care system, the board of education mandated, as of August 1, 1933, the apportionment of available beds among Iowa's counties on the basis of population.[19]

MEDICAL EDUCATION: THE COSTS OF AUSTERITY

Austerity also strained the abilities of the College of Medicine and the Department of Internal Medicine to carry out their educational missions. However, here they not only faced the problem of declining budgets combined with rising demands for service; their problems were also aggravated by the need to satisfy two distinct constituencies with competing and sometimes conflicting expectations. On the one hand, an Iowa constituency, including the legislature and elements of the public at large, demanded undiminished access to medical education; on the other hand, regulating and certifying bodies such as the Association of American Medical Colleges and the AMA's Council on Medical Education and Hospitals demanded adherence to hard-won educational standards.

In 1930, the University of Iowa College of Medicine lowered the size of its entering class from 148 to 100 by implementing higher academic standards on pre-medical work, dropping total enrollments from over 500 in 1929–30 to 402 in 1930–31. However, fiscal and political pressures made it impossible to hold down student numbers, despite Dean Houghton's worry that the state's sagging economy might reduce the pool of applicants.[20] Total enrollments bottomed at 355 in 1933–34 but crept upward in subsequent years, exceeding 400 once again in 1935–36. A concerted effort—bolstered by a 1937 edict of the Board of Education to cap beginning classes at 100—brought total enrollments down again beginning in 1938–39. By the fall of 1941, the student body had shrunk to just 282. Throughout the period, the college maintained its distinctive concentration of Iowa residents. Of the total enrollment of 354 in 1934–35, for example, all but ten were Iowa residents, and only 20 percent of all the Iowans studying medicine were enrolled in out-of-state schools.[21] When Abraham Flexner wrote in 1934 seeking a place for a German medical student, Acting Dean John T. McClintock reaffirmed the long-standing policy to "exclude practically all non-residents."[22]

Of course, there was more than a little irony in the concern about spending Iowa tax dollars to educate non-resident medical students. Like virtually all professional schools in Iowa before and since, the University of Iowa College of Medicine turned out far more graduates than the state could absorb. Its restrictive admissions policies notwithstanding, the college was still educating other states' physicians, as Iowa residents left the state in substantial numbers after completion of the program. For example, only twenty-four of the seventy-four graduates from the class of 1926 and forty-five of the ninety-eight graduates from the class of 1930 were practicing medicine in Iowa in 1933.[23]

Nationally, medical school enrollments rose steadily from 1920 to 1931, peaked in the early 1930s, and then turned downward in the latter half of the 1930s. However, the number of graduates nationwide continued its steady rise, climbing from 4,735 in 1931 to 5,377 in 1937, reflecting lower dropout rates.[24] That trend, in conjunction with the economic hardship of the Depression, once again sparked cries of "overcrowding" in the medical profession.[25] Those complaints came despite evidence that, in large part because of the ongoing specialization and urbanization of American medicine, significant segments of American society were poorly, if at all, served by the existing health care system. Certainly overcrowding was not obvious in Iowa, where the number of practicing physicians had fallen over 20 percent from 1918 to 1931 and the number of physicians per one hundred thousand population had declined some 40 percent since the turn of the century.

Sentiment within organized medicine to limit the physician population meshed with growing concerns among medical educators about the quality of American medical education. While, as one authority put it, progress in medical education since 1910 had been "phenomenal, unparalleled,"[26] there were many widely acknowledged problems. Most importantly, while boosters appreciated the work of the American Medical Association, the Association of American Medical Colleges, and the various state licensing boards in raising standards of medical education, the 1920s had brought proliferating complaints about the medical curriculum. One critic noted in 1926, for example, that the curriculum had become "a crazy quilt affair," a rigid, poorly coordinated collection of courses ill-adapted to the explosive growth in medical science and associated specialization.[27] Many observers argued the virtues of curricular flexibility, allowing experimentation to incorporate current educational concepts and to help overburdened students integrate the diverse elements of the curriculum.

In 1925, the Association of American Medical Colleges created a Commission on Medical Education to study the problem of medical education and the relationship between medical education and medical practice. The commission, led by A. Lawrence Powell, President of Harvard University, included President Walter Jessup of the University of Iowa and Walter Bierring, who had risen to national prominence with a stint as chair of the AMA's Section on Practice of Medicine and membership on the National Board of Medical Examiners. The commission's work and its conclusions paralleled in many respects that of the better known Committee on the Cost of Medical Care, an independent group made up of representatives of the professions and significant interest groups.[28]

Both organizations released their reports in 1932, but neither report did much to change the organization of health care or the essential nature of medical education. The call for a drastic reorganization of health care delivery from the Committee on the Cost of Medical Care met with entrenched opposition, not least from its American Medical Association representatives.[29] For its part, the AAMC's Commission on Medical Education offered a survey of current medical education, criticizing attempts "to provide instruction in too many subjects in too great detail" and the emphasis on "meaningless laboratory work as a method of instruction."[30] The commission's report was also sprinkled with a handful of recommendations for educational reform designed to prepare medical students for a lifetime of self-education. In all, the commission's report was little more than a reiteration of progressive ideals of education—neither the first nor the last time for that call.

Such criticisms did, however, prompt the Council on Medical Education and Hospitals to begin a detailed survey of American medical schools in 1934. Dean Herman G. Weiskotten of the Syracuse University College of Medicine led the study. Weiskotten found a surprisingly wide diversity of programs and facilities in America's medical schools. For example, thirty-six of America's seventy-seven schools required three years' college work for admission, four required a bachelor's degree, while thirty-two, including the University of Iowa, still required only two years' college work.

More generally, Weiskotten found that Flexner's "university department" ideal had saddled medical faculty with heavy responsibilities in teaching non-medical students, especially in the pre-clinical fields. For example, according to a 1940 survey at the University of Iowa, 59 percent of instruction in anatomy, 78 percent in bacteriology, and 75 percent in physiology was for the benefit of non-medical students.[31] Ironically, in light of the situation described in Abraham Flexner's 1910 report, Weiskotten noted, too, that the "best and brightest" in academic medicine were now attracted to full-time clinical positions rather than to the pre-clinical sciences.[32]

Weiskotten visited the University of Iowa College of Medicine April 2–4, 1936; however, university officials waited with rising anxiety into 1937 for his report. During the winter of 1936–37, there were hints that the report would not be favorable, and indeed it was not. When the Council on Medical Education and Hospitals report arrived in June 1937, Dean Ewen MacEwen notified President Gilmore that the college had dropped from the top 10 percent of the nation's medical schools to a middling position. Weiskotten had especially faulted the college for a too-high student-teacher ratio, a lack of scientific research by overworked pre-clinical faculty, and too many students and too little material on the clinical wards.

Weiskotten's criticisms, although disappointing, were certainly no surprise. While the university and the College of Medicine had labored under the budget-slashing effects of the depression, the costs of educating new physicians had continued to climb; in 1933–34, the College of Medicine estimated the cost per student at $815 compared to $531 in 1927–28.[33] A second factor in the College of Medicine's slide was evolving expectations about the best way to conduct medical education; Iowa was only one of many institutions criticized for failing to implement new educational schemes, such as self-paced instruction and smaller class sizes that would require either fewer students or more instructors, or both.

In short, the University of Iowa College of Medicine, and not least the Department of Internal Medicine, was caught in a pincers. Budgetary pressures and rising expectations of national regulatory agencies seemed to mandate a drastic reduction in enrollment, but that was unthinkable for a state-supported institution. Iowa legislators were inclined to think that Iowa needed more physicians rather than fewer, and they thought that the college should provide them. Thus, the college had done, and continued to do, what it could to accommodate two very different, and sometimes very difficult, masters.

INTERNAL MEDICINE AND THE GROWTH OF MEDICAL SCIENCE

Despite the harsh fiscal realities of the 1930s, internal medicine faculty at the University of Iowa increased their participation in the world of medical science. Fred Smith, a man with a taste for fine clothes and fast cars, was remembered by his colleagues as a "very personable man," "a fine physician," "and an excellent teacher,"[34] and his place in the history of research into myocardial infarction and the coronary circulation needs no elaboration.[35] Beyond that, Fred Smith played a highly visible organizational role in medical science as a charter member of the Central Society for Clinical Research, fellow of both the American College of Physicians and the Association of American Physicians, president of the American Society for Clinical Investigation, editor of the *American Heart Journal* from 1938 to 1945, and presenter of numerous papers at scientific conferences. And prior to his years at the University of Iowa,

Smith had worked with James B. Herrick in organizing a Chicago group modeled on the Association for the Prevention and Relief of Heart Disease of New York, one of the local efforts that culminated in formation of the American Heart Association in 1924.[36]

Fred Smith's chief gift, however, may well have been his ability to recruit and inspire young talent in his department. In the 1930s, he gathered around him, in addition to Horace Korns, whose 1927 hiring was described in the previous chapter, an unusually capable group of younger faculty that included Willis M. Fowler, a 1926 Iowa graduate, whose work in diseases of the blood led him to write a standard textbook on hematology;[37] Elmer L. DeGowin, a 1928 Michigan graduate, who became a pioneer in the preservation of whole blood and in blood transfusion; Kate Daum, a 1925 Chicago Ph.D., who gained prominence both as an expert in nutrition and metabolism and as a role model for women in the male-dominated world of academic medicine; James A. Greene, a 1925 Harvard graduate, whose interests lay chiefly in metabolic diseases, notably diabetes insipidus and hypothyroidism; and Clarence W. Baldridge, an Iowa native and 1921 Iowa graduate, hired as clinical assistant by Campbell Howard in 1923 and promoted first to assistant professor in 1927 and then to associate professor in 1930.

While Smith himself spent less time in laboratory work in the 1930s, he encouraged, and indeed expected, faculty members to keep abreast of current trends in science and held weekly scientific conferences in the department as well as the more traditional grand rounds. Smith also expected faculty members to participate in the larger community of medical scientists through research, through memberships in medical scientific organizations, and through attendance at conventions and conferences. James Greene and Willis Fowler maintained research laboratories, and Fowler enjoyed the services of a Ph.D. assistant. Meanwhile, junior and senior faculty alike routinely attended scientific meetings across the nation. "I am anxious," Fred Smith explained to Dean Ewen MacEwen in 1935, "that as many of our young men as possible have the privilege."[38] And they traveled, often in groups of four or five, to Atlantic City, Cleveland, St. Louis, New York, and Washington, D.C., to share their findings through papers and exhibits and to learn from others. In 1937, Elmer DeGowin received a certificate of merit from the American Medical Association for his convention exhibit on "Renal Damage from Blood Transfusion,"[39] and in 1939, at the AMA's St. Louis convention, DeGowin won a Gold Medal for his exhibit outlining the work of the University of Iowa Blood Bank.

Support for such activities came from a variety of sources. Although University of Iowa president Eugene Gilmore sometimes complained about expenses and always counted every penny, the university formalized its rules regarding reimbursement for faculty travel during the 1930s. Much of the money for travel and research came from interest accumulated on the Rockefeller grants from the 1920s, a sum that reached nearly $162,000 in 1929 and that the state board of education agreed to set aside to support medical research.[40] Under Dean Houghton, the proceeds from that fund became the Scientific Reserve Fund, and in 1929–30 amounted to some $28,500, with $2,500 of that amount allocated to internal medicine.[41] In 1932–33, despite the depression, internal medicine's share of the Scientific Reserve Fund rose to over $3,200.[42]

A second source of support for research and travel was the department's Medical Fee Fund. Modeled on the practice in full-time departments of using fees from private patients to underwrite research, the Medical Fee Fund in internal medicine was built up from a portion of the professional fees from private patients and was used for special projects at the dean's discretion.[43] In total, then, the department had roughly $5,000 at its disposal each year from the Scientific Reserve and Medical Fee funds, money used for a variety of research-related projects. Willis Fowler's laboratory assistant, Adelaide Barer, for example, was often paid from those sources.

Grants from corporate industry and from private foundations were another relatively new source of support for research in the 1930s.[44] During the depression years, the College of Medicine received grants from a variety of corporate sources, some of them sponsoring long-term research projects. National Oil Products Company provided $6,000 per year in the mid-1930s for metabolism research; S.M.A. Corporation provided $2,500 in 1935 for Vitamin A research; Mead Johnson provided $6,000 per year, later $7,200 per year, for research in pediatric metabolism; the John and Mary Markle Foundation awarded $10,000 in 1937 for blood clotting work in the Department of Pathology;[45] the National Foundation for Infantile Paralysis gave $13,500 in 1939 for the study of poliomyelitis; Quaker Oats provided $2,000 per year for an ongoing project in calcium metabolism, with Kate Daum as principal investigator; and Eli Lilly awarded the Department of Internal Medicine $1,200 in 1935 to support Willis Fowler's research in iron metabolism.

Outreach programs through which medical faculty took the latest in science and techniques to Iowa practitioners also became more varied and more formalized in the 1930s. Fred Smith and other internal medicine faculty were widely sought as consultants across the state. The college also continued its Annual Clinic for Iowa practitioners, and medical faculty offered graduate courses through the university's extension service. In 1934, for example, the Department of Internal Medicine offered a "survey of internal medicine," conducted chiefly by Fred Smith, Horace Korns, Willis Fowler, and Kate Daum.[46] In March 1940, the college conducted an American College of Physicians graduate course in cardiac and vascular diseases under the direction of Fred Smith.

While still strained at times, relations between the Iowa State Medical

Society and the College of Medicine improved. One factor in that was reduced conflict over private practice at the University Hospitals, as some departments switched to a full-time basis while others, like internal medicine, agreed to limit private patients to 5 percent of total beds, with professional fees commensurate with charges by private physicians. In addition, university extension courses gave a boost to intra-professional relations. The extension concept, one Waterloo physician enthused, made "university supporters rapidly." "Former neutrals and critics," he said, "are made dependable 'minute men.'"[47]

Medical faculty accomplished much the same fence-mending mission through participation in the speakers bureau inaugurated by the Iowa State Medical Society. Fred Smith, Horace Korns, Elmer DeGowin, and Willis Fowler did yeoman's work for the bureau in the 1930s, and in November 1934, Clarence Baldridge died in an auto accident on his way to Fort Madison to present a talk for the bureau. Finally, statewide specialty societies, many of them state affiliates of national organizations, made their first appearance in the 1920s and 1930s, bringing together faculty and private practitioners. For example, at an organizational meeting in Des Moines in May 1925, Fred Smith was elected vice-president of the Iowa State Heart Association, the second state affiliate of the American Heart Association.[48]

In many respects, then, the world of medical science, although far removed in scale from today's vast enterprise, had become impressively diverse and sophisticated by the end of the 1930s. So, too, had the mechanisms through which academic researchers communicated with one another, and the same was true of the means by which private physicians were apprised of the practical implications of the latest scientific knowledge, from the effect of the xanthines on the coronary circulation to the anti-microbial uses of sulfonamides and the unraveling mystery of vitamin K, prothrombin, and the clotting of the blood.

SPECIALIZATION IN ACADEME AND IN PRACTICE

As the institutional foundations of medical science grew, the degree of specialization—among academic and practicing physicians alike—increased as well, and the outlines of the modern system of specialization were clearly discernible by the end of the 1930s. The 1928 publication of the first co-authored general medicine text, Russell Cecil's *A Textbook of Medicine, by American Authors*, was one symbol of the trend toward specialization, and its title suggested something about the maturity of American medical science as well.[49] Another symbol of specialization was the proliferation of specialty journals. In fact, so great was the "increase in the number of periodicals ...

limited to single, special fields of medicine," the editor of the *American Heart Journal* noted in 1925, "that the appearance of still another seems to call for a word of explanation."[50]

In 1927, a survey of 1915 graduates from fifty-two medical schools showed just 22 percent engaged in general practice, while nearly 35 percent specialized to some extent and over 40 percent limited their practice to a specialty, almost half of those in internal medicine. Moreover, almost 68 percent of respondents in that survey hoped to limit their practice to a specialty in the future. Of the eighteen Iowa graduates who participated in the survey, nine were full-time specialists.[51] Nationwide, the number of specialists in internal medicine stood at 3,377 in 1929 and nearly doubled in the following decade, as it did in every decade after that.[52]

From the turn of the century to the 1930s, there was substantial change in the meaning of specialization. As Rosemary Stevens notes, the conventional wisdom early in the century was that specialized knowledge should broaden rather than narrow the physicians' capabilities; moreover, specialists, by virtue of their privileged knowledge, incurred additional social responsibilities as advocates of a special group. The emergence of several specialties—such as pediatrics, obstetrics and gynecology, and to some extent cardiology—reflected those expectations. However, by the 1930s, specialties had already become much more science-based, or science-driven, more and more "divorced from the public or social aspects of these fields." Social concerns and environmental factors appeared subjective and, as Stevens notes, "politically suspect,"[53] a position more in keeping with the mainstream of American culture but one that contributed to the depersonalization of medical care.

As specialties became more science-based, they also focused more and more on chronic rather than acute conditions. As has been many times noted, the existence of many modern specialties in fact depends upon the gulf between diagnostic technologies and therapeutics, the latter often consisting of what Lewis Thomas has called "half-way technologies" that are palliative rather than curative.[54] A major therapeutic breakthrough will often displace a disease condition from the hands of specialists into the hands of general practitioners, as happened, for example, with insulin therapy.[55]

The trend toward specialization profoundly affected internal medicine in the 1930s, as the accumulation of diagnostic technologies and drug therapies since the turn of the century, and the accelerating rate of accumulation in the 1930s, rapidly expanded the internist's armamentarium. The proliferation of diagnostic and therapeutic technologies also lent a more positive meaning to the term internist, no longer defined as a specialist who was not a surgeon, a pediatrician, or obstetrician. But with the advance of medical science the internist, especially the academic internist, was quite rapidly becoming not a specialist but a subspecialist in what had heretofore been the vaguely drawn field of internal medicine.

While the University of Iowa Department of Internal Medicine continued to emphasize the general nature of internal medicine in the 1930s, there was significant de facto specialization among faculty members, a harbinger of later divisionalization. Fred Smith's and Horace Korns' reputations rested chiefly on their accomplishments in cardiology, although Smith was interested, too, in gastrointestinal problems, notably irritable colon. Meanwhile, Willis Fowler and Elmer DeGowin focused their energies chiefly on studies of the blood and blood-related diseases. Hospital admissions in the internal medicine service reflected Korns' and Smith's special interests; the nearly 2,000 admissions in the 1930–31 fiscal year included 218 cases each of arteriosclerosis and irritable colon, along with 101 cases of cardiac decompensation and 59 cases of auricular fibrillation.[56]

One factor motivating the Council on Medical Education and Hospitals survey of American medical education in the mid-1930s was the problematic relationship between specialization, particularly academic specialization, on the one hand and medical education on the other. Many observers wondered how the student was to obtain a general medical education in an academic environment that was increasingly compartmentalized. Furthermore, since specialized practice seemed the wave of the future, what kind of education should the medical schools provide? Dean Weiskotten, however, like the Commission on Medical Education before him, had few concrete answers to such questions.

By the 1930s, the one-year, rotating internship had become a routine part of the basic medical education, an admission that clinical teaching in the schools did not produce a full-fledged physician. Ninety-one of Iowa's ninety-four graduates in the class of 1935 served internships,[57] and, in the 1930s, several hospitals in Iowa offered internship programs accepted by the American Medical Association's Council on Medical Education and Hospitals. Some internship programs, as everyone recognized, offered better learning experiences than others, but in all of them interns put in long hours for very little money. At the University of Iowa, interns received room, board, laundry service, and one hundred dollars payable at the end of the internship year. Housed on the fourth and fifth floors of the hospital tower, they were on call twenty-four hours a day, seven days a week.

More remarkable than the development of the internship was the emergence of the residency. The appearance of the residency during the 1920s was symptomatic of the movement toward specialization in medicine, the residency serving as "a period of sustained specialty training" following the general practical experience of the fifth-year internship. The AMA's Council on Medical Education and Hospitals published its first list of approved residency programs in 1927,[58] and residency programs multiplied rapidly through the 1930s, providing another source of cheap labor for hard-pressed hospitals and becoming more or less standardized at two or three years in length. In Iowa, the University of Iowa hospitals were the only facilities offering AMA-approved residency programs prior to World War II.

The University of Iowa Department of Internal Medicine offered a three-year residency program. First-year residents spent a part of their time in Fred Smith's private service, chiefly taking patient histories and performing routine laboratory work. They then moved to one of the three indigent wards—C-33 under Fred Smith, C-32 under Horace Korns, or C-31, the largest, under the combined charge of Willis Fowler and James Greene. Second-year residents served as senior residents on one of the wards and often did some scientific research in conjunction with one of the faculty. Like interns, first-year residents lived in the hospital and were on call twenty-four hours a day, but residents, as full-fledged physicians, were better paid, receiving twenty dollars per month in the first year and eighty dollars per month in the second.

The rate at which American medicine moved toward specialization, both in practice and in graduate education, intensified long-standing pressures for specialist certification, no less so in internal medicine than in other areas. As in other specialties, however, there was much uncertainty in internal medicine over who should take charge of specialty certification: licensing boards, state medical societies, specialty societies, the National Board of Medical Examiners, or some new agency created for the purpose. In 1935, after much vacillation, and facing the prospect of internal medicine's disintegration into a number of emerging subspecialties, the American College of Physicians, working with the Section on Practice of Medicine of the American Medical Association, took the lead in erecting a certification system for internists. Walter Bierring—president of the AMA in 1934–35, a regent of the ACP from 1930 to 1939, and chair of the ACP Committee on Certification of Internists—was a central figure in those negotiations and was chair of the new American Board of Internal Medicine from 1936 to 1939.[59] By 1940, the board was already recognizing subspecialties in gastroenterology, cardiology, allergies, and tuberculosis.

At the University of Iowa, two ambitious young residents were chiefly responsible for creation of a program designed to prepare residents in internal medicine for ABIM certification. In 1939, Lewis January, who graduated from Colorado College and the University of Colorado Medical College before coming to Iowa City for his internship and residency, and Robert Hardin, who had earned his M.D. degree and served his internship and residency at the University of Iowa, wrote the American Board of Internal Medicine for information about certification and, in conjunction with Fred Smith and Horace Korns, drafted a training program to meet the board's requirements.

Thus, locally and nationally, specialization was a dominant theme of the 1930s as internal medicine became an increasingly well-defined specialty, with formal certification procedures, both for academic physicians and for private practitioners. The same impulse to specialization extended to medical education with the spread of formal programs of residency training. Within internal medicine, subspecialization, too, had become a clear trend. The American Board of Internal Medicine early on recognized several subspecialties; and, although the formal divisionalization of the Department of Internal Medicine at the University of Iowa still lay well in the future, a degree of subspecialization was apparent by the end of the 1930s.

WOMEN IN INTERNAL MEDICINE

As internal medicine emerged as a well-defined specialty in the 1920s and 1930s, it was overwhelmingly a male preserve. Prior to the late 1950s, only one female physician—Julia Cole—appeared on the faculty roll of the University of Iowa Department of Internal Medicine and that for only a brief period in the early 1930s. In general, the reasons for women's limited presence in medicine—ranging from outright discrimination to far more subtle cultural and structural impediments—are well documented.[60] Moreover, feminist historians have argued that one result of women's exclusion was the gendered construction of medical science itself.[61]

The growth of first the internship and then the residency, like many earlier reforms in medical education, made it harder for women, and minorities as well, to maintain places in American medicine. While only a handful of medical colleges refused to enroll women in the 1930s, most colleges maintained formal or informal enrollment limits for women as well as for minorities. Female enrollment at the University of Iowa College of Medicine hovered around 4 to 5 percent, and minority students were virtually nonexistent. It is not at all far-fetched to suggest that administrators might well have welcomed non-resident male students before accepting more resident females.

Just 105 of 712 AMA-recognized internship programs accepted women as late as 1940.[62] In Iowa at that time, the University of Iowa Hospitals operated one of only three internship programs formally open to women; however, in this as in many things, appearance and practice could be quite different. The housing of interns in the general hospital after its opening in 1928, while obviously convenient for disciplinary and other reasons, was also a convenient rationale for the exclusion of women from internships. As hospital director Robert E. Neff explained to a female applicant in 1939, the question of appointing women to internships was "governed by the availability of residence quarters for women." In short, there were no quarters for women interns; therefore, there were no women interns.[63] There had been in fact a suite of three rooms reserved for female housestaff, but those quarters were seldom used and were, in the late 1930s, converted to staff office space.

At the residency level, just 49 of 195 internal medicine residency programs nationwide were nominally open to women in 1940. Thus, there was intense competition for the few available residency slots for women. While the University of Iowa's residency programs were among those advertised as admitting women,[64] in practice the situation with residencies in the University Hospitals was much like that with internships. According to a tabulation done for the university administration in 1939, there were no women residents in the University Hospitals in the 1930s outside of pediatrics and obstetrics-gynecology.[65]

WOMEN IN INTERNAL MEDICINE: THE NUTRITION PROGRAM

As specialized services and formal administrative hierarchies developed in hospitals in the first decades of the twentieth century, "efficiency" and "scientific management" became watchwords in hospital administration.[66] One obvious intersection of scientific hospital management and scientific medicine lay in nutrition, and by the mid-1920s most larger hospitals, and especially teaching hospitals, had established dietary departments supervised by skilled female dietitians, most of whom had received their training in departments of home economics. While forbidding obstacles stood in the way of women's advancement in academic medicine, nutrition, at least at the University of Iowa, provided an alternative path of entry for women into the male-dominated world of medical science.

Campbell Howard of internal medicine and Ruth Wardall of home economics were chiefly responsible for establishment in 1920 of a nutrition department in the College of Medicine combining teaching, research, and hospital service.[67] Ruth Wheeler, a well-known figure in the world of nutrition, came to Iowa to head the new department. Born in 1877, Wheeler had graduated from Vassar College in 1899 and had taken her Ph.D. under Lafayette Mendel at Yale in 1913. Wheeler was a charter member of the American Home Economics Association and was also a founding member of the American Dietetic Association in 1917, serving as association president for two terms from 1924 to 1926.[68]

In building the Nutrition Department at Iowa, Ruth Wheeler entered an institutional milieu tightly controlled by males whose vision of her department often differed from her own. Moreover, competition for money, space, and professional turf was intense and often bitter in the College of Medicine and

University Hospitals, and Wheeler's requests for space, equipment, and support personnel sparked bureaucratic squabbles between Wheeler and Dean Lee W. Dean of the College of Medicine, between Wheeler and the hospital superintendent, A. J. Lomas, and between Dean and Lomas.

The jurisdictional claims of Wheeler's department also provoked resistance. In particular, pediatric staff in the Children's Hospital were reluctant to surrender their control over dietary operations, particularly the preparation of infant formulas. "It is of the greatest importance," the head of pediatrics lectured Wheeler, "that we can feel that the worker in charge of the milk room is in sympathy and harmony with our ideas, willing and anxious to carry out every reasonable suggestion which we see fit to make." He also reserved the right to "outline the ward diets if we see fit."[69]

Ruth Wheeler's greatest difficulties lay in her desire to make the Nutrition Department more than the University Hospitals' "feeding machine," as she referred to the dietary service. Wheeler's first concern was her master's degree program—America's first—in hospital nutrition, a program that, in addition to thirty semester hours of graduate coursework in nutrition and related areas, required nutrition interns to work 48-hour weeks in rotation through several service areas in the department. Under the circumstances, Wheeler argued, her interns deserved the same "complete maintenance" [i.e., room, board, and laundry] provided medical interns. It would be "impossible to get desirable interns without complete maintenance," she claimed.[70] However, hospital superintendent A. J. Lomas objected that nutrition interns were not at all like medical interns who were on call around the clock and were, in any event, essential to the university hospitals' operation. In the superintendent's view, nutrition interns came simply "to get experience in their line, and as far as I can see [render] the hospital nothing in return."[71] Dean Lee Wallace Dean concurred. Nonetheless, Wheeler prevailed with President Jessup, and her second class of interns enjoyed the complete maintenance she had demanded.

Wheeler met similar resistance from male colleagues with regard to her goals for research. If hers was to be "a real department of Nutrition and not merely a hospital dietary department," she observed in 1923, it must have an ongoing research program that would include research opportunities for interns.[72] Again, Dean and Lomas would have none of that. In this case, Dean contradicted his and Lomas' earlier position, turning Wheeler's argument for equality of nutrition and medical interns against her. "Hospital interns," he charged in a letter to President Jessup, "are primarily appointed for service in the hospital and not for research work."[73] Once more, however, Jessup sided with Wheeler, enabling her, after an unsuccessful search in 1923, to hire a full-time research assistant the following year.

After four years of struggle and with the main outlines of the Nutrition Department in place, Ruth Wheeler received an offer to become Professor of

Physiology and Nutrition at Vassar College in the fall of 1925, and the promise of more money for less work at her alma mater prompted Wheeler to submit her resignation effective in August 1926. By 1925, both the Nutrition Department's original champions, Campbell Howard and Ruth Wardall, had left the university, and Wheeler's anticipated departure opened the way to an attack on the department from its enemies, especially Dean Lee Wallace Dean.

In the fall of 1926, the Nutrition Department in the College of Medicine disappeared, with control over the hospital dietary service passing to a new Nutrition Department organized within the University Hospitals. At the same time, the Department of Internal Medicine was allotted funds for a faculty position in nutrition. Ruth Wardall, viewing developments from the University of Illinois, saw the dissolution of Ruth Wheeler's Nutrition Department as a direct challenge to the institutional legitimacy of nutrition and to women's place in academic science and expressed her alarm—to no avail—in a letter to Dean.[74]

With the separation of teaching and service functions in nutrition, Kate Daum, who had joined the Nutrition Department as Wheeler's research assistant in 1925, became Assistant Professor of Nutrition in the Department of Internal Medicine. Ruth Wheeler had recommended Daum as her successor, noting that she was "not so young as she looks" and could "carry on the work without a break."[75] Born in Great Bend, Kansas, in 1892, Daum had entered the University of Kansas intent on majoring in mathematics, but she soon discovered that mathematics was "a man's field" and switched to home economics, earning bachelor's and master's degrees by 1916. In 1925, Daum received her Ph.D. in chemistry and nutrition through Katherine Blunt's graduate program at the University of Chicago. Before coming to Iowa, Daum had been instrumental in organizing the Nutrition Department at Columbia-Presbyterian Hospital.[76]

Florence Ross, recruited from Simmons College in Boston, became head of the Nutrition Department, now relocated to the University Hospitals. However, Ross' tenure was short and troubled, in part because of inherent ambiguities in the status of the graduate program in nutrition caused by the separation of the service function lodged in the hospitals from the teaching and research functions housed now in the Department of Internal Medicine. During the winter of 1926–27, one of Ross' interns abruptly resigned, unhappy with the operation of the program, and in March 1927, a concerned medical faculty discussed "at considerable length" the relation of the Nutrition Department to the hospital, the college, and the Graduate College. The faculty approved a motion that the "hospital continue to offer opportunities for graduate work in nutrition."[77]

In May 1927, Lee Wallace Dean's resignation, preceded by the resignation of the hospital superintendent, left the medical faculty holding unprecedented power in administration of the college and the University Hospitals. While few medical faculty favored reconstituting the Nutrition Department in its earlier form, thus investing another woman with Ruth Wheeler's status and authority as a department head in the College of Medicine, a majority was ready to combine responsibility for nutrition service, teaching, and research in Kate Daum, who had favorably impressed staff and students alike with her energy and abilities. The subsequent removal of Florence Ross cost the resignations of three nutrition interns but saved the hospitals Ross' $3,000 annual salary, and Kate Daum assumed direction of the hospital's Nutrition Department in addition to her duties as an assistant professor in internal medicine.

Kate Daum chafed at the removal of the Nutrition Department from the College of Medicine. Nutrition, she lamented, was "the neglected and forgotten child of medicine,"[78] and the problem was that "food is the chief commodity and the kitchen the important workshop of this department." As a result, she observed, the status of nutrition personnel was only "a little above that of the ward maid in the hospital caste system."[79]

Daum's observation accurately reflected the general ambivalence of physicians and hospital administrators toward women's participation in the world of health sciences research. Most often, men viewed women as helpmates. For example, when William H. Walsh, Executive Secretary of the American Hospital Association, enumerated the roles of the hospital dietitian in 1925, he included administration, therapy, and teaching, but said nothing of research.[80] Similarly, Russell M. Wilder of the Mayo Clinic, while acknowledging that dietitians commanded "special knowledge of the science of nutrition," saw the dietitian as only a "superior technical assistant" to the physician in nutrition research.[81] As a result, the rapidly expanding field of nutrition was partitioned by gender. Women's chief base in nutrition lay in departments of home economics and hospital nutrition, while men's base lay in laboratory sciences such as physiology and chemistry and, to an increasing extent, in medicine.[82] Separate male and female professional associations and related institutions reflected and heightened the gender division. The American Dietetic Association, for example, represented women in hospital nutrition, while the American Institute of Nutrition, founded in 1928 and reorganized in 1934, represented chiefly male laboratory scientists who operated at a safe remove from the kitchen. Indeed, the Institute's founder worried lest its organ, the *American Journal of Nutrition,* "become known as the 'Rat Journal.'"[83]

During the depression, Kate Daum's program, like the rest of the College of Medicine and the University Hospitals, faced reduced staff levels, longer hours of work, and lower pay scales, while graduates of the nutrition program found fewer jobs waiting. Later, during the years of World War II, staff and students faced shortages even of basic uniform components. One anxious student reported to Daum that she had "no luck whatever in finding white hose," and another complained that the local Ration Board demanded a letter from Daum "stating that white shoes were necessary."[84] Despite dim employment prospects in the 1930s, however, the number of nutrition interns in the graduate program crept upward, reflecting the reputation of Daum's department and perhaps also reflecting declining opportunities for women in other professional fields.

Much of Kate Daum's research and that of her students focused on child nutrition and on various aspects of diabetic metabolism, but some projects dealt with specifically female subjects, including nitrogen metabolism during menstruation and the metabolism of calcium and phosphorus in pregnancy. And in 1934, Kate Daum and Margaret A. Ohlson, a Ph.D. candidate in nutrition, published one of the early studies of iron metabolism in women, previous studies having been limited to either male subjects or children.[85] Daum and her colleagues also collaborated with faculty in the Department of Internal Medicine, most notably in studies of nutrition in arteriosclerosis and in treatment of cardiac failure.[86]

During the 1930s and 1940s, there was a monastic quality to the nutrition interns' experience. Segregated in Westlawn, the nurses' dormitory west of the Iowa River, interns were isolated from much of campus life. Moreover, Kate Daum continued Ruth Wheeler's demanding program, requiring 48-hour work weeks as well as a "B" average in graduate coursework culminating in a thesis and both written and oral examinations in major and minor areas of study. Daum set high standards of deportment for her interns. She and her staff regularly evaluated their students' integrity, disposition, and culture—the last defined as "refinement, polish, manners, [and] broad interests." Daum also prescribed a uniform "with long sleeves and with the hem fourteen inches from the floor," with "a collar arrangement not too low" and "white oxfords of a comfortable, businesslike design." Daum also advised against silk undergarments since "the laundry does not do any silk and you will not have the time to do much of this sort of thing." In short, Daum warned new students, "The work is here but very interesting."[87]

The monastic ideal was enhanced by the fact that virtually all interns were young and single and significant numbers were in fact nuns. In 1931, Daum suggested to one young mother that hospital nutrition might not be "a wise choice" for her. "Anyone engaged in food work," Daum warned, "is more tied down than any other person." Besides, she pointed out, "pay is such that in the majority of hospitals you still receive living instead of money," in which case "your children could not live with you or if they did conditions would not be very satisfactory for them."[88] Most graduates of the nutrition program remained in a community made up largely of single women, a circumstance reflecting both the widely held perception that hospital nutrition was women's work and the practical problems in combining marriage and family with a career. Kate Daum, for example, never married, and only one of her four chief administrative dietitians in the period from 1921 to 1956 married. Just eight of seventeen therapeutic dietitians in that period were married, two of whom apparently resigned at the time of marriage.

Kate Daum, like her colleagues in Department of Internal Medicine, invested a great deal of time and energy in professional activities, joining her interests to larger communities of science and practice. Daum maintained a high profile in the American Dietetic Association, for example, heading the Diet Therapy Section already in 1927. Daum was also important in formation of the Iowa Dietetic Association, inviting nutritionists from across Iowa to an inaugural meeting in Waterloo in February 1930.[89] In addition, Daum actively promoted the principles of nutrition in talks before civic associations and service clubs around the state.

Kate Daum, then, promoted professional goals and kept her nutrition program afloat through the difficult years of the Depression and World War II, notwithstanding the long decline from 1930 to 1945 in the University of Iowa health sciences complex, a decline that affected nutrition as it did other departments and services.

INTERNAL MEDICINE AND WORLD WAR II

During World War II, the work of internists in a variety of areas, from the control of infectious diseases to the storage and distribution of whole blood, validated the rise of internal medicine as a distinct specialty.[90] Internal medicine also benefited from the wartime marriage of science and government, an experience that "demonstrated that major scientific goals could be attained by spending large sums of money and by focusing attention on defined objectives" and one that carried profound implications for the postwar world.[91] The U.S. Army actively promoted internal medicine in the war years, effectively providing graduate education and a taste of specialization to a generation of young physicians; thus, the trend toward specialization in American medicine was, if anything, accelerated by wartime experience. In a June 1945 survey, 7,282 of a sample of 21,000 military physicians attested that they had been in specialty practice before the war while 12,627, or 60 percent, wanted to pursue specialty practice after wartime service.[92]

Death rates in the American armed forces are testament to the contributions of American medicine, and especially internal medicine, to the war effort. In all of World War I, the annual death rate among U.S. servicemen was 35.5 per 1,000, but during World War II that rate fell by more than two-thirds, to 11.6 per 1,000. Of more immediate relevance to internal medicine, non-battle deaths fell from an annual rate of 18.4 per 1,000 in World War I—more than half the total death rate—to just three per 1,000 in World War II. Even more striking, deaths from disease fell from 15.6 per 1,000 cases in 1917–19 to 0.6 per 1,000 cases in 1942–44. Thanks to sulfa drugs and penicillin, for example, the case fatality rate for pneumonia fell from 28 percent in World War I to 0.7 percent in World War II and for meningococcal infections from 38 percent to 4 percent.[94] In addition, demonstrating the fruits of interwar medical science, military internists identified and treated a variety of conditions—e.g., cardiovascular, gastrointestinal, and metabolic—that were not immediately life-threatening.

There was a widespread mood of preparedness in the United States long before December 7, 1941, and as the Army's authorized strength began to climb abruptly in late 1940, reaching 1.4 million in 1941, the Army's Medical Department faced the prospect of expanding its physician ranks from 1,200 to 9,100.[95] In response, the Office of the Surgeon General asked the American Medical Association to survey its members' willingness to serve and to tabulate their individual qualifications. By December 1, 1940, 79 percent of America's 175,000 physicians, including 92.6 percent of physicians in Iowa, had responded, with the information encoded on punch cards for later use.[96]

Voluntary preparedness movements, like that in organized medicine, reflected both patriotism and a concern to head off the intrusion of "big government" in social and economic affairs. The American Medical Association and the Association of American Medical Colleges, for example, both formed committees on military preparedness before America's formal entry into the war and sought to devise private and quasi-public solutions to the problems of medical education and the distribution and delivery of medical services in wartime—including, perhaps most importantly, the mobilization of physicians for military service.

In June 1941, the AMA's House of Delegates, acting on the advice of the Committee on Health and Medicine of the National Council on Military Preparedness, agreed, perhaps as the lesser of two evils, to a cooperative scheme involving organized medicine and agencies of government in coordinating wartime medical services, an arrangement put in place by executive order of President Franklin Roosevelt in October 1941. The new agency, the Procurement and Assignment Service for Physicians, Dentists, and Veterinarians, was part of the Office of Defense, Health and Welfare Services, and men drawn from organized medicine—e.g., the president of the AMA, the retiring president of the Association of American Physicians, and the dean of the University of Minnesota College of Medicine—dominated its governing board. The Procurement and Assignment Service served as a clearinghouse and coordinating agency for requests for medical personnel from various government agencies, including the armed forces, thus insuring organized medicine a voice in health-related matters during wartime.[97]

The voluntary conversion to a wartime footing extended also to medical education. Already in 1940, the Executive Council of the Association of American Medical Colleges, responding to an appeal from selective service officials, recommended that member institutions increase their entering classes by 10 percent and continue instruction of the junior class, the class of 1942, through the summer of 1941 so that its members would graduate three months early.[98] In the aftermath of Pearl Harbor—in striking contrast to the indecision displayed on the issue of continuous instruction in World War I—the AAMC amplified its position, recommending elimination of the summer vacation period for all medical students, collapsing the four-year course into three years for the duration of the emergency.[99] In response to AAMC appeals, the University of Iowa agreed to expand admissions from ninety to one hundred each year and began the accelerated instruction plan on July 1, 1942,[100] admitting a freshman class and graduating a senior class every nine months thereafter. Eventually internships, too, were curtailed, cut from twelve months to nine, and the "9-9-9 Plan" instituted in 1944 severely restricted residency deferments and shortened the length of the residency to nine months also.

America's organization for total war in the months after Pearl Harbor brought an inevitable trend toward centralization in both medical education and the distribution of physicians. By early 1942, independent army and navy recruitment efforts were already disrupting hopes for voluntary coordination through the Procurement and Assignment Service.[101] Furthermore, after the initial wave of physician call-ups and enlistments, the armed forces effectively controlled medical student selection and placement through the selective service system and through deferred service arrangements such as the Navy V-12 program and the Army Specialized Training Program. By 1943, the assignment of entering students to the University of Iowa College of Medicine was largely in the hands of Army and Navy Seventh Service District commands, in consultation with Dean Ewen MacEwen and other medical college officials. Of the college's total enrollment of 307 in 1944–45, 265 were Navy V-12 and Army ASTP placements.[102]

With the apparatus of medical education increasingly co-opted for military purposes, the number of places open to women changed little, despite the pressing need for more physicians and a shortage of qualified male students. Entering classes at the University of Iowa fell far short of the announced goal of one hundred students during the war years, but women continued to make up only about 4 to 5 percent of the student body—14 of the 307 in 1944–45.[103] Likewise, despite the loss of able-bodied men to the draft, the war did not open internship and residency positions to women. The three residents in the University of Iowa Department of Internal Medicine in 1942–43, for example, were all males.[104]

The military effectively controlled medical faculty as well as medical students. Prior to 1942, the army exempted many faculty reserve officers from the call to active service; Dean MacEwen—a Lieutenant Colonel in the Medical Reserve—was one such case. The Office of the Surgeon General warned, however, that after March 31, 1942, all reserve officers would be called to active duty, whether or not they were performing an essential civilian service. Thereafter, medical faculty holding reserve commissions either chose military service or resigned their commissions and accepted classification as essential civilian workers. A few months later, Dean MacEwen warned President Hancher of "rumblings" from around the state that many "of our faculty men are hiding behind the essential teacher qualification."[105] At the same time, however, local draft boards were almost universally reluctant to draft physicians. At the University of Iowa, wartime medical education, conducted on a year-round basis, was a catch-as-catch-can operation. The skeleton faculty in internal medicine consisted of Fred Smith, Horace Korns, Willis Fowler, James Greene, Elmer DeGowin, William Paul, and Kate Daum, with an ever-changing cast of junior faculty, part-time assistants, and short-term residents.

Prior to the war, the trends that had so changed the face of American medicine in the 1920s and 1930s were scarcely visible in the organization and aims of military medicine. The U.S. Army Medical Department, for example, was still organized chiefly around its traditional surgical mission. Despite that, the armed forces, conscious of their public reputation for turning concert pianists into truck drivers, subsequently displayed considerable sensitivity in utilizing physicians. However, internal medicine itself encompassed a wide variety of specialized knowledge and skills; consequently, internists performed diverse roles in military service.

In February 1942, the Office of the Surgeon General appointed the first commissioned consultant in internal medicine. Thereafter, the Professional Services Division, later the Medical Consultants Division, developed slowly and on a trial-and-error basis, but the system of specialty consultants eventually broadened outward and downward to provide consultants in internal medicine to all the domestic service commands and then to overseas commands as well. The consultants' primary functions were to evaluate therapy and to assist in assessing the qualifications of medical personnel, and in 1944, as the restrictions on residency deferments and the difficulties in drafting civilian physicians reduced the supply of trained internists to a trickle, the Surgeon General added civilians to the consultant ranks.

The consultants in internal medicine were only the most visible and perhaps the most glamorous of a very large group of internists in national service. Internal medicine made up a good part of the caseload at military hospitals, both domestic and overseas, and the organizational structure of the U.S. Army's Medical Department, although little specialized in 1940, came more and more to reflect civilian practice during the war years, ultimately classifying all physicians by specialty and proficiency. Indeed, as noted earlier, wartime experience introduced many physicians to the rewards of specialized practice, converting a good many into postwar specialists.[106]

The wartime experience of the University of Iowa's Lewis E. January was in many respects typical. After an internship at the University Hospitals, January had been drawn to internal medicine by the example of Fred Smith and Horace Korns, and when his three-year residency ended on June 30, 1941, he stayed on in the department as an assistant. As the pace of military mobilization quickened, Dean MacEwen included Lewis January among the college's essential personnel shielded from military service; however, January, who had joined the U.S. Army Medical Reserve while at the University of Iowa, petitioned MacEwen for release and joined the Army Air Forces Medical Department as a first lieutenant in May 1942.[107]

Lewis January's first assignment was to Davis-Monthan Field in Tucson, Arizona, but in 1943, after earning American Board of Internal Medicine certification, January was elevated to the rank of captain and served as Chief of Medicine at U.S. Army Air Forces hospitals in Moses Lake and then Euphrata, Washington. In 1944, another transfer took January to a similar position at a station hospital in McCook, Nebraska, and in 1945, newly promoted to major, January became Chief of Medicine at the Pyote Army Air Field hospital in west Texas, a regional facility at the center of a network of several base hospitals.

Behind that bare-bones description of station assignments lay internal medicine's growing capabilities, its increasing institutional recognition in military medicine, and the flow of young servicemen who were Lewis January's patients. January modestly summarized his wartime service as "busy and rewarding," and for physicians like him, despite the isolated locations of most Air Forces facilities (Pyote, for example, was known as "Rattlesnake Army Air Base"), military service could be a time of excitement, intense training in administrative as well as medical areas, and substantial fulfillment.

Internal medicine consultants in Lewis January's service commands— Walter Bauer of Harvard in the Ninth Army and Paul Starr of Northwestern in the Second Air Force—enjoyed national reputations, made frequent visits to the hospitals in their service areas and often brought along other respected internists to share their expertise. In 1944, for example, January heard lectures by Andre Cournand, who originated cardiac catheterization and would share a Nobel Prize in medicine in 1956.

In early 1945, Lewis January's first experience with penicillin in the treatment of subacute bacterial endocarditis was a striking instance of the incorporation of the new science and technology into the Army Medical Department. Presented with a 27-year-old bombardier exhibiting "malaise, anorexia, fever and petechial hemorrhages," with some clubbing of the fingers and characteristic heart murmurs, January recognized the symptoms of endocarditis, an almost universally fatal condition. January, who had read published reports of the use of penicillin in such cases, began a twenty-one day course of penicillin therapy, and in what he remembered as his most moving experience of the war years, his patient survived—an episode that was still a vivid memory forty-five years later.[108] Paul Starr, who was visiting the Pyote hospital at the time, was as excited as January and later defended him when January presented a case report to a sometimes skeptical audience at the San Antonio School of Aviation Medicine.

Another example of wartime service was that of Robert C. Hardin, who was, as previously noted, a resident colleague of Lewis January at the University of Iowa. Robert Hardin's work, demonstrating the potential for subspecialization in internal medicine, was oriented around the adaptation of civilian blood banking techniques to the care of battle casualties, a project for which Elmer DeGowin also warrants special credit and for which Everett D. Plass of the Department of Obstetrics and Gynecology at the University of Iowa deserves mention as well.

The Whole Blood Project, in the making from 1940 to 1944, was a cooperative endeavor involving a small but vocal element of the U.S. Army Medical Department and key medical advisory committees of the National Research Council: the Committee on Transfusions, on which Plass served, and the subcommittee on blood substitutes, where DeGowin was an influential voice.[109] Although research early in the twentieth century had resolved the basic mechanics of blood transfusion, including blood typing and the use of anticoagulants, there were yet many unanswered questions surrounding the collection, storage, transportation, and transfusion of preserved blood in the 1930s.[110] Elmer DeGowin—in collaboration with Everett Plass, Robert Hardin, and others—conducted a series of experiments in 1937–38 that led to the modern system of blood-banking at the University of Iowa.[111] The immediate fruits of DeGowin's work were, first, the Blood Transfusion Service and the Blood Bank set up late in 1938 and early in 1939 at the University of Iowa Hospitals and, second, a gold medal from the American Medical Association for his 1939 convention exhibit outlining his blood-banking work.

At the outbreak of World War II, few authorities appreciated loss of blood as the primary cause of shock in battle wounds, and in any event most were convinced that blood plasma, or some substitute product, was sufficient to restore lost blood volume. Furthermore, despite experience dating as far back as World War I, there was widespread skepticism about the practicability of providing whole blood to forward hospital units. Elmer DeGowin nonetheless argued, both in meetings of the blood substitute subcommittee and in print, that whole blood was vital to the treatment of wound shock, that it should be administered to casualties as early as possible, and that it was indeed possible to supply it to forward military hospitals.[112]

In the meantime, Robert Hardin, now Captain Robert Hardin, was one of the handful of voices pressing the same argument inside the Army Medical Department. Attached in August 1942 to the British Army Blood Supply Depot to observe the established British system of whole blood collection, processing, and distribution,[113] Hardin was, by the middle of 1943, overseeing the establishment of blood banks at U.S. general hospitals in Britain. Later in the year, when the 152nd Station Hospital at Salisbury, England, was converted into a central blood bank for collection and processing of whole blood, Hardin became its executive officer.[114] Hardin's blood-banking work was warmly remembered; the commander of one general hospital commended "the splendid blood bank control under Dr. Robert C. Hardin" that had nearly eliminated transfusion reactions.[115]

In February 1944, as Allied staff worked out the intricate plans for the cross-channel invasion, Robert Hardin became theater transfusion officer, charged with overall coordination of supplies of whole blood for the soon-to-be expanding European theater. However, Hardin and others, realizing the inadequacies of existing blood supplies, argued for an airlift of preserved whole blood from the United States. The blood bank at Salisbury, they pointed out, could supply no more than 700 pints per day to American forces in France, and barely a month after D-Day, the scarcity of blood forced a system of allocation.[116]

In August 1944, the Surgeon General, USA, after a troubling tour of medical facilities in Italy, approved a long-delayed plan to transport large quantities of whole blood from the United States to Europe. In all, the blood transfusion service delivered more than 266,000 pints of preserved whole blood—more than half of that provided by American Red Cross donor stations across the United States—to forward hospital stations on the continent from June 1944 to May 1945.[117] In November 1944, the airlift of whole blood was extended to the Pacific theater. Overall, the organizational and technical problems in that undertaking were staggering; typing such enormous quantities of blood quickly and accurately was a serious challenge in itself.[118] Douglas Kendrick may well have been correct in claiming that "if any single medical program can be credited with the saving of countless lives in World War II, ... it was the prompt and liberal use of whole blood."[119]

In many ways, then, internal medicine made its mark in World War II, its high visibility a consequence of both the advances in medical science during the 1920s and 1930s and the extension of civilian specialization into military medicine. Internal medicine owed its wartime success to many players: overworked educators like Fred Smith and Horace Korns, who supplied physicians to the military; patient medical researchers like Elmer DeGowin, who solved problems of critical importance to military medicine and helped to create organizational structures to translate scientific research into practice; and young internists, many of them—like Lewis January and Robert Hardin—just out of their residencies, who took their expertise to the field.

CONCLUSION: THE SHAPE OF THE FUTURE

In retrospect, the legacy of the years of depression and war was mixed. On the one hand, there was a sense of excitement and accomplishment surrounding the growth of medical science and its successful application to practical problems; certainly medical science had played a key role in the war effort from 1942 to 1945. On the other hand, academic medicine emerged from the war with facilities and programs suffering from a decade and a half of neglect and with an uncertain future.

At the University of Iowa, the quality of medical education had declined relative to many other schools since the late 1920s. Even worse, Dean Ewen MacEwen complained in 1940 that the departments—e.g., anatomy, bacteriology, and physiology—that had received "a very low rating" from the Council on Medical Education and Hospitals in 1936 had continued their slide. Present staff levels in those departments, he noted, put the university at a disadvantage compared to other Big Ten schools.[120] A year later, just on the eve of World War II and prior to the system of military placement, MacEwen observed that the entering class in 1940–41 had been, "from the scholastic standpoint, one of the poorest in the experience of the school."[121] The College of Medicine's attempt to reverse the slide by raising admission standards from two years' pre-medical work to three years' was undone by a return to the two-year standard on January 20, 1943, as a war emergency measure recommended by the Association of American Medical Colleges.[122]

Yet depression and war were not the only causes of the College of Medicine's problems; in part, too, the plight of the college was due to changes in key leadership positions. At the top, President Eugene Gilmore was a far less persistent champion of the College of Medicine than was George MacLean or Walter Jessup. Similarly, neither Henry Houghton nor Ewen MacEwen, whatever their gifts, seemed able to match Lee Wallace Dean, whatever his faults, as an institution-builder. Finally, Fred Smith, a man who possessed many admirable qualities to be sure, was not so aggressive in temperament as was Campbell Howard, a difference perhaps reflecting their backgrounds: Campbell Howard coming from a renowned medical family and Fred Smith coming from rural Illinois.

Despite all that, the future held far more promise than anyone would likely have foreseen in 1945. When Lewis January and Robert Hardin returned to the University of Iowa Department of Internal Medicine after the war, they, along with Elmer DeGowin, Willis Fowler, and William D. "Shorty" Paul were the nucleus of the faculty that carried the department into a second era of expansion, one built on the scientific advances as well as the specialization of the 1920s and 1930s and on the marriage of science, medicine, and government arranged during World War II.

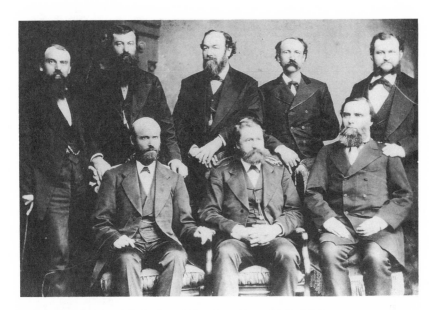

FIRST MEDICAL FACULTY, State University of Iowa, Medical Department, Iowa City, 1870-71. (*Standing*) Hinrichs, Shrader, Robertson, Middleton, Clapp. (*Seated*) Farnsworth, Peck, Dillon. *Photographs in this section courtesy of the Kent Collection, University of Iowa Archives.*

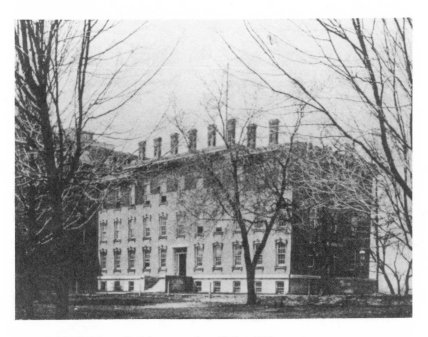

OLD SOUTH HALL, medical department from 1870 to 1883.

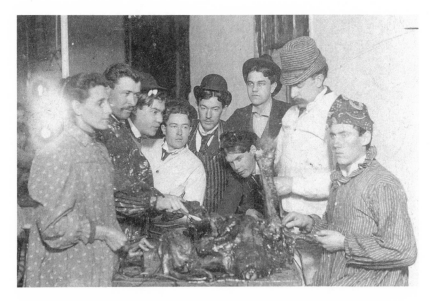

EARLY ANATOMY LABORATORY, 1893.

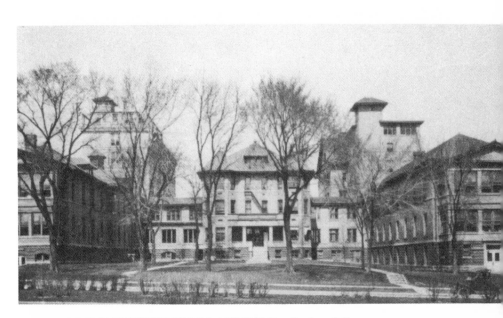

FIRST UNIVERSITY HOSPITAL, 1898-1928. Now Seashore Hall.

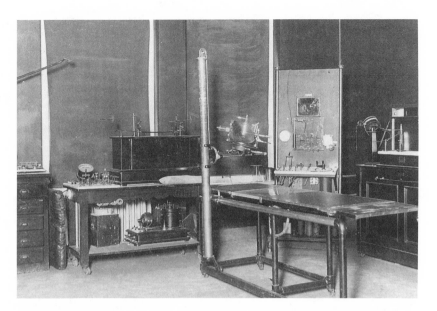

X-RAY ROOM, c. 1910.

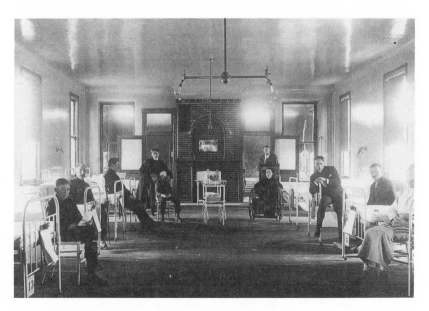

W. S. ROBERTSON WARD, old hospital (Seashore Hall), c. 1910.

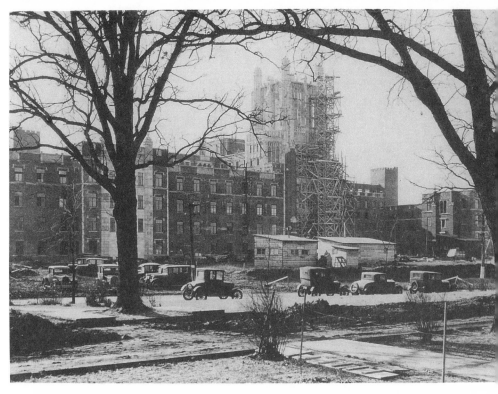

UNIVERSITY HOSPITAL gothic tower construction, 1927.

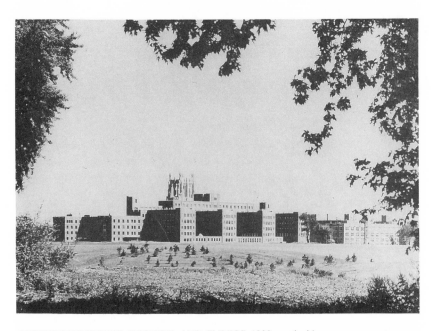

UNIVERSITY OF IOWA HOSPITAL AND CLINICS, 1928, south side.

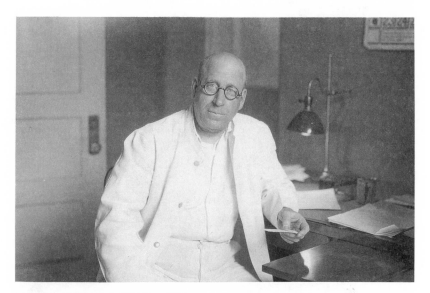

DEAN LEE WALLACE DEAN, c. 1925.

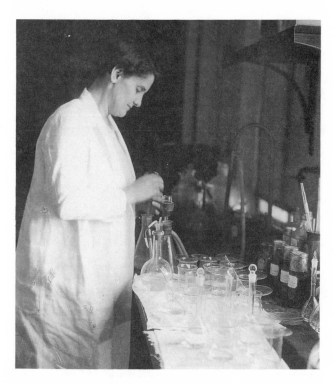

KATE DAUM, c. 1930.

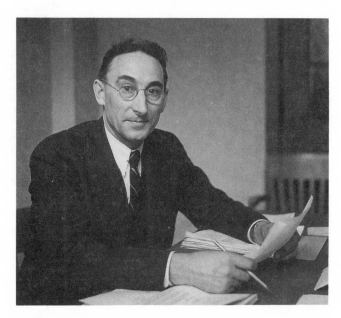

EWEN MacEWEN, 1937.

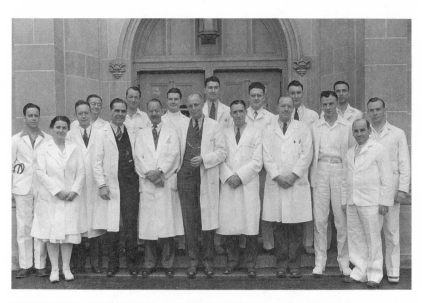

DEPARTMENT OF INTERNAL MEDICINE FACULTY, 1940s. (*From left*)
Robert Towle, Kate Daum, unknown, Lewis E. January, James A. Greene, Orrie
Couch, Horace M. Korns, Henry Zimmerman, Fred M. Smith, George Parkin,
Willis M. Fowler, L. W. Swanson, Elmer L. DeGowin, Lucian Ide, Ferrell Hamil-
ton, Raleigh Lage, William D. Paul, Forrest Coulsen.

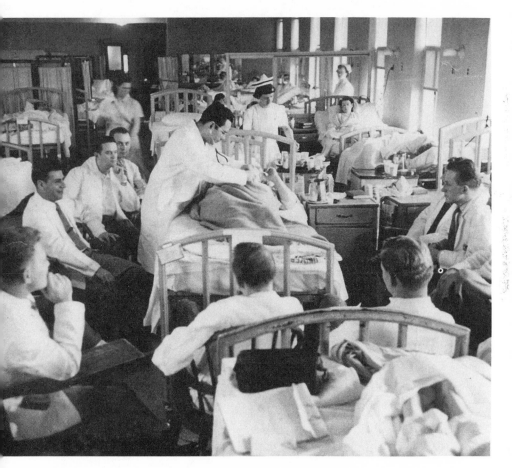

TEACHING PHYSICAL DIAGNOSIS to sophomores on C-32, c. 1950.

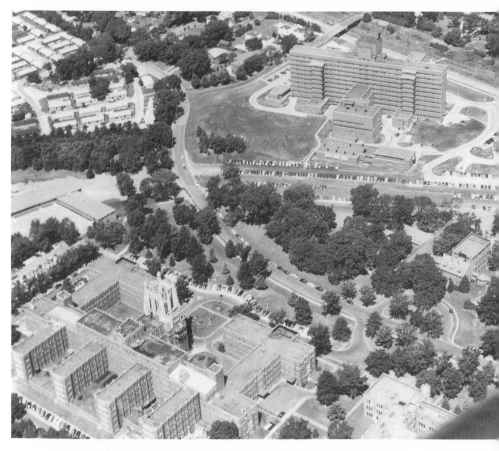

AERIAL PHOTO of UIHC/VA medical center, mid-1950s.

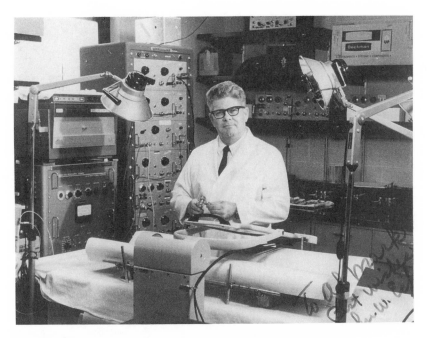

JOHN ECKSTEIN in the medical research laboratory, early 1960s.

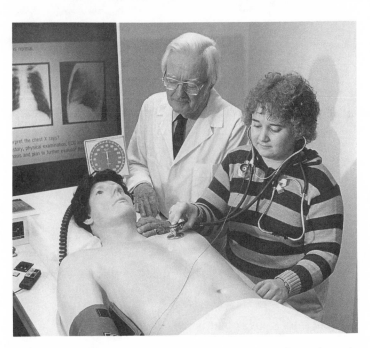

LEWIS E. JANUARY uses the cardiac patient simulator "Harvey" to teach a medical student, early 1980s.

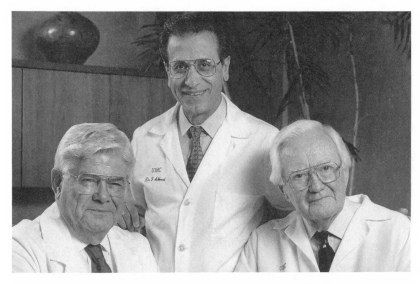

Three presidents of the American Medical Association. (*From left*) John Eckstein, François Abboud, Lewis January, late 1980s.

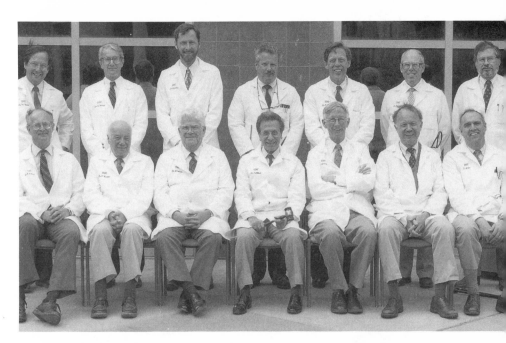

ASSOCIATION OF AMERICAN PHYSICIANS, 1990. (*Seated from left*) Robert Ashman, George Winokur, John Eckstein, François Abboud (president of the Association), James Clifton, Robert Clark, Robert Bar. (*Standing from left*) Michael Welsh, Donald Heistad, John Stokes, Gerald DiBona, Richard Wenzel, Phillip Schmid, Richard Kerber.

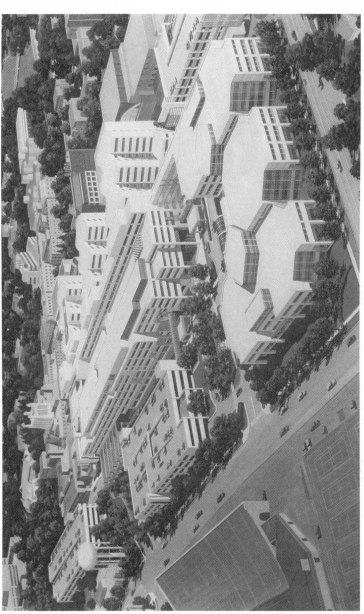

THE UNIVERSITY OF IOWA HOSPITALS AND CLINICS for the twenty-first century. Architectural rendering of the Roy J. Carver, John W. Colloton, John Pappajohn, and Pomerantz Family pavilions. These patient care and educational facilities represent the major phases of the UIHC program to replace early 1900-vintage nonconforming facilities with modern ones. The $47 million Carver Pavilion, $91 million Colloton Pavilion, and the $98 million Pappajohn Pavilion have all been constructed without state capital appropriations, as will the Pomerantz Family Pavilion.

II

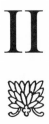

The Diffusion of Excellence

1945–1990

THE first seventy-five years of internal medicine at the University of Iowa mirrored in large part the fortunes of the College of Medicine as a whole: the grim years of the 1870s; the quiet, if somewhat provincial, optimism of the 1890s and the first years of the twentieth century; the crushing blow from Abraham Flexner in 1909; the near miraculous revival from 1910 to 1930 that, in the end, also owed much to Abraham Flexner; and the long decline through the years of depression and war. Given that backdrop, there were many unanswered questions about the future in the autumn of 1945.[1]

In retrospect, however, American medical science and education stood on the threshold of an era of unimagined prosperity at the end of World War II. Indeed, the succeeding two decades would constitute what John Burnham has called the "golden age" of American medicine, a period when the growth of faculty and facilities at American medical schools exceeded the expectations of even the most optimistic medical school deans, when the income of American physicians rose to unprecedented heights, when

97

the cultural authority of scientific medicine in American society often seemed beyond challenge, and when the leadership role of academic physicians in American medicine was widely acknowledged.

Clearly one key to the catalog of medical advances during that golden age—advances ranging from the spectacularly successful polio vaccines to the quiet strides in the treatment and prevention of hypertension—was a profound change in both the level of research funding and its sources. Despite the trickle of external funding in the 1930s, the chief weakness of the University of Iowa College of Medicine remained its heavy dependence on the state legislature to provide, in one form or another, appropriations for facilities and equipment and for faculty and staff. Whatever the attitudes of Iowa taxpayers and legislators toward the college, the Iowa economy—whether of the 1930s, the 1950s, or the 1970s—was a tenuous base on which to build and maintain a first-rate college of medicine, a fact that became only more obvious as medical science became more sophisticated and more expensive. Hence, just as the college's brief flirtation with eminence in the 1920s was fueled by an unexpected infusion of external funds, so, too, would its postwar future hinge on the constant flow of money from sources outside the state.

In the postwar era, financial support for both basic and applied research came in rapidly increasing amounts from a variety of sources. Funding from industry—a phenomenon first appearing in the 1930s—became a significant component of the Department of Internal Medicine's research budget by 1950. Research support from internal sources grew as well. For example, in the postwar years, funding from the College of Medicine's Central Scientific Fund grew substantially from the levels of the 1930s, while, from the early 1950s, returns from private practice in the department also contributed a significant share of research funds, a system regularized and expanded through the Medical Service Plan instituted in 1947.

It was, however, research funds from two quite different—and in some respects antithetical—sources that most profoundly affected American medical science and medical scientists as well as American medical schools and medical education in the postwar decades. The first of those sources was voluntary health agencies, of which the American Heart Association and the American Cancer Society were perhaps the most visible and most successful examples. The second major source was the various agencies of the federal government, particularly the National Institutes of Health.[2]

The increasing importance of voluntary agencies in medical research reflected the American preference for voluntarism, the suspicion of "big government," and the relative affluence of American society in the postwar decades. The expanding roles of the American Heart Association and American Cancer Society in particular also reflected the creation and fine-tuning of new organizational patterns, transforming once staid scientific organizations into dynamic fund-raising enterprises uniting medical and non-medical members behind an aggressive public service mission. The results were striking. In 1944, for example, the American Society for Control of Cancer, as it was then known, collected a modest $500,000 from contributors, while in 1949, its successor, the American Cancer Society, collected some $13,000,000, and collections continued to multiply rapidly through the 1950s.[3] Meanwhile, the American Heart Association, reorganized between 1946 and 1948, collected $2,650,000 in its first national campaign in 1949, and by 1964 the Association's annual income exceeded $26,000,000.[4] As voluntary agencies became major fund-raisers by the mid-1950s, fund-raising itself became extremely competitive, pitting the voluntary health agencies against one another to some extent and also matching the American Heart Association and American Cancer Society against the single-fund concept of the United Funds of America.

The federal government's postwar role in scientific research was an extension of the close working relationship forged between science and government during World War II. For obvious reasons, the Manhattan Project that led to production of the atomic bomb is the best known example of the wartime marriage of government and scientific research; however, the federal Office of Scientific Research and

Development supported a wide range of research projects during the war years, including many in medicine.[5] Furthermore, the highly visible wartime contributions of medical science and medical scientists lent credence to claims for the potential peacetime benefits of medical research pressed in the halls of Congress by a small but articulate lobby.[6]

Politics and economics, too, played important roles in justifying government support for medical research in the decades after 1945. In the context of the Cold War, American political leaders responded readily to the argument that national power was contingent upon national health. In addition, the specter of modern warfare raised specifically medical problems, especially in the areas of nuclear, biological, and chemical weapons. Meanwhile, the command of the American dollar over the global economy made it possible to pursue a variety of projects, from the "containment" of communism to the "space race" to medical research, in the name of national security.

A variety of federal agencies, including the United States Army, supported medical research in the postwar years; however, the National Institutes of Health, taking its present name and form as a collection of categorical—and often overlapping—institutes in the late 1940s,[7] swiftly became the major source of federal moneys, later augmented by the Department of Health, Education, and Welfare. From 1947 to 1960, HEW and NIH funding for medical research grew from $20 million to more than $400 million annually, and by 1965 their total research budgets exceeded $1.1 billion. In comparison, estimated total expenditures—both public and private—for medical research in the United States in 1941 came to only some $45 million. In medicine, the origins of "big science" as an enterprise fueled by federal dollars lay in the late 1940s and 1950s,[8] and the resulting revolution in academic medicine was arguably as important as that of the "Flexner era."[9]

The investment of previously unimagined sums—public and private—in medical research in the postwar decades not only spurred remarkable advances in medical science; it also led to a subtle but important change in the mission of American medical schools and in their internal governance as well. Whereas from the late nineteenth century through World War II the chief function of the medical school, as at the University of Iowa, was to train physicians for private practice, in the decades after World War II the schools' research function commanded increasing emphasis, in part because of the American Medical Association's vocal opposition to direct federal support for medical education as distinct from research. With the intensified focus on research, tenured faculty in some medical schools did little if any teaching. And as research and grantwriting became solidly entrenched as measures of worth in American medical schools, individual researchers became to some extent entrepreneurs,[10] a trend that—for better or worse—undermined the authoritarian administrative structures put in place in the 1920s and 1930s at American medical schools and reinstituted at least a faint echo of the collegial systems of the pre-Flexner era.

The history of the University of Iowa Department of Internal Medicine from 1945 to 1975 reflects all this and more, and that story constitutes the substance of the next four chapters. On the one hand, the convergence of resources and dedication produced an impressive story of accomplishment in the department that was at once both representative of national trends and yet uniquely local. What I have chosen to call the "diffusion of excellence" after 1945 played a crucial part in the raising of a major medical center from the Iowa cornfields. On the other hand, the sheer dynamism of the era carried a host of unforeseen problems, not least of which was the need to maintain an increasingly problematic balance among teaching, research, and patient care. Like earlier chapters in the department's history, then, this is a story of consensus and conflict, triumph and failure, opportunity and risk.

The concluding chapters of Part II carry the history into what might, by extrapolation, be called a "post-golden age" from 1975 to 1990. One of the hallmarks of that period was rising federal budget deficits that slowed enthusiasm for funding of medical research and raised complaints from some quarters that the massive federal investment in medical science and education had not worked. To some critics, the system had failed to produce enough physicians of the right sort, especially general practitioners willing to settle in small-town America. To others, medicine's failure lay in not having delivered an enumerated list of miracle cures. Still others charged that American medicine and medical science were racist and sexist. Such charges were closely related to a larger chorus of complaints about the quality, availability, and cost of medical care, proposed remedies for which had significant impact on medical education, medical research, and medical practice. In those years, too, the world of basic science research—like a variety of American institutions, from the military to the public schools—was invaded by business management attitudes and techniques that multiplied administrative rules and demanded demonstrable—that is, marketable—results.[11]

Despite that, the fifteen years from 1975 to 1990 saw a continuation of many of the trends of the previous quarter century. For example, the University of Iowa Department of Internal Medicine, because of the status achieved during the 1950s and 1960s, maintained its phenomenal rate of growth in the face of the increasingly competitive race for funding. Likewise, during those two decades an aggressive leadership in the University Hospitals supported an enormous program of construction, dwarfing even the expansion of the 1920s. Indeed, judging from this local experience, one might contest the common wisdom that American medicine's golden age sputtered to an end in the late 1960s and early 1970s.

4

Opportunity and Growth

1945–1960

THE University of Iowa College of Medicine entered the postwar era with a deteriorated and in some respects outmoded physical plant and a badly depleted faculty. "The situation on V-J Day," University of Iowa President Virgil M. Hancher conceded some years later, "was bad,"[1] and neither Hancher nor anyone else had any reason to expect a quick turnaround. In the Department of Internal Medicine, James Greene's departure for Baylor University, Horace Korns' September 1945 resignation in favor of private practice, and Fred Smith's death in February 1946 underlined Hancher's fears. In addition, resentments over private practice and the distribution of practice income had once again reached crisis proportions in the college, not only straining relations within departments, but also between the college and the university administration, and between the college and the state medical society.

Still, despite those obvious problems, the late 1940s marked the opening of a new era for the Department of Internal Medicine; in fact, the department's resurgence is the chief story of the postwar years. William Bean, who took over as department head in 1948 and whom President Hancher labeled "a brilliant young man,"[2] was a central figure in that resurgence, presiding over a period of unprecedented and unimagined growth. Under Bean's leadership, faculty ranks, departmental budgets and services, and faculty research multiplied several times over from the late 1940s to 1960. But the remarkable success of the Department of Internal Medicine in those years did not come without struggle. Nor was it just William Bean's story. Indeed, Bean's greatest contribution, as he himself suggested, may well have been his choice of supporting cast, many of whom also played prominent roles in affairs in the College of Medicine and in the larger world of medical science.

PRIVATE PRACTICE REVISITED: THE MEDICAL SERVICE PLAN

While the Procurement and Assignment policy of the war years had helped to keep at least a skeleton medical faculty in place, Hancher feared a mass exodus after the war unless he could find some way to settle the seemingly intractable problem of private practice.[3] During the war, Dean Ewen MacEwen and President Hancher had grappled at length with the problem, and Hancher had had conversations with several key faculty members on the issue. On the whole, those conversations had not proved very helpful. Fred Smith, for example, had noted cautiously that the college was "essentially a teaching and research institution," hinting that private practice might detract from those missions and perhaps from the image of the college as well. Clarence Van Epps, head of the Department of Neurology and long ago assistant to Walter Bierring and Campbell Howard, had likewise waffled in response to Hancher's inquiry, noting only that he was "very unsympathetic with the extension of private practice." And from Obstetrics and Gynecology, Everett D. Plass offered no concrete program but conceded that "it [i.e., private practice] is a disturbing matter and causes trouble among the younger men."[4]

In contrast, Nathaniel G. Alcock, head of the Department of Urology, was not a man to hide behind delicate ambiguity. In his history of the University of Iowa, Stow Persons notes that Alcock, while a widely respected surgeon, was also "an extremely aggressive and domineering man who ran his department with quasi-military discipline" and did not brook interference from anyone, perhaps least of all from university presidents.[5] That may have been an understatement; indeed, President Hancher once complained that Alcock was determined to run his department as he wanted and "the University could go to the devil."[6] Alcock, Hancher confided in a letter to Abraham Flexner, "has always been a law unto himself."[7]

As head of urology, Nathaniel Alcock enjoyed a very large surgical practice, a practice that boosted his annual income to near six figures, or so rumor had it, and allowed him to cement his modest empire through the distribution of patronage. Needless to say, Alcock was a principal champion of private practice, and he made plain to Hancher his conviction that the years from 1914 to 1924—before Lee Wallace Dean's limitations on private practice had taken full effect—were "the great period in Iowa medicine." The recent agitation over full-time, he charged, was "wrecking the College of Medicine" and was, moreover, just "one step toward socialized medicine."[8]

Based upon his estimation of local conditions and upon experience at other medical schools, Virgil Hancher toyed with several solutions to the private practice dilemma. First, with four departments already on a full-time basis, he could eliminate private practice in the remaining eight departments. However, the problem had not changed since the 1920s: How could the college pay high enough salaries to attract top-notch faculty? Second, and at the other extreme, he could authorize unlimited private practice for all faculty. But that option smacked too much of the days when physicians had sought academic connections in order to attract patients and inflate their fees, and Hancher did not care to lay the college open to charges of crass commercialism. The third option—perhaps the only viable one under the circumstances—was to devise a compromise system of limited private practice, confined to the University of Iowa Hospitals, for ranks of assistant professor and above combined with a scheme of income redistribution. Hancher called this "a near full-time plan,"[9] but the plan also embodied the principles of group practice, a concept that many, like Nathaniel Alcock, labeled "socialized medicine" and one that the American Medical Association had viewed with suspicion for decades.

Little respected by many of his part-time clinical chiefs, Dean Ewen MacEwen was in no position to force drastic change upon the faculty of the college. Hence, President Hancher's chosen vehicle of reform was a seven-member faculty committee appointed in January 1946 and known as the Committee on Status and Compensation. Five of the committee's seven members, including Fred Smith from internal medicine,[10] were department heads, but not all were part-time. Working with Hancher's guidelines and facing his threat of reform by fiat should the committee fail to produce an acceptable plan, the committee members fell into hopeless deadlock, rescued only by the intervention of ex-dean Henry S. Houghton.[11] It was Houghton who devised the details of the plan eventually endorsed by a five-to-two margin, with Nathaniel Alcock and Frank Peterson, head of the Department of Surgery, tendering a minority report.

In addition to providing junior faculty a share in the proceeds from private practice, the plan also provided a boost in basic salaries, setting a base of $4,000–6,000 for assistant professors, $5,000–8,000 for associate professors, $7,000–9,500 for full professors, and $8,000–10,000 for department heads. Salary supplements, known as commutation fractions, and maximum incomes likewise varied with rank. The plan entitled assistant professors to receive 50 percent of their base salaries as a share of private practice income, up to a maximum income of $9,000, while associate professors could receive an additional 75 percent up to a maximum of $15,000, professors 100 percent with a ceiling of $20,000, and department heads 100 percent up to $25,000.

Frank Peterson resigned rather than accept the new system, while Nathaniel

Alcock made an impassioned appeal to his faculty colleagues to reject the majority recommendations. Alcock warned that private practice funds in some specialties could not deliver the promised benefits. He argued, in particular, that internal medicine faculty, as "physicians to the poor," could not attract enough paying patients to make the plan work, and the department would wither relative to some other specialties. Nonetheless, the Medical Council made up of College of Medicine department heads, the full medical faculty, and the state board of education gave their assent, and the Medical Service Plan went into effect on July 1, 1947.

The smell of "socialized medicine" was too strong for many members of the Iowa State Medical Society to ignore. In its 1947 report to the House of Delegates, the Society's Committee on Medical Education and Hospitals, while sympathetic to the problem of faculty compensation at the college, viewed Hancher's solution as "clearly a form of socialized or communistic medicine,"[12] and rumor had it that Alcock and perhaps Peterson as well stirred those concerns. When the Webster County Medical Society passed a resolution in opposition to the Medical Service Plan, a local physician reported to President Hancher that the resolution represented both "a vote of confidence" in Alcock and Peterson and fears of the "bogey of 'socialized medicine.'"[13] Taking a more jaundiced view, Administrative Dean Allin W. Dakin warned Hancher of "an active campaign headed by Alcock and Peterson ... to sabotage the [Medical Service] plan."[14] In addition, Alcock continued his opposition to the plan from within the college, operating from his position as department head and from his place on the original Medical Service Plan Compensation Committee.[15]

Both Dean MacEwen and President Hancher were quickly disgusted by the guerilla warfare from within and without the College of Medicine. Hancher groused that his critics seemed to think "that you can have a single man at the head of a department and a lot of flunkies running around doing his bidding."[16] For his part, MacEwen showed his sentiment in a brief handwritten note affixed to a clipping from the *Minneapolis Star* lauding the tenth successful "blue baby" operation at the University of Minnesota. "This might happen to us," MacEwen noted bluntly, "if we had a dept [sic] of surgery interested in something besides making money."[17] Others, too, were dismayed; one alumnus noted that "our medical set-up [i.e., the College of Medicine] has deteriorated and what we have in large part is a group of eccentrics—to put it charitably."[18]

In internal medicine, despite Dr. Alcock's grave predictions, Medical Service Fund receipts rose rapidly from 1947 into the 1950s. Monies from the Medical Service Fund supported faculty salaries, while excess funds, transferred to the department's Medical Trust Fund, supported other activities as well, including travel to scientific meetings and a variety of research and teaching-related expenses. By the early 1950s, the Medical Service Fund contributed some 40 percent of the department's total operating budget, exclusive of research grants. Virgil Hancher's reorganization of private practice, then, provided a solid foundation for subsequent growth in the Department of Internal Medicine.

A NEW ERA: FROM FRED SMITH TO WILLIAM BEAN

The loss of James Greene, Horace Korns, and Fred Smith left just four members of the Department of Internal Medicine's wartime skeleton staff in place in 1946, a meager staff augmented by the return of Robert Hardin and Lewis January after wartime service.[19] Two days after Fred Smith's death, Dean MacEwen appointed Willis Fowler as acting head of the department, and Fowler understood from his conversations with MacEwen that the appointment would likely be made permanent. However, pressure to appoint an outsider to head the department came from heads of some clinical departments and from Carlyle Jacobsen, President Hancher's executive dean of health sciences and services.[20] The selection of Fred Smith's successor, these men argued, was an opportunity to bring in a figure of vision and ambition who could develop a major department of internal medicine at the University of Iowa.

Willis Fowler, then, was caught in a situation not of his own making and one that had little to do with either his potential as department head or his past record as researcher and teacher. In fact, his position was quite like that of Walter Bierring forty years earlier. In the previous two decades, Fowler's performance as a scientific researcher had exceeded that of Fred Smith and had been matched among his colleagues in internal medicine only by Elmer DeGowin. Moreover, Willis Fowler had many admirers in the College of Medicine. The decision to recruit outside the department was an indictment, deserved or not, of the leadership of Fred Smith and, some said, of the contributions of Horace Korns as well.[21]

Members of the Department of Internal Medicine were initially excluded from the recruitment process, a consequence of the concentration of power in the hands of the university's central administration, the dean of the College of Medicine, and department heads within the college. The selection process was well underway before faculty in the Department of Internal Medicine were even officially apprised of it. When rumor of impending action spread in the late summer of 1947, several department members resolved, as one of them remembered it, "to make their position known." At that point, Lewis January approached Dean Dakin and told him that if Fowler's appointment was not to be permanent, then Horace Korns should at least be solicited for his views on the subject of the new head. Dakin assured January, somewhat patronizingly, that responsible parties were giving "concentrated attention" to the appointment. However, Dakin did not address the faculty's central concern over lack of input.[22]

It was true that the selection committee was thorough in its approach, sifting some one hundred possible candidates. Among them was James A. Greene, who had been a favorite of Dean MacEwen's and whose departure for Baylor, President Hancher noted, had been "a severe blow to the Dean."[23] But because of the rapidly expanding opportunities in academic medicine and because of the relative decline of the University of Iowa College of Medicine in the 1930s and 1940s, the position at Iowa was far less attractive in 1947 than it had been in 1924 when Fred Smith, then a promising young clinician and researcher, had eagerly accepted the job.

Partly reflecting mounting frustration, the selection committee sent Carlyle Jacobsen and Nathan Womack—Frank Peterson's newly appointed successor as head of surgery—on an interview trip to the east in late January 1948. As a concession to internal medicine faculty, Lewis January was invited to accompany Jacobsen and Womack, an invitation that January understood initially as largely a matter of window dressing. Nonetheless, Jacobsen and Womack subsequently included January in all their meetings with prospective candidates and in associated deliberations, and in the end January did have major input into the selection process.

The Iowa delegation's first stop was Boston, where they talked with Robert Wilkins of Boston University. Wilkins commanded the conversation and made it plain that he was not interested in the Iowa position; however, he offered ready advice on what the department needed. Proceeding from Boston University to Harvard, Jacobsen, Womack, and January met with George Thorn, head of the Department of Medicine, who suggested that they talk to Louis Dexter, one of the pioneers in cardiac catheterization. Dexter was more personable than Wilkins, but he, too, expressed no interest in the Iowa position, despite January's private efforts to persuade him. The Iowa delegation then proceeded to New York, where Robert Loeb of Columbia suggested that they talk to Walsh McDermott, but McDermott likewise declined to be considered for the position at Iowa.

After several days on the road with nothing to show for their efforts, Jacobsen, Womack, and January arrived at the University of Cincinnati. There Marion A. Blankenhorn had arranged interviews with four members of his Department of Medicine: Morton Hamburger, Richard Vilter, Eugene Ferris, and William Bean. Of the four, it was Ferris who most impressed Jacobsen and Womack. Eugene Ferris was a dynamic young man seen by some as Blankenhorn's heir apparent as department head, but Ferris was skeptical of his future at Cincinnati. Clearly anxious to move on, he expressed a lively interest in the Iowa position.[24] Despite Jacobsen's and Womack's enthusiasm for Ferris, however, January was most taken with the last of the four, William Bean. William Bennett Bean's name, it turns out, had first surfaced in the fall of 1947, suggested to the University of Iowa selection committee by both Barry Wood and Carl Moore of Washington University and later seconded by Charles Doan, dean of medicine at Ohio State. From Cincinnati, Marion Blankenhorn had early on assured the committee that Bean was well qualified "in terms of clinical ability, investigative ability and administrative skill." William Bean's father had had a distinguished career in medicine, first in the Philippines, where the younger Bean was born, and then at the University of Virginia as Professor of Anatomy. William Bean was a Virginia alumnus, receiving his B.A. in 1932 and M.D. in 1935. Following graduation, he had taken an internship at Johns Hopkins followed by residencies at the Boston City Hospital and at Cincinnati General Hospital before becoming, in 1940, assistant professor and, after wartime military service, associate professor at Cincinnati.

But there was far more to William Bean than that. As Blankenhorn intimated to his Iowa visitors, William Bean was very bright, very ambitious, and also—in some respects—very different. Bean in fact arrived at his interview with the Iowa representatives dressed in U.S. Army issue parka and boots. Despite that, the conversation, mostly between January and Bean, was long and encouraging. January came away convinced that Bean—well educated, a voracious reader, and well connected—was precisely the sort of man the Department of Internal Medicine needed. In addition, Bean displayed a freshness of approach to basic problems. In his work on Army nutrition in World War II, for example, Bean had begun with the simple but innovative premise that the nutritional value of field rations hinged first and most importantly on whether or not the men would eat them.[25]

On their return to Iowa City, Jacobsen and Womack argued before the selection committee in favor of Eugene Ferris, while January, who was not formally a member of the committee, was unwavering in his support of William Bean. In subsequent committee deliberations, two factors elevated Bean's name to the top of the list: first, Jacobsen and Womack conceded that Bean was a strong second choice, and, second, the University of Washington was also courting Bean. Those factors led the selection committee to invite Bean for a campus visit February 28–March 3, 1948.

Bean's visit to the Iowa City campus was a smashing success, as Bean charmed his hosts. Subsequently, the Medical Council voted unanimously to offer Bean the position without interviewing further candidates. Although Bean reciprocated that enthusiasm, he did have reservations about the state of the department, the college, and the hospital facilities, which he outlined in a letter to Carlyle Jacobsen on March 10. He noted, for example, that the Department of Internal Medicine was woefully short of personnel and cramped for space; furthermore, he thought that much of the medical curriculum deserved "demolition and reconstruction [rather] than further interior decorating." Jacobsen was sympathetic to Bean's criticisms and extended his reassurance that these problems could be surmounted.[26] Bean then forwarded his letter of acceptance, noting that he was "looking forward with great enthusiasm and interest to the opportunities and possibilities for great development in the Department of Medicine."[27]

BUILDING FOR THE FUTURE: PERSONNEL

The fall of 1948 opened the William Bean era at the University of Iowa, and the expectation was that Bean would be a recruiter and builder, a man who could assemble the elements of a first-rate department and could do so in short order. Thanks in part to the benefits flowing from the Medical Service Plan, Bean began immediately to do just that. In light of the expectations of those who hired him, however, it was ironic that Bean did much of his recruiting from within the department, identifying promising medical students and residents and encouraging them to pursue careers in academic medicine. In 1955, Bean stated with satisfaction that "more than half of our senior staff have had their training in this Department of Medicine"[28]—a recruitment pattern that was a long tradition at Iowa when Bean arrived, was common at other schools as well, and has continued to the present.

The task of rebuilding the depleted department highlighted William Bean's chief strengths: his personable nature and his ability to attract and develop scientific talent. During the war, Bean had reason to reflect on the nature of leadership, and he saw the department head's role as chiefly one of cheerleader and mentor, a leadership style that he characterized as essentially democratic. "There is," he commented in 1954, "an increasing trend for departments to be led and guided rather than be run." During his tenure, Bean noted, weekly staff meetings had become a forum for "eager discussion of the most diverse topics."[29] And in 1958, on his tenth anniversary as department head, Bean's colleagues praised him for his habit of allowing staff "to develop in their own ways" and for his "encouragement of free discussion of departmental affairs," a remarkable testimonial at any time and in any department.[30]

The process of departmental expansion, however, also highlighted one of William Bean's admitted weaknesses: his distaste for administrative duties. While in Fred Smith's day a single secretary constituted the department's clerical staff and administrative routine commanded relatively little of the department head's time, the explosive growth of budgets and personnel—in internal medicine and in other departments as well—magnified the burdens of administration during William Bean's tenure. And it was not simply that the postwar department became larger; the increasing diversity of medical science imposed itself on the department as well. "The diversity of activities in the fields of research, teaching, and practice" was, Bean claimed in 1954, "one of the more attractive features" of his department,[31] but he did not welcome the associated administrative burdens. "My taste for routine administration is nil," he admitted on one occasion.[32] To a private correspondent, Bean conceded, "For administration in the ordinary sense, I not only have no taste but an active revulsion."[33]

Nonetheless, there were few complaints about William Bean's ability to recruit and inspire staff. Numbers alone tell an impressive story of the expansion Bean supervised between 1948 and 1960. In 1947, the year before Bean's arrival, the department consisted of eight faculty members, six of whom had been associated with the department in one capacity or another before World War II. In 1948–49, Bean's first year at Iowa, the faculty increased to eleven, including Mayo Soley, whose tenure as Dean of the College of Medicine and Professor of Experimental Medicine began July 1, 1948. The following year the number grew to fifteen. In the first half of the 1950s, the pace of expansion accelerated, taking the total of department staff to thirty-nine in 1955–56, including five clinical faculty associated with the nearby Veterans Administration Hospital. By the end of the decade, the total of internal medicine faculty stood at forty-three, an increase of 437.5 percent during Bean's tenure. In comparison, during the ten years from 1950 to 1960, total faculty numbers in the College of Medicine grew from 146 to 217, an increase of 48.6 percent, and internal medicine faculty increased from 10.3 percent to 19.8 percent of all medical faculty.

One thing, however, had changed little since the 1930s: the paucity of female faculty. In 1959–60, seven women were listed among department staff, but just two of those—June Fisher and Jeanne M. Smith—were M.D.'s. Three—Roberta Bleiler, Margaret Ohlson, and Ruth Lutz—were Ph.D.'s associated with the Nutrition Laboratory, and that, as we saw in the previous chapter, was an area traditionally open to women. The remaining two women in internal medicine were research assistants, one of whom—Adelaide Barer—had been with the department since the 1930s.

The small percentage of women in internal medicine at the University of Iowa was in keeping with national averages. Moreover, an unfortunate remark from William Bean regarding women in medicine reflected a widely held stereotype. "In my experience," Bean once wrote, "most women go into medical school to find a husband."[34] Still, Bean's sexism—perhaps like that of many other men who resorted to such clichés about women—appears to have been unreflective and inconsistent. He could be unstinting in praising his female colleagues; for example, his framed tribute to Kate Daum, who died in 1955 after thirty years with the department, hung in a departmental conference room for many years.[35]

A cursory glance at the recruiting classes of the late 1940s and early 1950s—including such names as Paul Seebohm, Henry Hamilton, Walter Kirkendall, Raymond Sheets, and James Clifton—suggests their critical place in the making of the modern department. Some of that group were Iowa graduates; many others completed all or part of their residency training at Iowa; and many were also veterans of World War II. In part because of their ambition and dedication and in part because of the department's rapid growth, promotions came quickly to the postwar staff, in contrast to the glacial pace of promotion before 1940. For example, while Frank Rohner had waited twelve years before promotion to associate professor in 1926, Robert Hardin, who joined the faculty after completion of his military service in 1945, was a full professor by 1953. Similarly, Henry Hamilton joined the faculty with the rank of instructor in 1949, rose to the rank of associate the following year, then to assistant professor in 1951, associate professor in 1954, and to professor in 1959. By 1960, there were eleven full professors and nine associate professors in a department that had had no more than two full professors or three associate professors at any one time prior to 1945.

Increased salaries were a key to the expansion in staff. By the mid-1950s, base salaries in internal medicine at the University of Iowa had risen to an average of $8,748 for full professors, $6,560 for associate professors, and $6,125 for assistant professors, the last representing a 100 percent increase since 1940.[36] And during the last half of the decade, base salaries rose further. In addition, as noted earlier, those salaries could be augmented from 50 to 100 percent by returns from the department's Medical Service Fund, and medical service revenues rose rapidly. In 1949, Medical Service Fund receipts totaled $64,176 with the commutation fraction, or departmental salary supplements, totaling $28,417. In 1955, total receipts reached $114,963 with $73,390 devoted to salary supplements. In 1960, collections topped $213,000 with a commutation fraction of $148,122,[37] and the total of base salary and commutation fraction put internal medicine salaries at the University of Iowa just below the national median of $18,824 for internal medicine faculty.[38] Private patient care, then, was one of the engines driving the growth in departmental personnel.

In the fifteen years after World War II, the numbers of residents rose roughly in proportion to faculty numbers, and residents played an increasingly larger role in patient care and teaching. However, the relationship between numbers of faculty and residents was not a simple one. While the department's normal wartime complement of three to four residents had jumped to eight in 1946 and to twenty in 1949, ten years later the number of residents still stood at twenty, despite the tripling of faculty numbers in the intervening decade.

In fact, much of the large increase in resident numbers from 1946 to 1950 reflected a demand backlog built up during World War II, when thousands of physicians had completed only a part, or none at all, of their residencies even as the wartime experience infected many more physicians with an interest in specialization. A 1945 American Medical Association survey indicated that as many as 17,000 physicians, military and civilian, awaited residency training at war's end, while residency programs had grown some 70 percent in anticipation of the postwar surge in demand.[39] As expected, young physicians flooded the still expanding residency programs in the late 1940s, with the result that participating hospitals, including the University of Iowa Hospitals, complained of the crush of numbers and expense.

The onset of the Korean War eased the pressure on residency programs, as many residents at the University Hospitals, for example, were called to active service. Five residents in internal medicine were called to active service in 1950–51 alone. The military draft also sharply reduced the number of new applicants for residency positions. Meanwhile, the number of hospitals offering internal medicine residency programs across America rose sharply by war's end, growing from 3,313 in 1949 to 4,862 in 1955 and 5,744 by the end of the decade.[40] In Iowa, the University Hospitals in Iowa City and Iowa Methodist Hospital in Des Moines had offered the only residency programs in internal medicine in 1949, with a total of 24 positions, but by 1959, there were forty-three internal medicine residencies in the state, twenty-six of those at Veterans Administration hospitals in Des Moines and Iowa City, an illustration of the impact of the VA's massive post–World War II construction program.[41]

Among the ranks of residents, as among faculty, the numbers of women were very small. Of the twenty-two residents in the Department of Internal Medicine in 1959–60, just two were women, reflecting both the small proportion of women among medical students, both at the University of Iowa and nationwide, and the tendency of female graduates, for whatever reasons, to opt for specialties other than internal medicine. The presence of two female residents was a striking contrast to the period from 1930 to 1945 when there had been none at all, but in light of the custom of recruiting junior faculty from among the ranks of residents, the scarcity of female residents portended little change in the proportion of female faculty in the immediate future.

THE DEPARTMENT AND COMMUNITIES OF SCIENCE AND PRACTICE

Overall, Department of Internal Medicine staff multiplied by a factor of eight from the end of World War II to 1960. Those numbers alone provide a measure of the profound changes underway in academic medicine in those years. But there was more to that transformation than numbers. Equally important were the remarkable, though still limited, growth in the volume of scientific research, the department's increased role in the national and international community of medical science, and internal medicine's increased service role in the University Hospitals.

The late 1940s and 1950s accelerated the trend toward an emphasis on research productivity in the evaluation of faculty performance. In comparative terms, research grants from external sources grew to a flood by the end of the 1950s; the volume of research publications increased proportionally; and more and more of those publications reflected basic research done in laboratory settings rather than reports of clinical observations. At the same time, department members developed ever more elaborate connections to the broader community of medical science; special interest conferences, conventions, and seminars multiplied; and more and more Iowa staff held offices in specialty societies and edited specialty journals.

As department head, William Bean provided the most striking example of the number and complexity of the links between Iowa City and the larger world of medical science. In 1948–49, his first year at Iowa, Bean held seats on the governing councils of both the Central Society for Clinical Research and the American Society for Clinical Investigation. He was editor of the *Cincinnati Journal of Medicine,* associate editor of the *Journal of Clinical Investigation,* and served on the editorial board of the *Journal of Laboratory and Clinical Medicine.* In 1949, Bean was elected to the American College of Physicians and the following year to the Association of American Physicians. In his first year in Iowa City, Bean also joined the Central Interurban Clinical Club, the Iowa Clinical Medical Society, the Iowa Heart Association, and the Johnson County Medical Society. Finally, in a continuation of the link between the department and government agencies forged during World War II, Bean became a consultant to the Veterans Administration and to the Iowa Selective Service as well, and he was a member of the National Research Council's Subcommittee on Relation of Stress and Nutrition in Industry.

Through the 1950s, William Bean's institutional connections multiplied in number and complexity. By the end of the decade, he was serving on the editorial boards of the *Journal of Laboratory and Clinical Medicine, Medical Education, Diseases of the Chest, Archives of Internal Medicine,* and *Medicine.* He was also a past president of the Central Society for Clinical Research and the Iowa Heart Association, had been elected a Fellow of the British Royal Society of Medicine, chair of the American Medical Association Section of Internal Medicine, chair of the General Medicine Study Section of the National Institutes of Health, and a member of the Board of Regents of the National Library of Medicine. He had, in addition, declined editorship of the *Journal of the American Medical Association* as well as offers from the Hearst papers and from the King Features Syndicate to contribute weekly medical columns for national distribution.[42]

The list of William Bean's memberships and offices provides only a glimpse of the maze of institutional connections binding department members to their colleagues in Iowa, the Midwest, and beyond. William ("Shorty") Paul, whose tenure at Iowa stretched back to the mid-1930s, was a fellow of the American College of Physicians, held memberships in other general interest societies, and served on the editorial board of *General Practitioner*. But Paul's chief interest lay in physical therapy, and he held a variety of positions in the Society of Physical Medicine, the American Physical Therapy Association, and the American Congress of Physical Medicine. Similarly, Lewis January, while he served as secretary-treasurer and president of the Central Clinical Research Club, also displayed considerable specialization in his professional connections. Through the late 1940s and 1950s, January was deeply involved with the Iowa Heart Association, serving at various times on the Association's executive committee, the board of directors, the program committee, and the lay education committee, as well as serving as editor of the journal *Topics*. By the end of the 1950s, January's participation and influence extended to the American Heart Association, where he held a variety of positions with the Council on Clinical Cardiology and served also as a member of the AHA's board of directors.

At a more local level, internal medicine faculty interacted directly with Iowa practitioners through a variety of formal and informal mechanisms. One source of interaction was through patient referrals, which made up the bulk of private practice patients on the department's services at the University Hospitals. "All but a tiny fraction" of the department's growing roster of private patients, William Bean noted, were "referred by physicians."[43] Interaction came also through memberships in county and state medical societies as well as voluntary associations, such as the Iowa Heart Association. Department members, in groups and individually, also contributed many hours to graduate education. The department, for example, offered a comprehensive graduate conference in internal medicine in June 1949, and department members also delivered dozens of addresses to local medical societies and civic groups each year. Finally, the department's Alumni Club, formed in 1951, was meant to maintain ties among the department's graduates and former residents.

Scientific publications were another mark of the department's expanding role in the medical science community. In 1948–49, William Bean published, alone or as co-author, fourteen articles in addition to dozens of book reviews and editorials. In total, department members contributed three dozen papers to a variety of journals in 1948–49. In 1955–56, Bean again led the department with fourteen scientific publications, including seven chapters in edited books, in addition to a variety of book reviews and editorial pieces, but a total of nineteen department members each participated in publication of an average of three original articles or chapters. Moreover, the department encouraged resident involvement in research and publication, and the department's 1948–49 *Annual Report* listed three papers published by residents, with several others in preparation.

THE GROWTH IN RESEARCH FUNDING

An influx of research funds, much of it in the form of external project grants, supported the department's growing role in medical science. Here the history of the University of Iowa Department of Internal Medicine paralleled the much larger story of the growth in funding of scientific research in American medical schools under the auspices of the federal government, corporate business, and voluntary agencies. In 1949–50, just five of the seventy-two American medical schools received more than $1,000,000 each in research grants and just seventeen received more than $500,000,[44] but by 1958–59, the average for all medical schools surpassed $1,000,000.[45] The University of Iowa College of Medicine reached that $1,000,000 mark in research grants for the first time in 1953–54, with funds drawn from more than a hundred sources,[46] and at the end of the decade the total stood in excess of $2,000,000, accounting for some 30 percent of total college revenues.[47]

In its *Annual Reports,* the Department of Internal Medicine recorded $43,700 in external funding for research in 1948–49, and while that was four times the level of the late 1930s, it was only a hint of what was to come. Also, nearly all those funds came either from agencies of the federal government (nearly 70 percent) or from industry (nearly 30 percent). In the next year, external funds for research support doubled, with the bulk of that funding coming once again from federal government and industry sources. However, in 1949–50, voluntary agencies had become significant actors, too, and through the 1950s, as the total of research funds available to the department multiplied, voluntary agencies—particularly the American Heart Association and American Cancer Society and their Iowa affiliates—played an ever larger role in research funding. Of the sixty-five grants awarded the department in 1958–59, for example, fifteen were from the U.S. Public Health Service and nineteen from the American Heart Association and Iowa Heart Association.

Surpluses transferred from the department's Medical Service Fund to its Medical Trust Fund also contributed to research, chiefly through the financing of research salaries and travel to conventions and conferences. In 1952–53, Trust Fund support amounted to nearly $15,000, a figure that remained more or less constant throughout the decade. Similarly, moneys from the College of

Medicine Central Scientific Fund, amounting to just over $12,000 in 1950–51, held constant during the decade, constituting 12 percent of the department's research budget at the start of the decade but falling to 1 percent or less by the end of the 1950s.

The state legislature's steadfast refusal to appropriate funds for medical research was an ongoing disappointment, both for the Department of Internal Medicine and for the College of Medicine at large. Initially, medical researchers assumed that the legislature's indifference could be overcome by education. In his first year as department head, William Bean suggested that the college make an effort "to educate the people" to the idea that "teaching and research are Siamese twins."[48] Surely the problem, Bean thought, was that the university administration was simply not delivering the message. However, the legislature's utilitarian cast of mind regarding higher education was unshakable, and state appropriations constituted an ever smaller proportion of the department's budget through the 1950s. Based upon prewar experience, few medical faculty could imagine continued growth in the research enterprise without "a specific adequate appropriation for this purpose ... from the legislature."[49] In the late 1940s and early 1950s, the possibility of rolling over "soft money" to build a first-rate teaching and research facility was not self-evident.

Even in the absence of state funding, scientific activity in the Department of Internal Medicine mushroomed in the 1950s. To suggest only a few examples, William Paul conducted studies of the metabolism of aspirin and the effects of buffering agents on tolerance and absorption, studies aided by grants from the Bayer Company and the Institute for the Study of Analgesic and Sedative Drugs. Elmer DeGowin expanded his researches in blood preservation with substantial ongoing grants from the U.S. Army. William Bean attracted funds from a variety of sources, including the U.S. Public Health Service, for his work in nutrition and metabolism. Willis Fowler, aided in the 1950s by Henry Hamilton and Raymond Sheets, continued work on blood coagulation and blood dyscrasias with support from the Iowa Cancer Society and American Cancer Society. Walter Kirkendall won grants from the American Heart Association for his work in renal and hepatic circulation. And Robert Hardin conducted his researches in diabetes with the help of grants from Baxter Laboratories and Eli Lilly and Company. By the end of the 1950s, grantwriting had become a significant part of the academic physician's job description.

BUILDING FOR THE FUTURE: THE SPACE RACE

With the multiplication of funding sources in the 1950s, money was not a major hindrance to departmental growth; rather, the chief impediment to expansion was a lack of space. Three factors heightened the problem: first, the physical facilities available to the Department of Internal Medicine and to the College of Medicine at large in 1950 were essentially those available in 1928; second, other departments also expanded rapidly in the late 1940s and 1950s, creating an intensely competitive space race; and, third, the college was largely dependent upon the state legislature for money for renovation and new construction of laboratory and hospital facilities.

Importantly, as the Department of Internal Medicine's patient load increased in the postwar period, space for patient service was as much a problem as for teaching and research. In 1949–50, the department's medical service admitted 2,579 indigent and clinical pay patients and treated over 3,000 patients in the outpatient clinic. In addition, department members saw 2,665 private patients, including 708 hospital admissions and 1,957 office visits. By 1952, the outpatient clinic alone recorded 8,400 patient visits, excluding hospital employees. At the same time, the private patient mix included 787 hospital admissions and 2,324 office visits.[50]

From the first, William Bean was outspoken on the inadequacies of the department's physical plant, and in 1953, he noted that the size of the department staff had tripled since his arrival in 1948, research activity had quadrupled, and the department's office and hospital practice had doubled, while the space available to internal medicine had in fact diminished.[51] Bean charged that staff were crowded more than one to an office; there were no rooms on the wards for residents and for small-group teaching; there was no research space for residents; and department secretaries occupied desks in the hallways. In January 1951, a College of Medicine faculty committee headed by Nathan Womack issued a report on hospital facilities that generalized Bean's complaints to all departments.[52] By 1954, Bean maintained that the lack of space was "currently the most important problem facing the department," and he warned of "a period of deterioration ... unless the space problem is solved."[53]

For the short term, the hospital administration and the department responded to the space shortage by shuffling people and services and by marginal renovations of the existing physical plant. In 1953, for example, the Blood Transfusion Service moved into new quarters on the hospital's seventh floor, and the Outpatient Clinic and Allergy Clinic received new paint and lighting. The next year brought rearrangement of much of the office space in the hospital's north tower as well; however, such stopgap measures did not address the fundamental problem.

In 1953, a College of Medicine faculty building committee chaired by William Bean began planning a new Medical Research Center to be added to the west side of the old Medical Laboratories building.[54] This, the first major building project since the 1920s, ultimately cost one-third as much as the original General Hospital and Medical Laboratories combined. Initial estimates placed the cost at $1,250,000, with $900,000 provided by a 1953 state appropriation and the remainder provided by the U.S. Public Health Service under the provisions of the Hill-Burton Act. However, by the time of completion, the cost had climbed to nearly $1,500,000, with the USPHS contribution increased to $436,000, the National Fund for Medical Education providing $34,000, and the College of Medicine adding $135,000 from interest accruing to the Rockefeller funds from the 1920s.[55] The opening of the Medical Research Center in November 1957 attracted state and local politicians and a cross-section of America's medical elite,[56] and in the next few years various Department of Internal Medicine service and research functions found homes in the Center.

BUILDING FOR THE FUTURE: SPECIALIZED SERVICE UNITS

As suggested earlier, much of the demand for space in the Department of Internal Medicine reflected the growth of an increasingly diversified complex of specialized service units,[57] all of them combining patient care with teaching and—to an increasing extent—research as well. Some of those units originated in the 1920s and 1930s, but the postwar years often brought significant changes in their mission and makeup. Other units appeared in the 1950s, reflecting new patient needs, the addition of new faculty to the department, the development of new technological capabilities, or, as was often the case, a combination of those factors. Whatever their origins, the specialized service units of the 1950s were precursors to many of the department's modern divisions.

Hematology

Hematology had been an established service and research field in the department since the 1920s, thanks to the work of first Campbell Howard and later Willis Fowler and Elmer DeGowin. DeGowin's Blood Transfusion Service maintained a steady rate of growth in the postwar years. The volume of whole blood collected and processed for patient transfusions rose 80 percent between 1948 and 1959, from 5,300 to over 9,600 pints, making the University Hospitals' Blood Transfusion Service the fourteenth largest such operation in the United States.[58] In addition, the service performed Rh testing on blood samples from across Iowa and also maintained the Intravenous Fluids Laboratory, which produced ten thousand bottles of pyrogen-free IV fluids each month by the end of the decade. In all, the operations under DeGowin's charge performed wide-ranging service and teaching functions within the college while continuing research into fundamental problems, such as erythrocyte survival, related to blood processing and storage.

Meanwhile, the Hematology Service, long directed by Willis Fowler, likewise performed a growing service function, particularly in examining bone marrow smears and conducting patient rounds. The addition of Raymond Sheets and Henry Hamilton, the latter noted in particular for his clinical skills and boundless energy, ensured continued strength in hematology. In 1951, the department organized a weekly hematology conference to publicize "current concepts and advances" to interns, residents, and staff, with contributions from radiology, pediatrics, and pathology as well.[59] Throughout the 1950s, the hematology unit maintained its established research work in hemorrhagic conditions and anemias. However, cancer and cancer-related blood disorders attracted increasing attention and resources. As early as 1950–51, Willis Fowler received a $5,000 grant from the Iowa Cancer Society for bone marrow studies related to leukemia, and over the course of the decade investigators in hematology received similar grants in increasing numbers.

Gastroenterology

The Gastroenterology Clinic was yet another established area of service and research. In the early 1950s, under William Paul's direction, the clinic was principally a patient service unit performing gastroscopic and sigmoidoscopic examinations. Through the 1950s, the total number of examinations grew slowly, from 840 in 1949–50 to 949 in 1959–60, but the nature of the work performed in the Gastroenterology Clinic changed considerably during those ten years. For example, sigmoidoscopies rose from 57 percent to more than 90 percent of endoscopic examinations by the end of the decade; moreover, the clinic's work expanded into sophisticated tests of intestinal absorption and pancreatic function.

The most striking change in gastroenterology, however, came in the expansion of research work accompanying the addition of younger staff with more specialized interests and training, notably James Clifton, who worked with F. J. Ingelfinger in Boston during a fellowship year in the mid-1950s, and also Harold Schedl, who earned a Ph.D. in organic chemistry from Yale before completing his medical studies at Iowa. By 1960, gastroenterology staff, under Clifton's general direction, were actively involved in a variety of areas of gastroenterology-hepatology research. In addition, the department had, with the cooperation of the Radiology Department, instituted a weekly Gastroenterology Conference as a teaching device and also organized a Gastroenterology Research Laboratory.

Allergy

In contrast to hematology and gastroenterology, active work in the field of allergy-immunology began in earnest at the University of Iowa only in the 1950s. While the study of "hay fever" and other allergies had drawn increasing attention in the medical-scientific world in the 1920s, the idea of establishing an allergy section at Iowa had surfaced only in the late 1930s and did not become fully operational until the establishment of the Allergy Clinic under the direction of Paul Seebohm in 1950. A Cincinnati graduate, Seebohm came to Iowa from a fellowship at the Cooke Institute of Allergy at Roosevelt Hospital, and under his guidance the Allergy Clinic quickly became an important center of research and service in the department. Meanwhile, Seebohm's activities in the rapidly expanding field of allergy-immunology carried him to a prominent position and varied offices in the American Academy of Allergy as well as in other specialty societies.

Through the 1950s, the bulk of Allergy Clinic services fell into two broad categories, work-up or diagnostic visits for new patients and subsequent desensitization visits. The Allergy Clinic saw steady growth in those functions through the decade. In 1950–51, staff reported 1,000 work-ups and 1,300 desensitization visits. By 1954–55, those numbers had doubled, and the Clinic's service function continued to grow in the last half of the decade.[60] Likewise, research activity at the Allergy Clinic grew in volume, much of it reflecting recent discoveries in steroid and pituitary hormone chemistry as well as Paul Seebohm's ongoing interest in emphysema, bronchial asthma, and rhinitis. Jeanne M. Smith, who became assistant director of the clinic in the late 1950s, contributed research in basic immunology. Like other service units, the Allergy Clinic was also a major training area. Residents, for example, served a two-month rotation in the clinic, and five of those went on to private practice as allergy specialists between 1949 and 1955.[61]

Endocrinology and Metabolism

The outlines of the modern Endocrinology and Metabolism Division were scarcely apparent in the 1950s. Despite the fact that endocrinology was by then a well-established field in internal medicine with roots extending back to the turn of the century,[62] endocrinology at the University of Iowa could draw upon only scattered service and research areas. Work in diabetes, for example, had begun early in the twentieth century, and, as noted earlier, Campbell Howard had introduced insulin therapy at the University Hospitals in the mid-1920s. In the post–World War II period, the Diabetic Service headed by Robert Hardin performed a broad service function, assuming responsibility for management of diabetic patients in all internal medicine units and in the services of other departments as well as conducting an outpatient clinic. In addition, the Diabetic

Service and outclinic were important training areas for residents, and staff associated with the service conducted research on the complications—e.g., vascular and retinal disease—accompanying diabetes and on metabolic studies of insulin preparations and oral hypoglycemic agents. Meanwhile, Robert Hardin earned a national reputation in diabetology and served many years on the board of state governors of the American Diabetes Association and would become the association's national president in 1969.

The Metabolism Ward and Thyroid Clinic were also related to the modern Endocrinology Division. The Metabolism Ward had been largely moribund until resurrected by William Bean, whose early reputation rested largely on his research in pellagra. Combining laboratory investigation with clinical facilities for the treatment and study of metabolic disorders,[63] the Metabolic Ward was the cite of a variety of investigations, including iron metabolism in hemolytic anemias, fructose metabolism, the action of vitamin C in scurvy, metabolic aspects of rheumatoid arthritis, and ongoing studies of pantothenic acid [coenzyme A] deficiency. Some of the work in the Laboratory touched upon endocrinology but much of it was also related to other subspecialties—for example, cardiology and gastroenterology.

The Thyroid Clinic, organized in 1950, was the last piece of the endocrinology puzzle at Iowa. The clinic was a cooperative venture among internal medicine, surgery, radiology, and physiology, and with Elmer DeGowin as chairman, offered diagnosis and treatment in a variety of thyroid conditions, chiefly goiter and myxedema.

By the late 1950s, there was some sign of the integration of scattered interests and resources in the broad area of endocrinology. An every-other-week Endocrine Conference was one integrating mechanism. The Endocrine Conference, in which Robert Hardin played a prominent role, was largely a teaching device, meant to help interns, residents, and staff keep abreast of recent developments in what was by then an increasingly complicated field. Another sign of integration was the fact that residents in the Diabetic Service also assumed responsibilities in the Thyroid Clinic and for diagnosis of all endocrine disorders presented at the Outpatient Clinic. Nonetheless, the formal organization of endocrinology lagged well behind many other emerging subspecialties in the department.

Infectious Diseases

Like endocrinology, infectious diseases was a late developing area, one in which the department lacked both an organized program and broad expertise in the early years of William Bean's tenure. It was not until 1955 that the department took the first steps toward the making of today's Infectious Diseases Division. First, Ian Smith's appointment as assistant professor, after two years at the Rockefeller Institute, brought the necessary specialized training in infectious disease to the department. Second, with a grant from the United States Public Health Service and funds from the Medical Trust Fund, the department organized an Infectious Diseases Laboratory. The primary focus of investigation in the laboratory lay in the natural history and treatment of staphylococcal infections and, appropriately enough in a rural environment, investigations of staphylococcal and other infections among rural populations and farm animals.

Physical Therapy

The Physical Therapy Division, headed by William "Shorty" Paul, was one of the department's largest and most productive service and research units in the early 1950s, but it was one whose development took an unusual turn. Paul's interests in physical medicine, physical therapy and rehabilitation, and sports medicine were wide-ranging, and his studies of the absorption and metabolism of various salicylate formulas, including buffered formulas, were perhaps his best remembered research contributions.[64]

While a number of factors boosted the status of physical medicine in the years immediately after World War II,[65] it was chiefly the alarming increase in the incidence of poliomyelitis in Iowa that fueled growth in Paul's Physical Therapy Division, making treatment of poliomyelitis patients the division's most visible service function. In 1950, Paul estimated that half of Iowa's polio victims were receiving treatment at University Hospitals,[66] and in the early 1950s his Physical Therapy Division saw 500–700 polio patients each year. Some 60 percent of those were children,[67] most of them admitted for short-term care but some confined to the division's eighteen respirators for weeks or more.

Polio also shaped a research agenda oriented around basic physiological and virological studies as well as treatment and rehabilitation. In addition to service and research, the Physical Therapy Division served an important teaching function in the hospitals, offering formal certification and a master's degree program in physical therapy. The exponential growth in Paul's Physical Therapy Division, along with physical medicine's national movement toward specialty status, led in 1954 to the transfer of Paul's program from the Department of Internal Medicine to a separate Physical Therapy and Rehabilitation Department.

Cardiovascular

Cardiology was the first of the modern subspecialties to receive special emphasis in the Department of Internal Medicine. When the College of Medicine held its ninth annual Medical Clinic in February 1920, one of the attractions was a demonstration of the "Electrocardiograph Station," precursor to the later Heart Station. With the arrival of Fred Smith and Horace Korns in the 1920s, both the Heart Station, under Korns' charge, and the broader field of cardiology became established elements of the department. For the future, the example of Smith and Korns attracted younger men into the field. Because of those historical foundations and because of continued technological advances, cardiology became the department's largest subspecialty in the post–World War II era.

When Horace Korns left in 1945, direction of the Heart Station fell to T. Lyle Carr; however, at Willis Fowler's suggestion, Lewis January took charge when he rejoined the department in 1946. At that time, the staff of the Heart Station included just one technician and the physician in charge. With the Station's single galvanometer electrocardiograph machine—standard until the advent of direct recording machines in the 1950s—the taking of tracings, including processing of photographic film, was a laborious procedure. The first major improvement in procedure came with institution of the unipolar theory developed by Frank Wilson at the University of Michigan, and in November 1947, Lewis January took a sabbatical leave in order to train with Wilson and returned, along with Henry Hamilton, for another session in late summer of 1948.

In 1947–48, the Heart Station processed over 3,700 electrocardiograms and added another full-time technician; in addition, four residents spent three months each at the station.[68] Through the 1950s, activities at the Heart Station expanded as did the station's technological capabilities and its medical and technical staff. In 1954–55, the station recorded nearly 5,600 electrocardiograms, and in 1958–59, over 7,300.[69] Early on the station included cardiac fluoroscopy among its services, thanks to the participation of Eugene Van Epps of radiology, and in 1954–55, the station initiated a program in vectorcardiography. Meanwhile, grants from several sources, including the College of Medicine Central Scientific Fund, the Iowa Heart Association, the American Heart Association, and the Iowa State Department of Health, still headed by Walter Bierring, encouraged the growth of the Heart Station and the research programs attached to it.

The first elective course in electrocardiography for senior medical students began in 1947. By 1954–55, the entire senior class was in attendance, and the fundamentals of electrocardiography had also been incorporated in the first-year physiology course. In the early 1950s, a Cardioscope Room, made possible by a grant from the State Department of Health, was the first specialized classroom in the College of Medicine. An oscilloscope and stethophones allowed up to fifty students to monitor heart sounds and rhythms both from live patients and from a library of magnetic tapes. Not only was the cardioscope facility used in training students and house staff, it was also the center for a weekly cardiology demonstration clinic organized by January, Walter Kirkendall, and Henry

Hamilton that brought together adult and pediatric cardiologists, cardiac surgeons, and radiologists. By the end of the decade, the station had, with contributions also from Ernest Theilen and June Fisher, become an important center within the College of Medicine for the teaching and study of cardiac disease.

The Cardiovascular Laboratory was a second major component of the department's expanding program in cardiology. A striking illustration of the central role of technology in the making of the modern internal medicine subspecialties, the Cardiovascular Laboratory organized in 1950 owed its origins to cardiac catheterization. First demonstrated in 1929, cardiac catheterization did not immediately excite interest among cardiologists who at first resisted such invasive techniques; however, in the late 1940s and early 1950s, cardiac catheterization was widely practiced, thanks at least in part to work in cardiac surgery during World War II.

In 1947, Dean Ewen MacEwen noted that the resignation of Horace Korns and the death of Fred Smith had left the Department of Internal Medicine's cardiology programs embarrassingly understaffed.[70] In addition, department members were generally agreed on the need of a cardiovascular diagnosis and research facility capitalizing on the catheterization procedure. William Bean hoped, as did Dean MacEwen, to recruit a major figure in cardiac catheterization to head the proposed laboratory. As might be expected, however, that proved easier said than done, and Bean instead chose a younger man, James Culbertson, just then finishing his training with Robert Wilkins in Boston.

When Culbertson joined the faculty in December 1949, the task of organizing and equipping the new Cardiovascular Laboratory on the third floor of the hospital was well underway, financed chiefly by grants of $14,000 from the U.S. Public Health Service and $15,000 from the Iowa Heart Association— the latter sum in fact borrowed from the Iowa Tuberculosis Association prior to the Heart Association's first Iowa fund drive. While administration of the Cardiovascular Laboratory was vested in the Department of Internal Medicine, the laboratory was from the first an interdepartmental enterprise, drawing also upon the resources and expertise of the departments of physiology, pediatrics, and surgery.

The organizers' initial goals were to train sufficient personnel to make the lab self-sustaining and to win a legislative appropriation to underwrite normal operating expenses. The latter hope in fact did not materialize; however, continuing support from the Iowa Heart Association, the American Heart Association, the USPHS, the Iowa State Department of Health, and internal medicine's Trust Fund—the last, much to Bean's chagrin—subsidized continually expanding laboratory operations. Already in 1953, the laboratory's staff consisted of five physicians and physiologists, two research associates, seven full-time research technicians, and two medical students serving as part-time research assistants. By the end of the decade, the laboratory was a base for seven full-time physicians as well as research fellows representing various specialties, supported by an expanding corps of technical workers. In the mid-1950s, with continued growth in personnel and diversity of research interests in medicine, surgery, physiology, anesthesiology, pediatrics, radiology, and biochemistry, Cardiovascular Laboratory staff inaugurated a weekly research seminar for the benefit of staff, research fellows, and residents.

Early work in the Cardiovascular Laboratory focused primarily on the diagnosis and surgical correction of congenital heart defects and problems resulting from rheumatic heart disease. In 1952–53, laboratory staff performed more than one hundred catheterizations, 75 percent of those primarily for research purposes, and by 1959–60, the number of catheterization procedures had risen to 176.[71] From the early 1950s, however, researchers also pursued work in other areas. For example, the discovery of hypertension as a widespread phenomenon in American society, combined with the first steps in diuretic therapy, led to work in renal studies. In addition, Iowa researchers investigated hepatic physiology, peripheral vascular disease, and pulmonary physiology.

In short order, the Cardiovascular Laboratory encompassed more or less free-standing renal and pulmonary units, each with its associated staff, patient clientele, and research and teaching agendas. By 1960, the interest in renal studies, nourished by advances in diuretic pharmacology, had fostered Hypertension Clinics both at the University Hospitals, under the direction of Walter Kirkendall, and at the Veterans Administration Hospital, under Mark Armstrong. In addition, a Pulmonary Research Laboratory performed routine clinical tests on pulmonary volume, ventilation rate, and blood gases.

An influx of young researchers insured the vitality of the nascent Cardiovascular Division. Ernest O. Theilen joined the faculty in 1951 after completing his residency at Iowa; Mark Armstrong joined the department and the Veterans Administration Hospital in 1955; George Bedell joined the department in 1952 and became a principal figure in the rapidly expanding area of pulmonary research in the late 1950s; David Funk—like Bedell a Cincinnati graduate—also joined the faculty in 1952 after completing his residency at Iowa. One of the fastest rising stars of the 1950s was John Eckstein, who joined the department and the Cardiovascular Laboratory staff as an assistant in 1953 upon completing both his medical studies and residency at Iowa. After a year's fellowship with Robert Wilkins in Boston in 1955–56, Eckstein very quickly built a scientific reputation that, before the end of the decade, earned him a five-year Established Investigator award from the American Heart Association.

When James Culbertson left Iowa in 1958, his resignation prompted in part by personal differences within the department, direction of the Cardiovascular Laboratory fell to Walter Kirkendall, who had been important in the growth of renal and hypertension studies.[72] By the time of Culbertson's departure, the vigorous expansion of the Heart Station and Cardiovascular Laboratory had cemented cardiology's place in the department and laid the foundations for the modern Cardiovascular Division. Indeed, in 1960, cardiovascular research already attracted some 40 percent of the grant money coming to the Department of Internal Medicine.

Nutrition Laboratory

The Nutrition Laboratory was another of the oldest units in the Department of Internal Medicine, dating to the opening of the new general hospital in 1928. Under Kate Daum's leadership, nutrition research had blossomed in the 1930s, and the Nutrition Laboratory also served as a training ground for the more than 270 women who earned master's degrees in Daum's nutrition program from the 1920s to the mid-1950s.

By the late 1940s, Kate Daum had achieved wide distinction in the field of nutrition. In 1949, she received the Borden Award for fundamental research in nutrition at the San Francisco convention of the American Home Economics Association, and in May 1951, Daum was at last elected to membership in the American Institute of Nutrition.[73] Furthermore, the coming of William Bean—whose chief interests lay in metabolism and metabolic disorders—to head the Department of Internal Medicine seemed to promise an even brighter future for nutrition. Indeed, into the 1950s, the Nutrition Laboratory contributed to a variety of studies conducted by internal medicine faculty, including investigations of blood cholesterol levels, lipid clearance, pantothenic acid deficiency, and metabolic aspects of rheumatoid arthritis.[74] Kate Daum and her colleagues in nutrition and physiology also published the "Iowa breakfast studies" in the early 1950s, a series of investigations supported by General Mills and the Cereal Institute to determine the efficacy of various breakfasts in different age groups, both male and female.[75]

Ironically, however, even at the peak of the Nutrition Laboratory's productivity and in the midst of the Department of Internal Medicine's extraordinary expansion, the laboratory's future was problematic. First, until the 1950s, the chief focus of nutrition research, as in the Iowa breakfast studies, had lain in defining and quantifying the constituents of an adequate diet,[76] but already by 1950, in nutrition as elsewhere in medicine, the focus of research was shifting from clinical studies toward laboratory research, and especially toward cellular and molecular biology—a trend for which Hans A. Krebs' 1953 Nobel Prize serves as a symbolic watershed. As a result, nutrition research became more technology-dependent and more expensive and the training of nutrition researchers was substantially redefined, trends that made it difficult for nutrition programs like the one built by Kate Daum to remain competitive in nutrition research.

Second, nutrition research had also become increasingly medicalized by the 1950s. The American Medical Association's creation of a Council on Foods and Nutrition in 1936 evidenced widening medical interest in nutrition, and during World War II, the U.S. Army sponsored considerable nutrition research by physicians such as William Bean, an experience that further broadened interest in nutrition within the medical community. In 1952, the *Journal of Clinical Nutrition* appeared with its editorial board of eight physicians, and at the end of the decade the journal became the official organ of the American Society for Clinical Nutrition, an organization whose charter membership, including William Bean, consisted entirely of physicians. On the whole, the medicalization of nutrition research did not bode well for independent research programs conducted by women Ph.D.'s in colleges of medicine.

Third, from Kate Daum's peers in nutrition research came charges that women were not aggressive enough in staking their claim in the research arena. Already in 1939, one outspoken critic pointed out that the majority of articles in the *Journal of the American Dietetic Association* dealt with administrative issues, while the nutrition research published in the *Journal of the American Medical Association* included no collaborating dietitians.[77] Meanwhile, Kate Daum's own graduate program, while it afforded students some limited research experience, produced only a handful of Ph.D.'s. The program's practical effect was to use science and technology to create careers for women that extended their traditional roles and relationships in the areas of meal planning and food preparation, but the graduate program did not train independent researchers. Meanwhile, women classified as hospital dietitians found it very difficult to shake the stigma of the kitchen and, in the context of male-dominated institutions like the University of Iowa Hospitals, to legitimize a professional-scientific language differentiating the dietitian's activities from those of the housewife.

To some extent, at least, Kate Daum was aware of those problems and especially of the need to separate nutrition research from the kitchen. In 1945, a former student, then in charge of the Dietary Department at Starling-Love University Hospital at the Ohio State University, wrote Daum of plans to elevate her department to academic status, in either the college of medicine or in the existing Department of Home Economics. Kate Daum was emphatic in warning of the pitfalls of association with home economics. "I quite agree," she wrote, "that your department should not be a part of home economics."[78]

More to the point, Kate Daum raised the issue of her own department's status with Dean Norman Nelson of the College of Medicine in 1953. After reviewing the history of the department, she noted that it would "be highly desirable if the original departmental status [i.e., in the College of Medicine] could be reestablished." Daum noted that, because of her academic rank in the Department of Internal Medicine, she was a member of the faculty of the Graduate College; however, none of her senior staff enjoyed academic rank in the university and could not, under university regulations, examine master's candidates in the nutrition program. Not only was that an embarrassment; it also complicated recruitment of staff. "In the next few years," Daum concluded, "I will want to discuss the question of the department with you."[79]

Kate Daum, however, died of cancer on December 31, 1955. Her successor, Margaret Ohlson, was a Ph.D. student of Daum's, a recipient of the Borden Award, and president-elect of the American Dietetic Association. However, by all accounts, the future of the Nutrition Laboratory was already in doubt when Ohlson assumed Kate Daum's place. By the early 1960s, according to the Department of Internal Medicine's Annual Report, nutrition graduate students spent the bulk of their laboratory time performing routine analyses for the Metabolic Ward.[80] In 1965, the Nutrition Laboratory closed, marking an end to what had seemed, in the 1920s and 1930s, a promising niche for women in academic medicine.

AN ASSESSMENT OF GROWTH

The growth of the University of Iowa Department of Internal Medicine from 1945 to 1960 was part and parcel of the larger postwar expansion of American medical science and education, but it was no less remarkable for all that. Nor was it any less surprising to those who participated in it. At the University of Iowa and elsewhere, one of the keys to postwar development—surely the one most often cited by medical historians—was the ability to tap new sources of funding for medical research, particularly federal agencies and voluntary health associations. A second key was technological advance; both improvements in existing technologies, as in electrocardiography, and the development of new technological capabilities, as in cardiac catheterization, were crucial factors in the expansion of the 1950s.

At a local level, two other factors were crucial to the department's development. One was history. On the one hand, the dynamic building program from 1910 to 1928 provided an essential institutional foundation for the postwar expansion; to a considerable extent, the modern Department of Internal Medicine reflects the dedication of George MacLean, Walter Jessup, William Boyd, Campbell Howard, and also Abraham Flexner. On the other hand, the unique constellation of personnel and interests that emerged in the 1920s and 1930s profoundly shaped the department's postwar growth. For example, the legacy of Fred Smith and Horace Korns was obvious in the department's expanding programs in cardiology, and Willis Fowler and Elmer DeGowin had much the same impact in hematology.

A second local factor in postwar development was the Medical Service Plan. Despite its early critics both inside and outside the College of Medicine, the Medical Service Plan enjoyed the wholehearted support of most faculty; for example, a September 1949 resolution of support introduced by Elmer DeGowin received faculty approval by a vote of sixty-seven to four.[81] Many who witnessed events of the late 1940s remembered the Medical Service Plan as a major landmark in the postwar history of the college. Defended by President Virgil Hancher against charges that it constituted "socialized medicine,"[82] and amended from time to time through the years, the Medical Service Plan has remained a key to the college's success in attracting and holding some of the best and brightest researchers and teachers. Furthermore, subsequent studies have suggested that in general the rewards for practice provided by such plans have been an important factor in maintaining clinical faculty involvement in patient care and teaching, countering the intensifying demands of research.[83]

Finally, William Bean's role as department chair deserves mention. While some critics suggested a lack of cohesion—indeed, some said, even coherence—in his department as issues of organization, coordination, and adaptation grew more pressing, it was also the case that the rapid pace of growth in the 1950s placed unheard of demands upon department heads, not just at the University of Iowa and not just in departments of internal medicine. Clearly, no one in 1950 was prepared for the transformation of the next decade. Clearly also, Bean's freshness of approach, his willingness to experiment, and even his penchant for whimsy were attributes that, in the main, served him and the department well in that dynamic era. At the same time, his passion for the natural history of disease and the importance of acute clinical observation were timeless qualities. In 1948, few doubted that Bean's appointment augured well for the future, and from the vantage point of the 1990s there are still few doubters.

5

The Department and the College

1945–1960

OR internal medicine faculty, the quickening pace of academic medicine in the 1950s meant a greater commitment of time to teaching and administration. Medical education became more labor-intensive in the postwar years, and the knowledge explosion in medical science coupled with the accelerating pace of specialization and subspecialization fed the continuing debate over the nature and substance of medical education. In administration, meanwhile, the evolution of medical education, the increasing complexity of medical science, and the rapid growth in faculty numbers throughout the College of Medicine led to new organizational patterns and new administrative structures. Overall, innovations in both medical education and administration meant a substantially increased workload for internal medicine faculty and a more visible role for the Department of Internal Medicine within the college.

The changing nature of medical education in the 1950s affected Department of Internal Medicine faculty in two ways. First, in contrast to the still largely didactic format of the 1930s and 1940s, medical education at the University of Iowa in the 1950s demanded increased faculty contact with students and brought an increased emphasis on small-group instruction. As a result, the time that individual internal medicine faculty spent in teaching increased in spite of the major expansion in faculty numbers and in spite of the fact that student enrollments remained virtually unchanged after an immediate postwar surge. Second, with more knowledge to pack into an already crowded curriculum, internal medicine faculty and their College of Medicine colleagues engaged in an extended debate over the essentials of medical education, even as fears of a physician shortage sparked external pressures to expand physician training.

In administrative areas, the growth and diversification within the College of Medicine opened opportunities and responsibilities for more direct faculty involvement in program assessment and policy-making. Most immediately, the greater faculty commitment to administration was obvious in the growth of the college's committee system and the multiplication of faculty committee assignments. However, just as important was an episode in faculty self-rule in the college in the wake of Dean Mayo Soley's death in 1949, an episode that extended to 1953 and one in which internal medicine's Willis Fowler played a central role. While only a temporary expedient, that four-year interregnum experiment signaled a fundamental shift in the power structure within the college, one that would lead to a major shakeup in the 1960s.

TEACHING: ENROLLMENT PATTERNS

The late 1940s saw a strong rebound in enrollments in the University of Iowa College of Medicine. GI Bill benefits were perhaps a factor in that enrollment surge; however, it appears to have marked chiefly a return to prewar enrollment trends and, to a lesser extent, widespread concern in the late 1940s over a physician shortage in Iowa and throughout America. Nationally, the postwar era began with a medical student population of 23,216 in 1945–46, compared to 22,888 in 1934–35. By 1949–50, student numbers stood at 25,103, over 60 percent of them veterans of World War II. Through the 1950s, enrollment figures continued their gradual ascent, reaching 28,583 in 1954–55 and 29,614 in 1958–59.[1]

At the University of Iowa, the early growth in enrollments was much more dramatic, a pattern reflecting both a modest decrease in enrollments in the last half of the 1930s and the military placement policies that brought small classes by the end of the war. In the fall of 1947, with junior and senior classes stunted by low wartime placement levels, there were just 278 medical students at the university, but in the fall of 1950, total enrollment had rebounded to 386. After that postwar recovery, enrollment gains at Iowa closely matched the national pattern, as the student population stood at 437 in the fall of 1958.

Behind the gradual rise in medical school enrollments nationwide from the late 1940s to the end of the 1950s stood a remarkable fluctuation in the number of applications for entry to medical schools, and it was here that the GI bubble was most noticeable. From 1947 to 1951, as veterans finished the mandatory three to four years of undergraduate studies preparatory to medical school admission, applications to medical schools reached record numbers, peaking in 1949–50 with 24,434 applicants filing 88,244 applications for admission, a ratio of 3.62 applicants for each place in the 1950 freshman class. Meanwhile, the percentage of applicants accepted fell to a record low at barely 32 percent. At the University of Iowa, the ratio of applicants to available places was 3.03. Over the next five years, as that bubble worked its way through the system, the number of applicants plummeted nearly 40 percent to 14,538 nationally, and by 1959 had recovered only to 15,170, just 1.86 applicants for each freshman place. In 1959, the University of Iowa again fell slightly below the national average with 199 applicants for 120 positions, a ratio of 1.66.[2]

With the influx of returning war veterans, American medical schools became more discriminating in their admissions policies. In 1945, women made up over 14 percent of the entering class in American medical schools. Even Harvard Medical School had admitted women for the first time. As a result, the numbers of female students and graduates peaked in 1948 and 1949, as women made up 9.5 percent of the medical student body in 1948 and 12.1 percent of medical graduates in 1949. However, by the mid-1950s, the number of female students and graduates had returned to their prewar levels of 5 to 6 percent.[3] Because the University of Iowa College of Medicine lagged behind the national averages in admitting women during the war years, the peak percentages of women students and graduates at Iowa fell significantly below national averages, standing at 7.6 and 11.1 percent respectively in 1949–50.[4] Moreover, by 1959, just three of the one hundred College of Medicine graduates were women.[5]

It may be that the most immediate obstacles facing women in medicine were cultural and structural, reflecting, for example, vocational tracking in secondary and post-secondary education, expectations about women's family responsibilities, and the disproportionate impact of the costs of higher education upon women's career decisions.[6] From 1929 to 1960, the acceptance rate among female applicants to American medical schools in fact closely approximated the rate among male applicants. In 1950–51, for example, as enrollments of women plummeted from World War II highs, medical schools accepted 31.3 percent of female applicants and 32.6 percent of male applicants according to American Medical Association figures.[7] For whatever reasons, then, it appears that the numbers of women applying to medical schools plunged during the 1950s, and in 1959, there were just four women among the 199 applicants for admission at the University of Iowa College of Medicine.

The question of discriminatory practices of course went beyond the issue of female enrollment and graduation rates. Many American medical schools and hospitals maintained informal quotas on Jewish and other minority medical students, interns, and residents. The University of Iowa College of Medicine's long-established habit of restricting admissions to Iowa residents—an overwhelmingly white, Christian population—meant that the college was no haven for minority students. The college had just nineteen black graduates in its first century of existence.[8] It is suggestive also that when Meier Steinbrink, chair of the Anti-Defamation League, argued in 1947 that equal opportunity was the most important issue facing American medical education, Dean Ewen MacEwen was casually dismissive of Steinbrink's concerns.[9]

The overall quality of the medical students admitted to the University of Iowa in the postwar years is difficult to judge. Annual MCAT reports to the university suggested that the mean score of Iowa students routinely fell in the middle of the nationwide performance range. Fewer than 30 percent of the University of Iowa College of Medicine graduates in 1949 held bachelor's degrees, compared to the national average of over 48 percent. As late as 1959, only forty-three of 120, or 36.7 percent, of entering freshmen at the college held bachelor's degrees.[10] Also, 17 percent of the record total of applicants for admission in 1950 had had undergraduate grade point averages below 2.20 and were not even considered by the College of Medicine's Admissions Committee.[11] Yet in some respects at least the Department of Internal Medicine considered its programs superior to those at some other schools. In 1953, for example, Elmer DeGowin conducted a ten-day "cram" course in physical diagnosis for transfer students "in order that they may keep up with their [Iowa] classmates."[12]

On the whole, it appears that the quality of the student body may have lagged behind the quality of the faculty recruited during the 1950s. Based upon statistics provided by the Association of American Medical Colleges, a 1952 *New York Times* article argued that residence restrictions like those at the University of Iowa generally lowered the quality as well as the size of the pool of applicants.[13] However, the combination of political pressures from the legislature and existing pressures on facilities at the college made the adoption of a more open admissions policy unlikely.

POLITICS AND ENROLLMENTS:
THE GENERAL PRACTICE CONTROVERSY

In Iowa and across America, the late 1940s brought an outcry over a physician shortage. That physician shortage, however, was largely a problem of physician distribution prompted by the increasing urbanization of American society and the associated trend toward specialization in medical practice. As a higher proportion of physicians chose specialty practice and as more and more Americans moved from rural areas to urban, the proportion of rural general practitioners declined.[14] As such, the physician shortage was a problem whose roots lay in demographic and economic trends that were widely noted and well documented already in the 1920s.[15]

Nationally, a 20 percent decline in medical school graduates from 1947 to 1949—a product, again, of small wartime entering classes—sharpened debate over the shrinking pool of rural general practitioners. At the University of Iowa, the graduating class of fifty-seven in 1948 was the smallest in two decades and sparked considerable alarm in the state legislature and in the Iowa State Medical Society. In 1949, there were 2,403 practicing physicians in Iowa, of whom more than one quarter were at least sixty-five years of age. A College of Medicine study estimated that some seventy physicians were needed in Iowa each year for replacement alone, a figure well above the fifty-seven graduates in 1948.

The low proportion of Iowa graduates who normally remained to practice medicine in the state made the situation appear even more bleak. In the period from 1926 to 1940 just 45 percent of Iowa graduates had actually practiced medicine in Iowa,[16] and in the years immediately following World War II it appeared that situation was apt to worsen. While some 20 percent of College of Medicine graduates normally sought internships at the University Hospitals before the war, that number fell precipitously in the postwar years, bottoming at less than 2 percent in 1948—just one of the fifty-seven graduates.

President Virgil Hancher claimed that the problem arose from "the unhappy experience our school, like many others, had with students assigned to the school under the Army and Navy training programs."[17] Although Hancher ignored the obvious negative impact of the Depression on enrollment figures,[18] he was nonetheless justified in pointing the finger at the significant distortions produced by wartime placement procedures. Moreover, entering classes had substantially recovered the losses of the previous decade already in 1946, and by 1950 graduates from the first of those classes—made up once again almost entirely of Iowa residents—were ready to join the ranks of Iowa practitioners, more or less re-creating prewar placement patterns.

Still, the debate over the feared physician shortage simmered on. In 1949, the state legislature demanded that the college increase the size of its entering class from ninety-three to 120, but legislators promised no additional funds to accomplish that ambitious goal. In testimony before the legislative interim committee in June 1949, university officials warned that meeting the legislature's enrollment goal by 1951 would add $310,000 per year to operating expenses and would necessitate some $1.6 million in new construction in coming years.[19] Meanwhile, the Iowa State Medical Society—embroiled at the same time in the Medical Service Plan controversy—played both sides of the issue. The society's official position was that the state was in fact adequately served by physicians; yet a February 1950 editorial in the *Journal of the Iowa State Medical Society* castigated medical schools for limiting enrollments in opposition to the wishes of the profession at large.[20]

Such friction between the college and the medical profession of course built on a rich tradition. One Iowa physician of that era noted the common opinion among private practitioners "that those who did research [i.e., academic physicians at the university] were just a degree above the moron," while many academic physicians thought "that only doctors of poorer mentality ... were practicing on 'the outside.'"[21] Understandably, President Virgil Hancher saw the hand of Nathaniel Alcock, president of the Iowa State Medical Society in 1949–50, behind the state medical society's complaints against the College of Medicine. In Hancher's estimation, Alcock had "used his office more or less consistently to embarrass the College of Medicine and more particularly to embarrass me."[22]

President Hancher was among those who argued that federal aid to medical education was likely essential to any dramatic expansion in enrollments. Moreover, Hancher was highly critical of the medical profession's vocal opposition to federal aid to medical education. It was hypocritical, Hancher charged, for physicians to cry "socialized medicine" at the mention of federal aid to medical education while simultaneously castigating medical schools for failing to educate more physicians. Whether or not the physician shortage was as serious as often said, the public believed it existed, Hancher pointed out, and the image of the medical profession would suffer if physicians' only contribution to the debate was to obstruct potential solutions to the problem.[23]

In 1947, Dean Ewen MacEwen suggested setting up residency programs to train general practitioners for Iowa's rural communities, a plan that paralleled a national movement toward recognition of a general practice specialty.[24] MacEwen claimed that there was interest both among medical students and among medical school deans of his acquaintance, but, he charged, "the laissez faire attitude of the physicians is [a] stumbling block." In short, in MacEwen's uncharitable view, practicing physicians, while complaining of the decline of general practice, were too lazy to supervise general practice residencies.[25]

In September 1949, an Iowa State Medical Society Committee on General Practice met with the College of Medicine Executive Committee to discuss a proposed program of general practice residencies, and in mid-December, the college's Subcommittee on General Practice Residencies, chaired by William Bean of internal medicine, presented the outline of such a program to the faculty at the college. Just two weeks later, however, another medical society committee issued a report again blaming the college for the dearth of general practitioners. "It is imperative," the report read, "that the emphasis in medical education at our State University Medical College must be changed." After all, the report continued, "the primary function of the Iowa Medical School is to turn out doctors."[26]

Robert Tidrick, then head of the College of Medicine Executive Committee, responded that the college was already implementing the general practice residency plan put together chiefly by Raymond Sheets of internal medicine, and residencies would begin on July 1, 1950. Tidrick was, he said, "slightly disturbed" at the tone of the medical society report, especially because copies had been sent to the governor and other state officials as well as President Hancher. Despite the friction, and at William Bean's behest, college and medical society committees met again on January 22 to work out their differences.

The general practice residency program began on schedule under the chairmanship of William Bean, and in 1950–51, there were two general practice residents at the University Hospitals. The program provided a diverse training experience, as residents divided their time among pediatrics, dermatology, obstetrics-gynecology, otolaryngology, radiology, anesthesiology, and internal medicine. The following year, in another attempt to foster an interest in general practice, the college joined the increasing number of medical schools requiring students to serve a preceptorship between their junior and senior years, observing firsthand the work of a practicing physician.[27]

The substantial increase in enrollments and in numbers of graduates in the early 1950s, along with innovations such as the general practice residency and preceptorship programs, quieted the physician shortage controversy for a time. Indeed, the *Des Moines Sunday Register* in February 1952 celebrated the remarkable recovery of the College of Medicine from recent turmoil.[28] Yet higher enrollments and more graduates did not address the fundamental problems in physician distribution. First, there was no guarantee that physicians trained at the University of Iowa in the postwar years would choose to practice medicine in the state in any greater numbers than had been the case in the past. Second, in light of the trend toward specialization in medical practice and the decline in Iowa's rural population, it was highly unlikely that even a dramatic increase in physician numbers in Iowa would put doctors back in Iowa's small towns. And in that regard, the general practice residency, "calculated to produce well trained general practitioners so sorely needed in Iowa,"[29] was a disappointment, discontinued in the mid-1950s because of a lack of student interest and because of the nagging tendency of residents to defect to one of the specialties that made up the program rotation.

By the end of the 1950s, the declining appeal of general practice once again fired debate over the shortage of rural physicians. Despite the fact that nearly all the students at the University of Iowa College of Medicine were Iowa residents in 1958 and half came either from farms or from towns of fewer than 10,000 population,[30] the relatively low income, long hours, and limited facilities and technologies awaiting rural practitioners were strong disincentives to small-town practice. Nor was Iowa alone in that. Nationwide, nearly 48 percent of medical college graduates had chosen general practice in the period from 1900 to 1924, but that number fell to just 24 percent among graduates in the years from 1940 to 1954 and was well under 20 percent for graduates of the late 1950s.[31]

Whatever the facts of the situation, the University of Iowa College of

Medicine was often blamed for failing to train enough physicians or to bend would-be physicians toward general practice in Iowa's smaller communities. "The University of Iowa Medical School," charged one such critic, "is a high grade institution, but it is more interested in turning out Specialists, Research Technicians and Ph.D. scholastic types than country Doctors."[32]

TEACHING: THE CHANGING NATURE OF MEDICAL EDUCATION

One of the most pressing issues facing medical educators in the 1950s was the need to fit both the exploding universe of scientific knowledge and at least the rudiments of increasingly divergent practice specialties into the traditional framework of two years of basic science instruction and two years of clinical experience. Since the days of Abraham Flexner, the often-touted ideal in medical education had been to teach students scientific habits of thought, thus inspiring a taste for lifelong learning, rather than to stuff them with "facts" that might soon be obsolete. In practice, however, the content of medical education had become increasingly factual. That trend continued in the 1950s, making it more and more difficult to organize and present all the relevant science in a four-year curriculum. In practical terms, "for any course in the four years of medical school," William Bean moaned, "It would be well if everything else had come previously."[33]

William Bean was also very much aware of the limits of curricular reform, dismissing as "earnest furniture arrangers" those who sought to place too fine an adjustment on curriculum and student evaluation. Bean, like many others, argued that "the most important part" of learning "is informal."[34] In addition, Bean—himself well educated in the classical sense—was an earnest champion of the liberal arts and an opponent of too much emphasis on the strictly scientific-vocational in medical education. He laced his publications with dry wit and literary references, and he distributed what he took to be classic essays in medicine to staff in his department. "In contemporary American life," he noted in 1949, "there is generally a fear of culture as though it were a perversion of normal." In fact, he argued, since language is the basis of professional training and practice, "the thoughts and words of the finest members of the human race" had practical as well as esthetic utility.[35]

During the 1950s, perhaps the most striking change in the clinical curriculum was a sharp reduction in the time students spent in lecture situations and an extension of time spent in hands-on patient care and related activities. In 1954, William Bean claimed that the College of Medicine had accomplished an 80 percent reduction in lecture time since World War II, "the time gained [being] devoted to the clerkship" as a means of expanding clinical experience, especially in specialty areas.[36] As part of that emphasis on learning by doing, clinical instruction also began earlier in the curriculum, with the sophomore schedule including an introductory course in clinical medicine.

With the growth of specialized knowledge in internal medicine came the demand for more specialized instructional time, making it more and more difficult for the department to coordinate its clinical instruction with that of other departments. Indeed, College of Medicine departments became increasingly competitive in their claims to discrete blocks of students' time. One result was the demise in 1950 of the correlated clinical course, an interdepartmental project begun in the early 1940s with the intention of making clinical instruction more efficient and fostering cooperation among the specialties.[37] William Bean, as a member of the College of Medicine Curriculum Committee, was pleased "to witness its death and help arrange a decent burial."[38]

The reorganization of clinical training in the Department of Internal Medicine included substantially revamped courses in laboratory diagnosis and physical examination, the building blocks of clinical practice. The course in laboratory diagnosis, dating back to the turn of the century, expanded continuously in the 1950s, incorporating a growing array of tests, bringing students into the laboratory for longer periods of time, and demanding more faculty time in laboratory instruction. However, for William Bean, the course in physical examination directed by Elmer DeGowin was the more important, first, because its combination of readings, lectures, demonstrations, and actual patient examinations served as "the chief means of transition from the preclinical laboratory to the bedside,"[39] and, second, because Bean was skeptical of the too enthusiastic embrace of technological approaches to diagnostics. Bean was fond of saying that often in his teaching he would ask students to approach a diagnostic problem as if "the electric current were shut off."[40]

The junior and senior clerkships were the center of undergraduate clinical training, with much of the previous lecture format replaced by small group instruction on the wards. In groups of four or five, junior and senior students rotated through the wards on a five- to six-week basis, following assigned patients under the guidance of staff in internal medicine, neurology, and surgery. Clerks gained additional experience from assignment to the Outpatient Clinic, supervised by Robert Hardin, Paul Seebohm, and James Clifton, from teaching rounds conducted by senior staff in the department, and from departmental staff conferences, such as the Thursday afternoon medical-surgical conference.

One of the more interesting innovations in the undergraduate curriculum of the 1950s was William Bean's effort to introduce "a more comprehensive approach to the patient" through his "Psychosomatic Program,"[41] a program reflecting both Bean's concern over the increasingly specialized and technological nature of medical practice and the innate tension in medicine between reductionist and holistic approaches to disease.[42] Bean's aim was to inculcate in students a broader appreciation of the concepts of health and disease as well as promoting understanding of the mental and social parameters in disease. As part of his appeal for humanism in medicine, Bean argued for consideration of what he called "spirit" in medical education, medical research, and medical practice. Medical science, he charged, showed a "perverse inability to deal with nonmaterial, nonobjective phases of existence," phases which were very real and very objective to patients.[43] In short, William Bean proposed—in abstract philosophical language meant to command respect from his male colleagues—the reintroduction of the female concept of "caring" in medicine.

Aided by Bernard I. Lewis, recruited in 1950, Bean provided junior students a psychosomatic course combining lectures and clinical seminars. Despite his initial optimism, however, Bean admitted early on that "the results of such a program defy quantitation [sic]," leaving him to hope "that at least some of the students will have developed the attitude of considering the whole patient."[44] Bernard Lewis's departure a few years later and the increasing demands of "hard science" on valuable curriculum space caused the demise of the experiment in 1958, but William Bean no doubt derived a good deal of satisfaction from the arguments about holistic approaches to health care that surfaced in the 1970s and 1980s.

The second of the Department of Internal Medicine's teaching responsibilities lay in internship and residency programs. The one-year rotating internship program at the University Hospitals brought interns to the internal medicine wards and specialized services for a few weeks of training, a pattern little changed since the standardization of the internship in the 1920s. The residency, however, was the major focus of graduate training in the department, and here, too, the 1950s saw significant change, much of it stimulated by the growth of the special service units described in the previous chapter.

William Bean emphasized that the aims of residency training were fourfold: to foster teacher-pupil relationships akin to an apprenticeship, to allow residents to assume as much responsibility in patient care as soon as possible, to base subspecialty training on broad exposure in internal medicine, and to encourage resident participation in research.[45] In the postwar years, residents still worked long hours for little pay. As a first-year resident in 1946–47, Raymond Sheets earned $480; in that same year, as a second-year resident, Henry Hamilton earned $720; meanwhile, Walter Kirkendall earned the princely sum of $1,000 as a third-year resident; and all received room, board, and laundry in addition to their stipends.[46]

The department's residency program was "tightly organized," and William Bean held firmly to "the idea that sound training in internal medicine cannot be offered in 'cafeteria style.'"[47] More than once, Bean expressed his concern about residents who preferred to become superspecialists before becoming doctors.

Residents gained experience on internal medicine wards, in outpatient services, and in a variety of specialized service areas; also, much of the department's structure of specialized conferences was aimed at resident instruction. In addition, the department subsidized residents' attendance at regional and national meetings of professional societies, and in the late 1950s, recognizing the growing importance of basic laboratory research in internal medicine, the department began a trial program offering one or two second-year residents assignments of six to eight months in a basic science department. Finally, a major innovation of the 1950s was the recruitment of internal medicine residents from as far afield as Britain, Turkey, China, Japan, India, and Australia.

As a whole, the instructional innovations of the 1950s, particularly in the undergraduate program, only intensified the half-century old debate over the mission of the medical school and the essentials of medical education. The formalization of the internship in the first two decades of the century followed by the inception of the residency in the 1920s had implied that the function of the medical schools was less to make doctors than to provide the scientific and technical foundation for later practical training in graduate programs. In fact, however, medical schools in the 1950s expanded students' exposure to hands-on work in the wards and clinics, while trying desperately to cram more and more science into an increasingly crowded and in some respects jerry-built curriculum. That institutional response was conditioned in part by the schools' reluctance to surrender the physician-training function to other agencies; it was also conditioned in part by the general practitioner controversy and the continuing public perception of medical schools as doctor factories.

TEACHING: TIME AND RESOURCES

Despite ongoing attempts to reform the curriculum during the 1950s, several obstacles hampered instruction, both undergraduate and resident, in internal medicine. For example, the focus on hands-on teaching experience intensified the chronic scramble after suitable clinical material, and both the ongoing transition toward "secondary care" in the University Hospitals and a nursing shortage further aggravated that problem. In addition, with the diminished lecture format, department staff found that teaching commanded a larger portion of their time, and in clinical instruction as in other areas, the department faced a serious problem in providing ancillary teaching space. Finally, underlying most other concerns was the fiscal burden imposed by larger enrollments and the increasing tendency toward student-oriented teaching.

Patients were the basic material of clinical instruction, and in the 1950s problems in the supply of patients in many respects resembled those at the turn of the century. The department of internal medicine had at its disposal 113 indigent patient beds, but many of those were routinely taken up with the overload of private patients. And the average indigent patient stay of more than sixteen days further reduced effective capacity. At the same time, the limited range of clinical conditions presented by the indigent patient population limited the breadth of clinical instruction, a problem that had worsened since the 1920s,[48] while the lack of chronic illness, mild illness, or acute minor conditions presented in the Outpatient Clinic only exacerbated the problem.

Also, in 1952 and 1953, the hospital closed one of the internal medicine wards because of a lack of nursing staff, costing the department 25 percent of its patient beds. William Bean saw the combination of fewer patient beds coupled with expanded student enrollments as a near disaster. A part of the nursing problem lay in competition from the new Veterans Administration Hospital, which offered nursing salaries as much as 20 percent above those at the University Hospitals.[49] A further contributing factor, as Bean saw it, was the late 1940s conversion of the university's nurse training program to a baccalaureate basis; the extension of the nursing course, Bean growled, meant only a "reduction in the time spent in the practice of nursing before marriage."[50]

A further problem in clinical teaching arose from the increased demands on staff time that came with the emphasis on small-group teaching in clinical areas. In 1958, William Bean noted that at Washington University in St. Louis the ratio of teaching faculty to the total of second-, third-, and fourth-year medical students stood at 0.7, or seven faculty for every ten students, and at the University of Chicago the ratio was 0.21. At the University of Iowa, however, the ratio was one tenth that at the University of Washington and one third that at Chicago: 0.07, or one teaching staff member for each fourteen students.[51] And since only a part of clinical teaching took place at the bedside, physical facilities were similarly burdened, prompting Bean to complain repeatedly and at length about the need of rooms for small group conferences and consultations.

The Veterans Administration Hospital that opened next to the health sciences campus in March 1952 supplied additional teaching staff and facilities as well as clinical material for junior and senior clerks and for residents. One of the postwar "Dean's Hospitals," so named because the dean of the College of Medicine was formally charged with supervision of its medical services, the hospital at first seemed a mixed blessing, as it recruited two of the Department of Internal Medicine's most promising young staff—Walter Kirkendall and Richard Eckhardt. However, despite William Bean's "great concern" over the loss,[52] VA staff subsequently received adjunct clinical appointments in the College of Medicine, quickly blurring the distinction between Veterans Administration and College of Medicine staff, and the VA hospital became a valuable "adjunct to the teaching of medicine."[53]

The problem of funding was perhaps the most intractable of the obstacles to effective teaching, whether in the clinical areas or in the basic sciences. A 1951 Iowa study placed the cost of medical education at $11,180 per graduate, while noting that just $82,829 of the College of Medicine's $865,462 annual budget came from tuition and fees.[54] At the same time, although various federal agencies invested ever larger sums in medical research, and although Hill-Burton moneys fostered new hospital construction across America in the 1950s, there were no federal programs in direct support of medical education except for limited grant-in-aid programs. When the University of Iowa's Medical Research Center was built in the mid-1950s, for example, the U.S. Public Health Service calculated its contribution from Hill-Burton moneys on the percentage of the total cost apportioned to patient service as distinct from teaching and research. Meanwhile, Iowa legislators were far more enthusiastic in demanding expanded enrollments at the College of Medicine than in appropriating additional funds for instruction.

Across America, the growth in enrollments and rising costs of equipment and facilities in the immediate post–World War II years sparked talk of a crisis in the funding of medical education, a situation not unlike that of the early twentieth century and one that no doubt reflected the long drought of the depression and war years. In a 1948 survey by the Association of American Medical Colleges, two-thirds of medical school deans thought federal aid to medical education either desirable or necessary in the face of their funding problems, even though most admitted that such a proposal was "fraught with potential difficulties and dangers."[55] In contrast, the American Medical Association—adamant that there was no physician shortage and seeing federal aid to medical education as a step on the slippery slope toward "socialized medicine"—stood firmly against federal aid to America's medical schools.[56] In the late 1940s and early 1950s, the issue of federal aid to medical education surfaced routinely in the United States Congress but met stiff resistance, from the AMA and from other quarters as well.

As suggested previously, the national debate over federal aid to medical education had its echo in Iowa. In his presidential address to the Iowa State Medical Society in 1950, Nathaniel Alcock unleashed a loosely reasoned diatribe at the "socializers in the federal government." Alcock conceded that the threat from national health insurance schemes was obvious to his physician colleagues; however, "the danger," he warned, was "most insidious and deceptive" in the area of federal aid to medical education—a back-door approach to socialized medicine.[57] Ohio senator Robert Taft—a principal sponsor of legislation to provide federal aid to medical education—would surely have been astonished to be labeled a "socializer," and Virgil Hancher, in any event, confided to one correspondent, "I am not the least bit afraid of Federal support of medical education as a step toward socialized medicine." In fact,

Hancher continued, physicians were "becoming somewhat hysterical on the topic." If the federal government could subsidize agricultural education, Hancher asked, why not medical education?[58] Likewise, the *Des Moines Register,* hardly a hotbed of socialist sentiment, noted that "aid is sorely needed."[59]

The National Fund for Medical Education, founded in 1949, was the first major national effort to ease the funding crunch in medical education. As a private institutional response to a public problem, the National Fund was typically American, and it was perhaps fitting that Herbert Hoover served as honorary chairman. The motivating idea was that the fund, energized by prominent trustees such as Alfred P. Sloan of General Motors, Robert Lovett of the Washington power elite, and William S. Paley of the Columbia Broadcasting System, would solicit donations from major corporations and distribute the proceeds to American medical schools. And by the end of the 1950s, the National Fund for Medical Education was distributing some three million dollars annually, at the rate of $15,000 plus $60 per student to each four-year medical school.[60] Substantial though such sums were, they were hardly a sufficient answer to funding problems in American medical education. The $43,080 that the University of Iowa College of Medicine received from the National Fund in 1957 amounted to scarcely 3 percent of the college's budget.[61]

By the late 1950s, hopes grew for federal support for medical education. First, for several reasons, AMA opposition to direct federal aid to medical education had waned. Second, the National Defense Education Act of 1958— one of the products of the post-Sputnik anxiety—made it seem that broad federal support for education was a matter of national security. Nonetheless, those changed attitudes did not bear fruit in the area of medical education until the early 1960s, and even then federal support for medical education was limited to matching grants for construction and direct aid to students through loan programs in the health sciences. As the costs of medical education spiraled upward through the 1950s, then, medical schools like the University of Iowa College of Medicine were hard pressed to find additional revenues. Over the years, student tuition and fees covered a shrinking proportion of costs; erratic state appropriations provided an uncertain base for future planning; and the potential of federal aid to medical education was more promise than reality.

ADMINISTRATION: THE EXECUTIVE COMMITTEE

In the postwar years, the faculty's increasing share of administrative duties was in part a simple consequence of the increasing size and complexity of the

College of Medicine, but it was also evidence of a trend toward democratization in the college, a trend that grew in part out of the internal turmoil of the late 1940s. The sometimes bitter conflict engendered by the Medical Service Plan was only one symptom of the deep divisions over the power structure and the distribution of rewards within the college. In fact, the 1947 majority report of the Committee on Status and Compensation that contained the outline of the Medical Service Plan also included a section—suppressed by the university administration—on faculty participation in medical college governance.[62]

Dean Ewen MacEwen's death in 1948 and the suicide of his successor, Dean Mayo Soley, in June 1949 created a power vacuum in which the College of Medicine faculty pressed its claims for administrative reform. In a letter to President Hancher two days after Soley's suicide, faculty members noted that MacEwen's and Soley's deaths were evidence of the "need for change in the management of the duties of the office of the dean." And the faculty, they argued, should "be given the opportunity to present its recommendation relative to these changes."[63] Badly shaken by Soley's suicide and concerned that recent problems in the college might indeed have been a contributing cause, President Hancher hesitated. After pondering for five days the question of the deanship and the faculty's initiative, Hancher circulated to faculty members a proposal to appoint an Executive Committee of five members to administer the college pending appointment of a new dean.[64]

It was never Hancher's intention that the Executive Committee—headed in its first year by Robert Tidrick of the Department of Surgery and subsequently by Willis Fowler of the Department of Internal Medicine—serve as anything more than a brief stopgap, and Hancher immediately organized a search for a new dean. Within two months, a selection committee had compiled its short list of candidates, a list headed by Joseph T. Wearn, dean of medicine at Western Reserve.[65] However, it soon became obvious that no one on the selection committee's list wanted the job. Two years earlier, during the search for Ewen MacEwen's successor, it had not been easy to attract suitable candidates; in fact Mayo Soley, then an associate professor at the University of California, had been the selection committee's sixth choice.[66] After Soley's suicide, the deanship at the University of Iowa College of Medicine had sunk even further in the estimation of prospective candidates.

At that early date, Robert Hardin's name surfaced as a possible candidate for the deanship. With his background in blood banking, Hardin had left the University of Iowa to take a position with the American Red Cross in Connecticut in 1949; however, with the College of Medicine already having charge of medical affairs at the Veterans Administration Hospital in Des Moines and with an Iowa City VA Hospital in the planning stage, President Hancher sought to bring Hardin back to the College of Medicine in 1950 as Assistant Dean for Veterans Administration Affairs. At that time, Hancher and others toyed with the idea of recruiting Hardin for the deanship.[67]

Generally, though, the search for a new dean sputtered, and the faculty continued to assert its independence. In July 1949, the Compensation Committee in charge of the Medical Service Plan, expressing its concern for the welfare of Mayo Soley's widow and three children, voted to pay Mrs. Soley $15,000 annually for two years for "research work" in anesthesiology to be conducted in California. President Virgil Hancher was, to say the least, astonished at the proposal, questioning Mrs. Soley's qualifications to do such research, the level of remuneration, and the non-resident nature of this research. Despite the fact that Mrs. Soley was a medical graduate of the University of California, Hancher suspected that the Compensation Committee's action had little to do with research. Chiefly, he thought, the plan was a gesture of defiance aimed at the university administration, an illustration that the committee could apportion Medical Service Plan monies as it saw fit. The Faculty Committee of the State Board of Education backed President Hancher, ruling that the Compensation Committee's proposal went well beyond its authority as outlined in the regulations governing the Medical Service Plan.[68]

The faculty also pursued fundamental administrative overhaul along more conventional tracks. In September 1949, Elmer DeGowin introduced a resolution before the medical faculty expressing satisfaction with the work of the Executive Committee, a resolution that passed with just one dissenting vote.[69] And in February 1950, Executive Committee Chair Robert Tidrick transmitted to Hancher a faculty document entitled "Organization of the Deanship," a detailed proposal dealing with the deanship's relationship to the faculty, the hospital, the university administration, and outside institutions. At the heart of the proposal were plans to resurrect the faculty's formal advisory role that Dean Houghton had buried in the 1930s and to continue the executive committee whose function in the proposed system would be to "advise and aid the dean."[70]

In the spring of 1950, faced with such demonstrations of faculty intent and the lack of progress in recruiting a new dean, President Hancher resigned himself to the continuance of the Executive Committee. Hancher conducted a confidential survey of faculty opinion about the workings of the Executive Committee and found that, indeed, the committee enjoyed overwhelming faculty support. Only Nathaniel Alcock was forthright in his preference for a new dean, or as Alcock put it, "a dictator."[71] At the same time, Hancher solicited faculty advice on committee membership. In reply, William Bean reiterated his support for his colleague Willis Fowler, while excusing himself and also the heads of pediatrics and surgery from committee service on the basis of the workload in those major clinical departments.[72] Fowler's name appeared on several other lists as well, one respondent noting that Fowler had for years "been a rock of strength in the Department of Internal Medicine."[73] Not only did Willis Fowler have many admirers in the college; he was also well regarded outside the college. In May 1950, a Mason City physician praised Fowler as "a most excellent salesman for the College of Medicine" and went on to suggest that Fowler would be an excellent choice for dean.[74] In June 1950, Hancher agreed to continue the Executive Committee as originally constituted, with Willis Fowler taking over as chair in place of Robert Tidrick.[75]

In 1950, the search for a new dean was for all intents and purposes moribund and continued so until mid-1951, by which time the state board of education was prodding the university administration for action, obviously displeased by the eruption of democracy in the College of Medicine. "The College of Medicine should be headed by a competent Dean, and not by a Committee," board members complained to President Hancher. Moreover, they added, the dean "should not be required to have an advisory committee." In August 1951, Hancher responded to the board's complaints, sketching the long and complicated history of the situation at the college and pointing out the practical problems in the deanship search. Hancher noted that he and the search committee members had reviewed dozens of names, and he provided a list of five outside candidates as well as four current faculty members then under consideration. He also warned the board that the meager salary of $14,000 carried in the university budget for the deanship was "no inducement to an outstanding clinician." In January 1952, Hancher forwarded to the board a list of seventy-three names that had been considered in the preceding two years and cautioned that "there are fewer qualified men desiring medical deanships than the layman might think."[76]

In fact, only two of the outside candidates on Hancher's August 1951 list had been at all interested in the position, and both made campus visits in the late summer and fall of 1951. The first was Harold C. Leuth, Dean of the University of Nebraska College of Medicine, but Leuth was noncommittal in the weeks and months after his visit. The other candidate was Hamilton Anderson, then Professor of Pharmacology at the University of California and previously Dean of the School of Medicine at American University in Beirut. Hancher, however, was uncertain whether Anderson was the right man for the job. In a personal letter to Hancher, President Stephen Penrose of American University had expressed concern about Anderson's administrative abilities, although Penrose had also allowed that given the cast of "international dilettantes" at American perhaps Anderson's failures were understandable. Hancher, too, was concerned about Anderson's abilities as an administrator, adding that he might be too much like Mayo Soley, "an excellent doctor" who had made "a grave mistake when he decided to go into administrative work."[77]

Twice in 1951, university provost Harvey Davis had polled faculty preference on the deanship issue, always with the understanding that faculty should not consider the administration bound by the outcome. First, in June,

Davis asked whether faculty members preferred to see the college function under a dean with advisory committee or under the present Executive Committee. According to Davis and Hancher, faculty sentiment had swung toward appointment of a dean by a three-to-two margin. Later, in December 1951, Davis asked whether faculty preferred an outside or inside appointment to the deanship. Not surprisingly, the faculty preferred elevation of a current faculty member to the post, with Robert Tidrick and Willis Fowler as heavy favorites.[78]

President Hancher appears to have been more than willing to consider appointment of either Tidrick or Fowler, no doubt increasingly willing as the selection process dragged on. Hancher had in fact raised the idea of the deanship on more than one occasion with Tidrick and had assured Tidrick of his willingness to support his candidacy before the state board of education. However, by February 1952, no one had yet approached Willis Fowler directly about the deanship, and at that time Hancher instructed Provost Davis to do so.[79] Yet the problem in promoting an insider was much the same as the problem in recruiting outside the college: the most likely candidates, in this case Tidrick and Fowler, were reluctant to take the job.

President Hancher's turn to Tidrick and Fowler had come on the heels of yet another unsuccessful recruitment effort early in 1952. The candidate on that occasion was Roscoe Pullen of the University of Washington, who subsequently withdrew when offered the deanship at the University of Missouri. With Pullen, Tidrick, and Fowler out of the picture, another candidate, Myron M. Weaver, dean of the newly established Faculty of Medicine at the University of British Columbia and previously of the University of Minnesota, came to Iowa City in February 1952. Although Weaver expressed interest in the Iowa job, he too declined the position, citing his desire to finish his work in building the new school at Vancouver.[80] One more possibility surfaced in April when Hancher informally courted Dean Joseph C. Hinsey of Cornell. However, officials at Cornell looked with disfavor on this attempted raid, and it, like all the rest of Hancher's efforts, came to naught.

By the fall of 1952, the pressure on President Hancher was mounting, and not only from the state board of education. In July 1952, the Iowa State Medical Society had proclaimed that "a strong dean from outside the present faculty is essential to the best interests of the State University of Iowa College of Medicine."[81] But by fall the university's search was at a standstill for want of candidates; however, two new names surfaced in December: Donald G. Anderson, Secretary of the AMA's Council on Medical Education and Hospitals and ex-Dean of the Boston University School of Medicine, and Norman B. Nelson, then Dean of the School of Medicine at American University. Anderson was the first choice, visiting the campus and meeting with the Board of Education in early January 1953. Noting the "many opportunities for growth," Anderson commended the potential of the College of Medicine, but he then withdrew from consideration in early February.[82] That left Norman Nelson as the last hope when he came to Iowa City to tour the campus and meet with members of the Board of Education. When Nelson expressed his willingness to take the job, Hancher and the Board wasted no time in making a formal offer, and in July 1953, Norman Nelson began his tenure as dean.

At the end of the long and frustrating effort to fill the deanship, President Hancher congratulated the Executive Committee for having "done very well." However, he added, "it is tired of the job."[83] While Hancher's assessment of committee members' attitudes may have been right, the Executive Committee experiment had nonetheless whetted the faculty's appetite for a greater voice in administration, and the old authoritarian structure crafted by Dean Lee Wallace Dean and President Walter Jessup and finalized by Dean Henry Houghton was visibly weakened. Also, for the Department of Internal Medicine, the four-year interregnum was especially important. Willis Fowler's role on the Executive Committee, especially his three years as chair, was a mark not only of the widespread admiration for Fowler in the college but also evidence of the department's growing stature. Indeed, Fowler's chairmanship was a precedent for Robert Hardin's subsequent elevation to the deanship in the early 1960s.

ADMINISTRATION: THE GROWTH OF COMMITTEE ASSIGNMENTS

The Executive Committee experiment in collegial administration was only the most dramatic symptom of a sometimes subtle, yet significant, shift in the power structure of the College of Medicine and in the university as a whole. During and after the Executive Committee experiment, faculty participation in administration and policy-making functions in the college expanded in several directions, including the formation of standing and ad hoc committees that addressed a multitude of issues, from curricular revision to administration of the Veterans Administration Hospital. Those changes, too, directly involved Department of Internal Medicine staff in the ordinary governance of the College of Medicine.

Even as head of internal medicine, William Bean had few administrative duties outside his department in 1948–49. Most obviously, he was, ex officio, a member of the Medical Council, the department heads' advisory body created by Dean Henry Houghton in the early 1930s. Beyond that, Bean's official role in the college at large was limited to service on the Admissions and Curriculum Committees. Moreover, because of the centralization of authority in the office of the dean and secondarily in department heads since the 1920s, there were virtually no roles open to other department staff in administration of the college in the late 1940s and early 1950s. The two major exceptions—the Compensation Committee of the Medical Service Plan and the Dean's Committee in charge of medical services at the Des Moines Veterans Administration Hospital—reflected recent innovations.

However, during the years that the Executive Committee directed the college, there was a major expansion of the committee system. In 1950–51, for example, William Bean held places on five College of Medicine committees and three advisory committees of the University Hospitals; in all, Bean's responsibilities ranged from the Curriculum and Admissions Committees to the Library Committee and the Committee on Nursing Education. Likewise, Elmer DeGowin served on eight College of Medicine committees, chairing five of those. In addition, both Lewis January and Robert Hardin served three-year terms on the Medical Service Plan Compensation Committee in the early and mid-1950s. Robert Hardin also served on the Dean's Committee for the Iowa City Veterans Administration Hospital, and Willis Fowler served on Dean's Committees for both Des Moines and Iowa City VA Hospitals.

Although Dean Norman Nelson generally took little notice of it, an enlarged Executive Committee survived his appointment to the deanship in 1953 and became an ongoing part of the administrative structure of the College of Medicine. Willis Fowler continued his work on the Executive Committee through the 1950s and into the 1960s, and Walter Kirkendall of internal medicine joined him on the committee in 1959. Robert Hardin, as chair of the Dean's Committee for the Iowa City VA Hospital, was also an ex officio member of the Executive Committee in the late 1950s. Moreover, Dean Norman Nelson relied on Hardin in a number of ways—both formal and informal—to perform a variety of administrative duties in the college; during Nelson's prolonged illness early in 1960, Hardin—who was also a favorite of President Hancher—acted effectively as dean.

Department of Internal Medicine staff served as well on a variety of ad hoc committees, perhaps most importantly on search committees organized to select new department heads. In 1950–51, for example, Elmer DeGowin chaired the committee charged with choosing a successor to Robert Gibson as head of the Biochemistry Department, and in 1958–59, Robert Hardin chaired the committee to select a new head of the Department of Obstetrics and Gynecology. Although both DeGowin and Hardin were full professors and both were widely respected in the college at the time of their respective committee appointments, the fact that selection committees were headed by faculty who were not themselves department heads was a telling indicator of the changing power structure within the college.

It is worth noting in passing that the medical faculty unrest in the late 1940s and early 1950s was symptomatic of unrest among the university faculty as a whole, unrest directed at President Hancher's preference for authoritarian leadership at the university level as well as at the level of colleges and departments.[84] For example, much as was the case in the College of Medicine, university faculty had no formal voice in university affairs until 1948, when Hancher grudgingly consented to formation of an elected University Council with advisory powers. Robert Hardin and Raymond Sheets of internal medicine served on the Council at different times in the 1950s, and in 1959–60, Hardin served also on the Council's Committee on University Senate which tried unsuccessfully to achieve a compromise with Hancher on the constitution of a full-fledged faculty senate. On the whole, medical faculty may have been more successful in widening their administrative roles within the College of Medicine than they and their colleagues outside the college were in attaining a stronger voice in the university at large. Nonetheless, the steps toward administrative reform in the College of Medicine in the late 1940s and 1950s were only the opening phase in a far-reaching process of change in administrative structures in the coming decade.

CONCLUSION

As suggested in this and the previous chapter, the late 1940s and 1950s brought profound and in some respects revolutionary change in American medical education, much of it directly related to the changed economic and political environment of postwar America. Between 1945 and 1960, Americans' per capita incomes rose nearly 50 percent, and the proportion of American families whose incomes fell below the poverty line dropped from 40 percent in 1950 to just 10 percent in 1960. Meanwhile, a combination of economic prosperity and Cold War jitters sparked an extraordinary investment in education; expenditures in the public schools alone rose from six billion dollars in 1950 to fifteen billion dollars a decade later.[85]

With the expansion of incomes and educational opportunities, more and more Americans found higher education, including medical education, within their grasp. Meanwhile, for the first time in American history, a clear majority of American consumers commanded sufficient resources to gain access to professional medical care. Personal spending for private health insurance, for example, rose from $602 million in 1950 to $1.377 billion in 1960, while personal spending in private hospitals rose from $1.959 billion to $5.096 billion in the same period.[86] Rising personal incomes, then, had the power to transform the health care market in terms of both supply and demand.

Within American medical schools, as at the University of Iowa, the political and economic environment of the 1950s brought dramatic opportunities to expand student enrollments, staffing levels, research activities, and patient care. However, as we have seen, the rapid pace of expansion in that much celebrated "golden age" destroyed the relatively quiet, closed world of medical education created in the 1920s and 1930s, forced major changes in curriculum, in organization, and in administrative structures, triggered controversies over the quality and quantity of medical graduates, and highlighted serious weaknesses in the funding of medical education. Far from being permanent, the changes instituted in the 1950s were only the first steps in an ongoing process that shaped much of the debate over the quality and availability of health care services as well as the nature and accessibility of medical education for the next three decades.

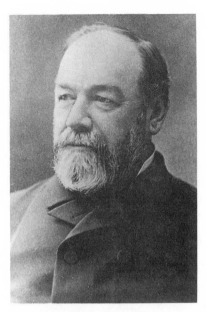

WILLIAM S. ROBERTSON,
department head, 1870-1887. *Photographs
courtesy of the Department of Internal
Medicine, University of Iowa Hospitals and
Clinics.*

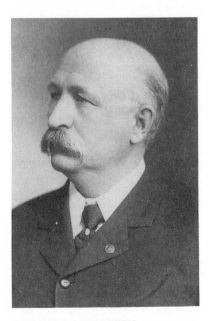

WILLIAM D. MIDDLETON,
department head, 1887-1891.

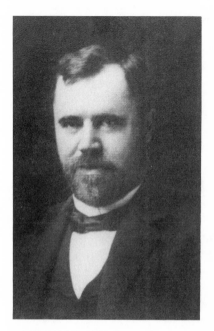

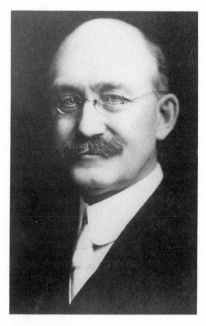

LAWRENCE W. LITTIG,
department head, 1891-1903.

WALTER L. BIERRING,
department head, 1903-1910.

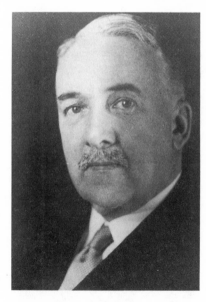

CAMPBELL P. HOWARD,
department head, 1910-1924.

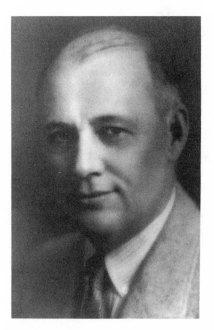

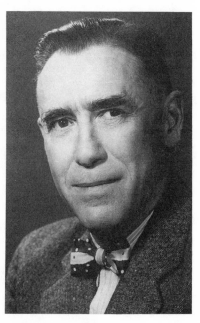

FRED M. SMITH,
department head, 1924-1946.

WILLIS M. FOWLER,
department head, 1946-1948.

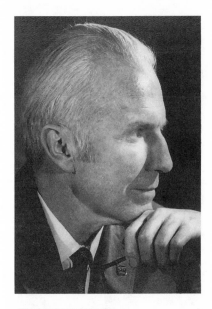

WILLIAM B. BEAN,
department head, 1948-1970.

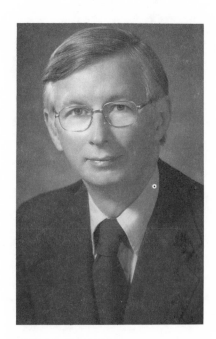

JAMES A. CLIFTON,
department head, 1970-1976.

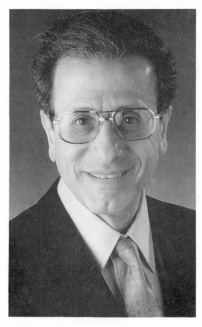

FRANÇOIS M. ABBOUD,
department head, 1976-.

6

Growth and Change in a
Technological Age

1960–1975

ANY of the patterns set in the Department of Internal Medicine in the
1950s continued through the 1960s and into the 1970s. The
demand for patient service continued its steady growth; the department's commitment to research intensified; faculty numbers continued to
grow; and the department's graduate programs expanded. However, the 1960s
and 1970s also brought important changes to the department, many of them
reflecting major innovations in federal policy, the impact of new technologies
on medical research and on medical care, and significant shifts in public
expectations of the health care system.

In the 1960s, federal agencies took a leading role in shaping the medical
research agenda, spurred in part by the Great Society vision of the Lyndon
Johnson years. As the total of federal research funds expanded rapidly into the
late 1960s, granting agencies adopted an increasingly categorical approach to
research funding, and legislative initiatives, such as the heart disease, stroke, and
cancer legislation of 1965, reinforced the targeting of research funds on specific
problem areas. Granting agencies also sought to develop interdisciplinary
approaches to research problems, an approach exemplified in the University of
Iowa's Clinical Research Center and Cardiovascular Research Center. By the
early 1970s, however, inflation and ballooning federal budget deficits slowed
the rate of growth in appropriations for research and heightened the competition
for available funds, contributing to a growing sense of crisis in the world of
academic medicine.

Similarly, the 1960s and early 1970s brought new federal initiatives in the delivery and regulation of medical services. The Medicare and Medicaid programs established in 1965 provided access to health care to the elderly and indigent and transformed much of the indigent population of teaching hospitals into paying patients. Less obvious, perhaps, but just as important to the development of academic medicine were federal programs designed to foster closer ties between teaching hospitals and community health services, widening access to the complex technologies and expertise available at institutions such as the University of Iowa Hospitals. Again, however, fiscal concerns were important determinants of federal policy by the 1970s, shifting the emphasis from broader access to health care toward containment of health care costs.

Also in the 1960s, technology assumed a paramount role in the development of medical science and medical institutions and of public expectations of medicine and physicians as well. The marriage of scientific medicine and technology was not new; after all, the most celebrated medical advances of the nineteenth century were related to the appearance of new technologies and to the refinement and adaptation of older technologies. Nonetheless, the bond between medicine and technology intensified and also diversified in the twentieth century, particularly so after World War II. By the 1970s, medical technology had become a multibillion-dollar business, and corporate research and development coupled with aggressive promotional strategies added to the pace of technological change.

Meanwhile, the late 1960s and early 1970s provided the setting for a pervasive challenge to traditional authority relations in much of American society, a challenge exemplified most visibly in the civil rights, antiwar, and women's movements. Medicine, too, attracted its share of scrutiny and criticism. On the one hand, dramatic advances in medical science and technology heightened public expectations of modern medical care; on the other hand, dramatic rises in the costs of physicians' services and hospital care from the mid-1960s to the mid-1970s,[1] coupled with concerns over quality and availability of health care services, sparked a significant shift in public attitudes toward medicine and the medical profession.

The relationship between internal medicine and those varied developments was a complex one. Certainly internal medicine contributed much to the scientific and technological advances of the 1950s and 1960s, advances that for a time at least seemed to foster an unprecedented public confidence in medical science. Likewise, as skepticism and disillusionment set in during the 1970s, internal medicine took its share of the blame. At the same time, the extraordinary volatility in political, fiscal, and technological environments left departments of internal medicine, like that at Iowa, facing a rapidly changing constellation of problems with no readily apparent solutions. Indeed, by the mid-1970s, the pace and complexity of academic medicine had become causes of both astonishment and concern to many of the department's old hands. Younger staff, some senior members remarked wistfully, seemed to find little time for fun.

PRACTICE INCOME AND THE LIMITS OF GROWTH

As noted in Chapter Four, the Medical Service Fund had been an essential element in the building of the Department of Internal Medicine in the 1950s. However, by the early 1960s, the Medical Service Fund was stretched to the limit, and William Bean noted in 1961 that "for the first time in thirteen years the total income [i.e., practice income] of the department declined."[2] From the first, the system had relied upon faculty, especially senior faculty, to contribute more to the fund than they received in salary supplements; the surplus revenues then subsidized salaries for the expanding roster of entry-level positions in the department as well as underwriting sundry expenses associated with departmental research and educational programs. As William Bean described it, it was a "bootstrap" operation.

By 1961, again according to Bean, "the work saturation point had been reached" in terms of faculty commitment to patient service, particularly since research and teaching responsibilities had increased as well.[3] Furthermore, the weak economy meant that there was little chance of augmenting revenues by charging higher fees. The result was stagnating faculty contributions to the Medical Service Fund. To make matters worse, grade creep within the department had increased the claims of higher faculty ranks on the fund, an effect magnified by successive increases in maximum salaries approved in 1952 and 1957.

As red ink threatened the Medical Service Fund, only creative bookkeeping kept the department "just about at the break-even level." But it was no longer feasible, William Bean warned in 1962, to expect "medical practice to provide as large a proportion of the departmental income as it has in the past."[4] More and more, it seemed, the maintenance of the existing structure of faculty salaries depended on appropriated funds from the state legislature and on grants from the federal government, industry, and voluntary health agencies, leaving few resources for further departmental expansion.

By the mid-1960s, however, two factors eased pressures on the Medical Service Fund. The first of those was the growing variety of career development and career investigator awards from the National Institutes of Health and from voluntary health agencies. In part because of such awards, the commutation fraction distributed as staff salary supplements in the department fell from nearly $139,000 in 1961 to just over $103,000 in 1964.[5] At the same time, private medical insurance plans, largely a product of collective bargaining agreements, boosted Medical Service Fund revenues by providing more paying patients. Spending for private health insurance in the United States doubled between 1950 and 1960 and nearly doubled again between 1960 and 1970,[6] and ultimately "the broader coverage of patients with hospitalization and medical insurance" significantly changed "the complexion of the hospital as a service and teaching facility."[7] In part because of private insurance payments, Medical Service Fund revenues in the Department of Medicine grew nearly 30 percent from 1961 to 1964.

The impact of Medicare and Medicaid programs on Medical Service Fund income was even more pronounced. On July 30, 1965, President Lyndon Johnson signed the three-part legislation to provide compulsory hospital insurance for the elderly, a voluntary program for the elderly offering government-subsidized insurance for physicians' fees, and assistance to the states for medical care for the poor.[8] At a stroke of the president's pen, most of the indigent of all ages effectively became paying patients, with profound, if unimagined, effects upon the American health care delivery system, including teaching hospitals and clinical departments associated with American medical schools. By 1975, all third-party programs funded two-thirds of America's estimated $116 billion bill for personal health care, and federal expenditures accounted for nearly 27 percent of the third-party total.[9]

The combined effect of private insurance and federal health care subsidies on medical service plan income at American medical schools was dramatic. While total medical school revenues from all sources rose 15 percent annually in the decade 1962–72, medical service plan income rose at a 27 percent annual rate and reached an aggregate of nearly $200 million in 1975. In the early 1970s, practice income provided over 15 percent of American medical schools' total operating income.[10] For the University of Iowa Department of Internal Medicine, the effect of third-party payments, especially Medicare and Medicaid, on practice income was just as dramatic. While Medical Service Fund income rose a modest 5 percent annually from 1963 to 1966, income jumped 34 percent in 1967 and another 39 percent the following year. In the 1974–75 fiscal year, the department's practice income exceeded the million-dollar mark for the first time.[11] During that period from 1967 to 1975, the faculty commutation fraction charged to the Medical Service Fund rose only a third, leaving a large share of practice income for other departmental uses.

The revenues derived from patient care were essential in maintaining many of the department's programs, but there were drawbacks to that dependence. There was no apparent limit on the demand for patient care or on departmental uses for practice income, and the budgetary stringency of the early 1970s only worsened those concerns.[12] As a result, the maintenance of an appropriate balance among patient service, teaching, and research responsibilities became increasingly problematic, and some feared that practice expectations could be an obstacle in recruitment of promising faculty.[13] William Bean suggested to University of Iowa President Howard Bowen in 1967 the possibility of employing part-time clinical teachers, arguing that such a "clinical yeomanry" would relieve full-time faculty of some of the burden of clinical teaching and patient service.[14] Nothing came of Bean's suggestion even though such practice was common at American medical schools.

DEPARTMENT PERSONNEL: A NEW PHASE OF GROWTH

The concerted recruiting efforts of the late 1940s and 1950s had brought together a highly regarded corps of internal medicine faculty. However, that period of rapid expansion was over by the mid-1950s, and faculty numbers grew very little in the last half of the decade. At the time, those with an eye for history might have discerned a pattern unsettlingly like that of the 1920s and 1930s, when a period of exuberant growth led to a prolonged period of stagnation.

However, there were several reasons for the slower rate of growth in the last half of the 1950s, none of which suggested a lasting downturn. First, teaching need was still the most immediate factor governing faculty size, and student enrollments remained essentially steady through much of the decade. Second, few observers at the time assumed a future of more or less continuous expansion. Certainly, nothing in past experience would have encouraged such expectations, and a 1959 national survey of departments of internal medicine revealed modest expectations for future growth.[15] Third, the flow of financial resources slowed, owing to economic recession, to limitations on the department's practice income, and to the widely held perception among Iowa voters and legislators that the chief functions of the College of Medicine were—in order of importance—to train physicians for Iowa communities, to provide health care for Iowa's indigent population, and to offer all Iowans access to sophisticated health services unavailable elsewhere in the state.

Nonetheless, teaching and service created pressures for a gradual expansion in departmental staff. As we shall see in the next chapter, the 1960s brought another push toward more labor-intensive teaching methods, while, as suggested above, the demand for patient service appeared to be virtually without limit. Thus, by 1964, the department's annual report claimed that "staff growth has not kept with [sic] the demands for service and teaching."[16] In addition, by the middle and late 1960s, the department had become noticeably top heavy with senior faculty, reflecting the ambitious recruitment during William Bean's first years as department chair. The rising age of the faculty, coupled with the impending retirement of two of the department's mainstays, Willis Fowler and Elmer DeGowin, provided much of the impetus for a second major faculty recruitment drive.[17]

In 1965, the department numbered forty-seven faculty, only four more than at the end of the 1950s. But with a major recruiting effort begun in 1967–68, the department comprised fifty-four faculty in 1968–69, sixty-five the following year, and eighty-eight in 1975. That pattern closely mirrored national trends in departments of internal medicine. In 1965, there were some 2,500 full-time faculty in internal medicine nationwide, a number that swelled to nearly 4,000 by 1970 and to more than 6,600 in 1975.[18] Likewise, the pattern in the Department of Medicine paralleled experience in other clinical departments of the College of Medicine, where total faculty numbers grew from 263 to 437, or 85 percent from 1965 to 1975.

The rapid growth in faculty ranks in the Department of Internal Medicine was accompanied by a like expansion in the department's residency program. The number of internal medicine residents remained stable through much of the 1960s, rising from twenty-six in 1961 to only twenty-seven in 1969; however, the number subsequently blossomed to thirty-two in 1970 and then to sixty-eight in 1975. To some extent, the increase in the early 1970s reflected the demise of the internship, but it also reflected substantial real growth in resident numbers.

The increase in internal medicine fellows in the late 1960s and early 1970s surpassed the growth in both faculty and resident ranks, as the fellowship became an entrenched part of graduate medical education. In 1960–61, the University of Iowa Department of Internal Medicine had seven research and clinical fellows. The number rose only modestly in the first half of the decade, reaching ten in 1965, but thereafter, thanks in large part to expanding programs of training grants, the ranks of department fellows increased sharply, numbering thirty-three in 1970 and forty-eight in 1975.

The rapid expansion of internal medicine staff numbers raised some significant problems and issues. One of the most troublesome of those was the lack of female and minority staff, a pattern carried over from the 1950s and one affected neither by the growing women's movement nor by inchoate affirmative action plans. Just three of the fifty-four faculty in 1969 were women and just four of the eighty-eight in 1975. Beyond that, the total of 204 department staff—including faculty, fellows, and residents—in 1975 included just eleven women. Nationwide, women accounted for just 8.6 percent of all internal medicine faculty in 1975 and only 6.8 percent of faculty with the M.D. degree.[19] While there was as yet no concerted attempt to recruit women at Iowa, it was also true that the low level of female medical school enrollments in the 1950s and 1960s made the recruitment of women to residency programs, fellowship programs, and faculty positions problematic at best.

The recruitment of ethnic minorities to the department faculty was a somewhat more complicated story. From the 1950s to the late 1960s, the appointment of foreign residents and fellows was commonplace, and their subsequent elevation to faculty positions was not uncommon. At the same time, the absence of African American faculty in the College of Medicine had become a cause of some concern by the late 1960s. The Executive Committee of the college recognized the problem in 1968 but asserted that there should be "no special considerations," "no lowering of standards" in making such appointments.[20] Here, too, the University of Iowa Department of Internal Medicine was, for better or worse, no different from the norm. A 1975 Association of American Medical Colleges survey of departments of internal medicine reported only fifty-four African American faculty, excluding schools at Meharry, Howard, and Puerto Rico. African Americans constituted less than 1 percent of the 6,300 faculty counted in the survey.[21]

Rapid expansion in the Department of Internal Medicine combined with the increasing emphasis on research, the growing demands of patient service and teaching, and the trickle of Ph.D. research scientists recruited to the department also raised troubling questions surrounding faculty promotion policies. Should research productivity, especially the ability to attract grant funds, be the chief qualification for promotion? Should faculty who contributed more than their share to patient service or teaching be rewarded, or should they be penalized? What were appropriate promotion policies for Ph.D. scientists? Such questions were the stuff of repeated studies and committee reports, both in the Department of Internal Medicine and throughout the College of Medicine, but they were questions for which there were no ready answers.[22]

Finally, departmental expansion could not go unnoticed in the competitive atmosphere of the College of Medicine. The fact that the Department of Internal Medicine was, in the mid-1960s, already by far the college's largest department further heightened sensitivities. At a November 1968 meeting of the college's Executive Committee, some representatives questioned the department's justification for its aggressive plan of faculty recruitment,[23] and it seems a safe assumption that that formal expression of concern reflected considerably wider discussion of the matter in the corridors and offices of the college.

RACING FOR MONEY AND SPACE

The 1950s had been a decade of wonder in academic medicine, and it was chiefly money—for normal operating expenses and for sponsored programs—that made it so. The 1960s delivered even more of the same. If the rise in expenditures at American medical schools from $69.5 million in 1947 to $439 million in 1960 was extraordinary, the further rise to $884 million in 1965 and to over $1.7 billion in 1970 was staggering. Moreover, sponsored programs—consisting chiefly of research and training grants, mostly from federal agencies—contributed $217 million to college of medicine budgets in 1960–61 and nearly $700 million in 1970–71.[24]

In general, the University of Iowa College of Medicine held close to that national pattern. The college's total budget rose from $8 million in 1961–62 to $22 million in 1969–70. Expenditures from the general university fund—money appropriated by the state legislature—doubled in those years, yet university funds declined from 48 percent to 39 percent of the college's total expenditures. During the same period, federal grants rose from 24 percent to 34 percent of College of Medicine expenditures, and General Research Support Grants and overhead charged to research grants became a significant factor in departmental and college budgets.[25] While many critics charged, as they had in the 1950s, that outside grants undermined the university's autonomy, weakened the institutional loyalty of faculty, and left the university vulnerable to the withdrawal of grant funds, University of Iowa President Howard R. Bowen championed vigorous growth built on such soft money. The university, Bowen charged, "should aggressively seek outside sources of research funds." Reliance upon state funding alone would reduce research to a "relatively minute" enterprise.[26]

At a national level, the early 1970s brought a slowdown in the growth of federally sponsored program funding, a response to persistent federal budget deficits, to political turmoil in Washington, and to a wave of skepticism about the medical research enterprise and about medical education and health care delivery. Although operating expenditures of American medical schools doubled in the five years between 1969 and 1974, sponsored program expenditures grew just 62 percent, and, more important, the total of federal research contracts and grants grew only 26 percent.[27] That development was particularly worrisome because colleges of medicine were chronically underfunded at state and local levels and had relied heavily upon federal funds for the explosive growth of the post–World War II era.

The University of Iowa Department of Internal Medicine's remarkable ability to pursue its expansion plans in the early 1970s in the face of the sluggish growth in federally sponsored programs was a critical factor in the department's history. As described earlier, practice income was an essential element in that expansion, but the department's harvest of research and training grants also grew over 300 percent from 1968 to 1975, rising from $1.3 million to $5.5 million, a striking contrast to national trends. The department and individual faculty members won grants from industry, from voluntary health agencies, from the National Institutes of Health, from the Veterans Administration, from private foundations, and from private memorials from wealthy Iowa individuals and families.[28]

Despite that success, the climate of the time nurtured anxiety. In 1975, internal medicine's John Eckstein, then dean of the College of Medicine, pointed out that the sheer multiplication of programs and goals at the federal level since the mid-1960s, whatever the benefits to colleges of medicine, was also a cause of confusion and uncertainty. From the Social Security Amendments [Medicare and Medicaid] and the Heart Disease, Cancer, and Stroke Amendments of 1965 to the National Cancer Act of 1971 and VA Medical School Assistance and Health Manpower Training Act of 1972, the universe of funding had become extraordinarily complicated. Moreover, any program could be, and many were, Eckstein noted, reduced without warning, either by executive impoundment or by legislative failures to appropriate amounts previously authorized.[29]

By the mid-1960s, university and College of Medicine officials envisioned substantial expansion of physical facilities on the medical campus to provide much-needed space for research, teaching, and patient service. This, too, was consistent with national patterns, as expenditures for medical school construction in the United States increased from $56 million in 1965–66 to a peak of nearly $400 million in 1973–74.[30] At the University of Iowa, as baby boomers moved into institutions of higher education, the years from 1965 to 1975 brought a frenzy of construction in both liberal arts and health science areas. During his five-year tenure from 1964 to 1969, President Howard Bowen oversaw the funding of a total of $125,000,000 in new construction projects on the University of Iowa campus.[31]

Robert Hardin, whose term as dean of the College of Medicine from 1962 to 1969 is discussed in the next chapter, played a major role in the new construction that changed the face of the health sciences campus. Hardin not only participated in the planning and design of new projects; he also encouraged innovations in large-scale fund-raising in the face of declining subsidies from state and federal sources. The earliest of the health sciences projects, the Basic Science Building, for which bids were let in early 1969, was financed in what had become a conventional fashion, that is, through a combination of National Science Foundation and Health Manpower grants and appropriations from the Iowa legislature. In contrast, two million dollars in private gifts from alumni, faculty, private foundations, and corporations accounted for nearly half the cost of the new Health Sciences Library begun soon after the Basic Science Building. Somewhat later, a $2 million gift from Muscatine, Iowa, businessman Roy J. Carver and proceeds from revenue bonds entirely financed a major addition to the General Hospital, an experience that set the pattern for several subsequent hospital additions.[32]

Those construction projects, while important to the College of Medicine as a whole, afforded limited immediate relief to the Department of Internal

Medicine. In 1960, the department commanded some 46,000 square feet, of which 50 percent was devoted to patient care and 20 percent to research. William Bean routinely noted the shortage of space for teaching, research, and faculty offices. In addition, the department had pressing need of expanded outpatient facilities. From the late 1940s to the 1970s, outpatient visits were the department's fastest growing service sector, yet there had been no major change in the department's outpatient facilities since the 1920s.

Bean delegated to John Eckstein and James Clifton the primary responsibility for the assignment and utilization of departmental space. Theirs was a thankless, if not hopeless, task. In fact, the chief prerequisite for the assignment may well have been an aptitude for mollifying, while rarely satisfying, a variety of competing demands in a rapidly diversifying department. Although the department's administrative offices moved in 1973 to the new "Southeast" addition to the General Hospital, the next year's annual report noted the "shortage of hospital beds" and the inadequacies of "available clinic space."[33] It was only completion of the Boyd Tower addition in 1975 that provided much needed outpatient clinics, inpatient beds, and office space.

In the meantime, the Veterans Administration Hospital provided unexpected ground for departmental expansion in the late 1960s. Although the integration of operations at the VA Hospital and the College of Medicine had begun in the 1950s, progress had been slow and haphazard. In 1963, for example, William Bean observed that the voluntary system by which faculty had previously conducted rounds at the VA had foundered because "volunteers have ceased to present themselves."[34] Bean then instituted a formal schedule for faculty rounds. Moreover, although planners had originally envisioned significant coordination between the Veterans Hospital and the College of Medicine, the VA Hospital was specifically designed for patient care, not for teaching and research.

A major reorganization and renovation of VA facilities began in 1968 under the guidance of John Eckstein. In August 1968, Eckstein became vice-chair of the Dean's Committee of the College of Medicine and subsequently became Associate Dean for Veterans Affairs. With the encouragement of three internal medicine colleagues—Dean Robert Hardin, Executive Associate Dean Daniel Stone, and VA Chief of Staff and Assistant Dean for Veterans Affairs Richard Eckhardt—Eckstein effected a whirlwind of improvements in physical facilities, personnel, and organization at the VA Hospital. Working also with the Veterans Administration Central Office, Eckstein won VA funding for training grants, for new staff positions, and for remodeling projects to provide research space. In less than a year, "despite some political rumblings," as the Department of Internal Medicine's annual report put it, the Veterans Hospital was well on its way to a much more meaningful integration with the College of Medicine. That integration, the department maintained, benefited VA patients as it strengthened the College of Medicine's, and particularly the Department of Internal Medicine's, teaching and research programs, providing research funding and facilities to clinical faculty and additional learning opportunities for medical students and residents. As William Bean commented, longstanding plans for integration of the VA "are now facts, not just dreams."[35]

COMMUNITIES OF SCIENCE AND PRACTICE

Like many other facets of the department's history in the 1960s and early 1970s, the relationship of the Department of Internal Medicine to national and international communities of medical science and to Iowa's practicing physicians blended continuity and change. Senior faculty assumed national leadership positions in a variety of professional organizations, while a steady stream of scientific publications flowed from the department. At the same time, the interactions of department staff with practicing physicians across Iowa took on new forms, chiefly the result of attempts at closer functional integration of the University of Iowa Hospitals and Clinics with local health care delivery systems and the growth of third-party payment plans that sharply reduced the internal medicine staff's traditional role as "physicians to the poor" and increased the number of referral patients.

Those faculty who had joined the department in the years immediately following World War II were well advanced in their careers in the middle and late 1960s, and several made significant marks in their specialized areas. As examples, Lewis January became president of the American Heart Association in 1966, the first department member to serve as president of such a prominent national agency and an event that William Bean recognized as a milestone. January later served on the editorial boards of *Circulation* and *American Heart Journal* as well. In 1969, Robert Hardin became president of the American Diabetes Association and played a central role in transforming the ADA from a professional association into a voluntary health organization. Paul Seebohm was president of the American Academy of Allergy in 1966–67, received the Academy's Distinguished Service Award in 1974, and served on the American Board of Internal Medicine's allergy subspecialty board in 1967–69.

By the early 1970s, a second postwar generation had also come to the fore. James Clifton, who had joined the department in 1953, became a Regent of the American College of Physicians and was later ACP president and also president of the Gastroenterological Association. Clifton was also an American Board of Internal Medicine member, chair of the gastroenterology subspecialty board from 1972 to 1975, and later headed the ABIM. By the early 1970s, Harold Schedl and William Connor, both of whom had joined the faculty in the mid-

1950s, were co-editors of the *Journal of Laboratory and Clinical Medicine,* and John Eckstein—who was the department's first Cardiovascular Laboratory Fellow and subsequently joined the faculty in 1954—won an American Heart Association Career Development Award and a Research Career Award from the National Heart Institute. Eckstein was also secretary-treasurer 1965–70, vice-president 1972–73, and president 1973–74 of the Central Society for Clinical Research.

Meanwhile, a third postwar generation had begun its rise. François Abboud, who joined the faculty in 1961 after completing his fellowship in cardiology, held a NIH Research Career Development Award from 1962 to 1970, was president of the American Federation for Clinical Research in 1971–72, and also served on editorial boards of *The Journal of Clinical Investigation* and *Circulation* in the early 1970s. John C. Hoak, who came to the department as a fellow in 1961–62, spent a year as an Advanced Fellow of the American Heart Association at the Sir William Dunn School of Pathology at Oxford University, and went on to serve the American Heart Association and several other scientific associations and publications in a variety of capacities.

In the 1930s and 1940s, Fred Smith's encouragement of conference attendance by faculty was an indicator of the department's growing integration into the scientific community, but such attendance was sporadic, and institutional support was often grudging. By the 1960s and 1970s, such attendance was the norm. In addition, department members' service on program committees for various specialty organizations and their work in organizing ad hoc conferences on a variety of clinical and research topics indicated a far greater degree of participation in the scientific enterprise.

Another, more general measure of the department's contribution to academic medicine was the ever wider distribution in American medical schools of faculty with an "Iowa connection." In a 1960 survey of full-time faculty in American medical schools, the University of Iowa Hospitals were the sixteenth most often mentioned site of residency training.[36] Also in 1960, 4.5 percent of the M.D.'s who had graduated from the University of Iowa between 1934 and 1958 held full-time faculty appointments, ranking Iowa twenty-third among American medical colleges.[37] By the mid-1970s, the University of Iowa had likewise become more than just a source of faculty candidates for other institutions; in an increasingly competitive market for new faculty, the Department of Internal Medicine displayed an ability to attract candidates from America's most highly regarded schools.

By the early 1970s, the department had redoubled its efforts, albeit with mixed results, to foster positive interactions with the community of Iowa physicians. In 1969, William Bean echoed the long history of ambivalence in that relationship, commenting that "our image is not projected to the state as it should be."[38] Nonetheless, in the 1960s and 1970s, the department continued a number of traditional mechanisms and inaugurated some new programs to bridge that gap. Formal and informal continuing medical education programs remained the centerpieces of departmental efforts to serve Iowa physicians. That focus was in keeping with the national displacement of continuing education functions from state medical societies to medical schools,[39] and it also reflected the movement toward continuing education requirements imposed by state legislatures and physician licensing boards.

Through the 1960s, the department hosted several American College of Physicians graduate courses on current topics in internal medicine. Those offerings routinely attracted 100–150 physicians and were well received, but a good share—sometimes a majority—of the audience came from outside Iowa. The department also held graduate conferences in conjunction with state agencies and organizations. The 1963 Cardiac and Respiratory Disease Conference sponsored by the Iowa Heart Association, Iowa Tuberculosis and Health Association, Iowa Thoracic Society, and Iowa State Department of Health was a typical example. Aimed specifically at Iowa audiences, such offerings were designed explicitly "to maintain a closer liaison with physicians throughout the state."[40] The department also staged special events for its Alumni Club and for specialty organizations such as the Iowa Clinical Medical Society. The *Journal of the Iowa Medical Society* became an informal organ of continuing education as well, with one issue each year designated the College of Medicine issue, filled with scientific papers written for a practitioner audience.

In addition to such educational approaches to improvement of staff-practitioner relations, there were also attempts to effect closer relations at a grass-roots, operational level. One simple example was the Wide-Area Telecommunications [WATS] line installed in the University Hospitals in 1968. Referring physicians had long complained of delays in forwarding of formal reports from university medical staff, a situation that left local practitioners to reconstruct as best they could the diagnoses, procedures, and therapies of returning patients. The WATS line, college and hospital administrators hoped, would facilitate communication, and they encouraged staff to pick up the phone and provide needed information to referring physicians.

The Iowa Regional Medical Program—advertised as a means "to unite the worlds of scientific research, medical education, and medical care"—was a major innovation in the Department of Internal Medicine's relations with Iowa's practicing physicians. Becoming operational in July 1968, the regional medical program grew out of the 1964 report of a Presidential Commission on Heart Disease, Cancer, and Stroke [the DeBakey Commission] and took shape in federal Heart Disease, Cancer, and Stroke Legislation [PL 89-239] of 1965. By 1970, the Regional Medical Program's legislative mandate had broadened to include "all other major diseases and conditions,"[41] and local programs and sponsoring medical schools had begun to experiment with organizational innovations in health care delivery systems in local communities, including multispecialty group practice arrangements.[42]

For many in the College of Medicine, not least in the Department of Internal Medicine, the Iowa Regional Medical Program afforded a mechanism to publicize the practical value of the College of Medicine's research and to address long-standing grievances over Iowa's vanishing rural health care services. Moreover, from the first the program's supporters were concerned to win "the acceptance and trust of Iowa's major providers of health care,"[43] and in the main they were able to do so despite an early warning from the Iowa Medical Society that the program might well effect a "complete revolution in the practice of medicine."[44]

The original mission of the Iowa Regional Medical Program was essentially one of continuing education, disseminating information and conducting training programs for physicians and other health care professionals, activities in which the Department of Internal Medicine was intimately involved. In addition, the department's Willard Krehl resigned as Professor of Medicine in 1967 to become the regional medical program's first coordinator, and Paul Seebohm of internal medicine served on the program's board of directors, the Iowa Regional Advisory Group.

The Mississippi River town of Muscatine was the site of the most ambitious project to grow out of the regional medical program concept. Muscatine, like many other Iowa communities, faced a potential crisis in medical services in the early 1970s, as the number of physicians fell from twenty-five to eleven between 1960 and 1972, seven of the latter beyond the age of sixty. In the fall of 1970, a local steering committee headed by John Parks, president of the Muscatine County Medical Society, and a College of Medicine Advisory Committee, including Paul Seebohm and Raymond Sheets from internal medicine, pieced together a project—the Muscatine Project—that would create a multi-specialty group practice to bring "high quality, comprehensive, personalized, modern health care" to area residents "at reasonable cost."

Working with funding from private and public sources, including a grant from the Iowa Regional Medical Program, planners established the Muscatine Community Health Center as a showcase for the latest in health care organization and appropriate technology, coordinating the work of a pediatrician, an internist, two to three family practitioners, physician's assistants, nurse clinicians, and a supporting cast of technicians. The center was also a site for educational programs, offering an elective senior clerkship for undergraduate medical students, a training rotation for residents in pediatrics, internal medicine, and family practice, a clinical elective for physician's assistants, and a variety of continuing education projects for local health professionals.[45]

Despite the apparent success of such projects, fiscal constraints and repeated rumors of the program's imminent phaseout undercut much of the potential of the Iowa Regional Medical Program to bring the resources of the College of Medicine to bear on the needs of local communities. The program began life in 1968 with a three-year grant of $1,260,000, an amount far smaller than planners had envisioned and one that resulted in elimination of some planned projects and sharp reductions in others, and throughout its lifetime the program suffered chronic underfunding. Its demise in the mid-1970s was evidence of the growing attention to cost control efforts in the determination of federal health care policy. The aim of the National Health Planning and Resources Development Act of 1974, for example, was to rationalize the allocation of health care resources while minimizing both government expenditure and government interference with the fee-for-service, free-choice structure of existing delivery structures.

In the 1960s and early 1970s, then, through traditional avenues such as scientific research, participation in professional organizations, and continuing education programs and through new initiatives, such as the Iowa Regional Medical Program, Department of Internal Medicine faculty intensified their contacts with colleagues in private practice as well as in academic medicine. Moreover, as the fate of the regional medical program suggests, those extended opportunities for interaction, whether with national and international colleagues in medical science or with Iowa colleagues in the practice of medicine, were to a considerable—and sometimes worrisome—extent dependent upon the department's ability to tap external funding sources.

TRANSITION: FROM WILLIAM BEAN TO JAMES CLIFTON

In the fall of 1968, William Bean marked his twentieth anniversary as head of the Department of Internal Medicine, and, not yet sixty years old, Bean notified College of Medicine Executive Associate Dean Daniel Stone of his intention to vacate the department chair as of July 1, 1970.[46] Bean had been discussing retirement from the chair for at least a year, and his resignation appears to have been prompted, first, by the increasing burden of administration in the department and, second, by his ambition to pursue his interests in the medical humanities. In fact, Bean submitted his resignation after taking a leave of absence from February to August 1968 to conduct research at the University of Virginia on his biography of Walter Reed.[47] James Clifton, who was then the department's newly appointed associate chair, had taken charge of department operations in Bean's absence.

The transition from William Bean to James Clifton took place under far different circumstances from those of 1948, when Bean had been chosen to head the department. First, during Bean's twenty-year tenure, the University of Iowa

Department of Internal Medicine had become—in terms of faculty numbers, research grants, patient service, and graduate education—a major department of medicine and had grown to a position of leadership in the University of Iowa College of Medicine as well. Second, an insider, James Clifton, was an obvious choice to succeed William Bean. Third, upheavals in the administration of the college itself—a subject addressed in the next chapter—meant that the choice of a head of internal medicine was not the center of attention in 1968 as it had been in 1948.

An affable man, his gentle demeanor sometimes masking his firm convictions, James Clifton was highly regarded locally and nationally and had demonstrated the requisite political and organizational skills both in directing work in his own area of gastroenterology and in his administrative role in the department at large. Moreover, despite occasional differences in philosophy and outlook, Clifton enjoyed William Bean's confidence and support, as well as that of President Bowen. James Clifton also had other suitors. In the spring of 1969, shortly after Bean gave formal notice of his intention to retire, officials at the College of Medicine and the university were particularly troubled by an offer to Clifton from Vanderbilt University. William Bean warned President Bowen that Vanderbilt's offer amounted to "a prince's ransom."[48] Clearly concerned, Bowen wrote that same day to Associate Dean Daniel Stone, chief executive officer of the College of Medicine. "I assume," Bowen began, "that Jim Clifton is the logical successor as head of the Department of Internal Medicine." That being the case, Bowen went on, perhaps an offer of the department chair might convince Clifton to stay at Iowa.[49]

The search for medicine's new head took place at a time when insiders warned that serious disruptions in the college's administration made it difficult to recruit candidates for vacant chairs in the college.[50] However, if that was true, there is no evidence that it was important in the Department of Internal Medicine search. With the unwavering backing of William Bean, President Bowen, and Bowen's vice-president for academic affairs and successor as university president, Willard L. "Sandy" Boyd, the real question seems to have been whether James Clifton would accept the position. While outside candidates visited the campus, all concerned seem to have shared the opinion that Clifton was the best candidate, and, in his formal offer in February 1970, Acting Dean William O. Rieke noted that Clifton had been the unanimous choice of the selection committee.[51]

Within the administration, there was concern also that William Bean should, by some means, be enticed to stay at Iowa. Already in the summer of 1967 Robert Hardin had raised with President Bowen the possibility of creating a distinguished professorship for Bean upon his retirement from the department chair. President Bowen endorsed the idea, and in 1970 Bean became Sir William

Osler Professor of Medicine.[52] Nonetheless, William Bean did leave the university in 1974, for a stint as director of the newly established Institute for the Humanities in Medicine at the University of Texas Medical Branch in Galveston.

TRANSITIONS IN ADMINISTRATION AND ORGANIZATION

The expansion of departmental operations in the 1960s and early 1970s added significantly to the complexity of administration and fostered significant bureaucratization in the Department of Internal Medicine. By the mid-1960s, an executive secretary headed the department's growing clerical staff and shouldered much of the responsibility for day-to-day supervision of department operations. A departmental advisory committee served as liaison between the faculty and the executive secretary and department head. Into the mid-1970s, the department's administrative support staff continued to grow in numbers and complexity, and an administrative assistant superseded the executive secretary, a change in title suggesting the larger scope and increasing functional differentiation in departmental administration.

The department's rapid growth and diversification also led to the formalization of relations among faculty and between faculty and the departmental administration. In 1974–75, the department's first Policies and Procedures Faculty Manual drew together departmental policies governing teaching, research, clinical practice, and promotion. In the early 1970s, the department also began to expand and formalize its internal committee system and to designate associate department chairs charged with specific areas of responsibility. In 1973, Lewis January became Associate Chair for Clinical Practice and coordinated the department's broad program of patient services in conjunction with a Clinical Practice Advisory Committee. At the same time, the department designated an Associate Chair for Education, a position held for several years by Richard Freeman. Through Freeman's efforts, the department's residency program became nationally competitive, attracting 400 applications for the twenty-three available openings in 1973.

In the 1950s and 1960s, many departments of internal medicine across America adopted a divisional structure that granted some measure of administrative autonomy to the subspecialties. However, William Bean stubbornly opposed divisionalization on political and philosophical grounds. Rejoicing that his department at the University of Iowa was able to hold together "numerous lusty siblings," Bean once noted that the enthusiastic embrace of subspecialization as symbolized in divisionalization had some similarity to "a state of medical anarchy with some remote analogies to juvenile delinquency."[53]

Bean's resistance to the demise of the Renaissance man in internal medicine seemed impractical to many of his colleagues. Yet, while Bean may have appeared to his critics to exhibit a stubborn conservatism in refusing to yield to the apparently unavoidable consequences of the explosion of knowledge and technology in internal medicine, his aversion to subspecialization was rooted in his philosophical objection to what he perceived as a largely unchallenged and sometimes spurious scientism in modern medicine. Moreover, his objection to subspecialization and divisionalization, his interest in psychosomatic medicine, and his often expressed skepticism of medical technology were all of a piece.

Throughout his career, William Bean complained that modern medicine too often lost sight of the patient at the center of medical care. Illness, Bean understood, was a complex phenomenon, one imbedded in personal experience and culture as well as in the technical-scientific parameters taught in the medical schools. For that reason, Bean decried the trend toward what he called "Medicine 1984" in which machines intruded between physician and patient.[54] For the same reason, he was uneasy with the eclipse of clinical research by laboratory technology.[55] "Medical science," Bean charged, "tends to overvalue precise measurement and mathematical treatment of data," and that, in his view, reflected the lack of a critical intellectual tradition in medicine.[56] In Bean's telling, it was his desire to air this critical perspective that led him to accept the position of book review editor for *Archives of Internal Medicine*.[57]

William Bean also warned of the political pitfalls in the scientific and technological trends in modern medicine. In "trying to solve complexity we have achieved isolation," he charged,[58] an isolation that risked fragmentation of departments of internal medicine and the consequent loss of departmental influence in colleges of medicine. Beyond that, Bean pointed to the larger political danger of a restive public, its expectations encouraged by a "groundless but boundless faith that science can accomplish any objective." Whatever the triumphs of medical science, Bean reminded his colleagues, "man still must die, a fact generally overlooked."[59]

Still the systemic pressures toward subspecialization in internal medicine were powerful. First, it had become patently impossible for any individual to keep abreast of developments in all of internal medicine, a fact that seemed to justify granting a measure of autonomy to the subspecialties. Second, academic reward systems favored subspecialization; whatever the contributions of the generalist, one critic notes, they were "not always rewarded in the currency of academia"—i.e., promotion and tenure.[60] Third, the flood of research funding loosed in the years after World War II increasingly favored categorical, peer-reviewed, laboratory research projects over more generalized clinical research. Fourth, both inside and outside academia, third-party payment plans fostered specialization by offering higher remuneration to high-technology specialists than to low-technology generalists.[61]

One of James Clifton's first acts as department chair was to implement a divisional plan in the department. The reorganized department comprised seven divisions, each with its own director: Infectious Diseases, Hematology, Gastroenterology, Endocrinology, Clinical Pharmacology, Renal-Hypertension-Electrolyte, and Cardiovascular. Three subspecialties—Allergy-Immunology, Pulmonary Disease, and Rheumatology—were represented as sections that soon became divisions in their own right. Of the department's divisions and sections, three—Cardiovascular, Renal, and Pulmonary—were the constituent parts of the old cardiovascular complex, but the new Cardiovascular Division nonetheless remained the largest of the department's subunits.

The seeds of the department's divisional structure were already apparent in the 1950s; in fact, several subspecialty areas already operated much as divisions, grouped along functional lines by research interests and by teaching and patient care responsibilities. To that extent, the department's formal divisionalization brought administrative structures into line with *de facto* functional arrangements. Still, divisionalization was a bold move, the most important organizational change in the history of the Department of Internal Medicine, and divisionalization was also a major factor in the department's continued growth. Yet most would concede that William Bean's warnings about the impact of specialization and technology on the practice of medicine and upon the image of medicine and medical institutions in American society retained much of their force.

PATIENT SERVICE: TECHNOLOGY AND COMPETITION

In 1960, according to the department's annual reports, the four internal medicine wards in the University Hospital recorded 2,610 patient admissions totaling 36,313 patient days. Department staff also saw 4,548 outpatients. In addition, department staff were responsible for the 215 beds on the four general medical wards of the Veterans Administration Hospital, with 2,529 patient admissions. VA outpatient clinics attracted another 2,532 patients. By 1974–75, patient admissions in medical services of both the University and VA Hospitals had more than doubled, reaching 5,425 and 5,533 respectively. Meanwhile, combined outpatient visits at internal medicine clinics in the two facilities exceeded 49,000. The University Hospitals' General Medicine Clinic and the VA Hospital's Primary Care Clinic together attracted more than 11,500 patients, while internal medicine specialty clinics recorded over 37,600 patient visits.

Much of the growth in patient service came in established areas. EKG tracings at the Heart Station, for example, rose from 8,600 in 1960–61 to 25,000 in 1974–75, and in the latter year, the Veterans Administration Hospital reported an additional 11,500. Also by 1975, the Gastroenterology-Hepatology Division, having grown to eight permanent staff with James Christensen as director, maintained separate Gastroenterology and Hepatology consultation services as well as outpatient clinics. Similarly, the Pulmonary Disease Section, its staff reduced to just two in 1968, grew to a half-dozen in 1975, with responsibility for a growing array of inpatient and outpatient services, including the Pulmonary Function Laboratory.

Such older service areas and subspecialties also expanded in significant new directions, driven by new faculty and new faculty interests, by new technologies, and by new patient populations. By 1975, for example, the Cardiovascular Division offered pacemaker clinics, coronary bypass procedures, treadmill exercise stress testing, angiography, and echocardiography. In hematology, the growing interest in oncology in the 1950s led to the establishment of a bone marrow laboratory in the Hematology Service and, by the mid-1970s, to plans for a bone marrow transplant program as well, and, with divisionalization, the new Hematology-Oncology Division contained both Hematology and Oncology Sections. In endocrinology, where work had long focused on diabetes, an influx of new faculty enlarged and diversified service and research areas; the new Endocrinology and Metabolism Division of the early 1970s conducted endocrine clinics and a general endocrine consultation service in addition to the long established Diabetic Clinic. Finally, basic research in immunological mechanisms begun in the 1950s transformed the Allergy Section into the Allergy-Immunology Section and ultimately the Allergy-Immunology Division, which for a time also included the department's Rheumatology Section.

Medicine, at least in its public image, was virtually inseparable from modern industrial technologies by the 1960s, and in many respects the intensive care units that blossomed in the 1960s were a metaphor of the new technological medicine. The Department of Internal Medicine opened its Medical Intensive Care Unit in September 1964 as a pilot three-bed unit under the direction of François Abboud. Despite its modest size, the ICU accommodated 166 patients in its first year of service. The unit was an important training ground for third-year residents in charge of day-to-day operations and for nursing staff who created the specialty of intensive care nursing.

The department's experiment with the intensive care concept led to the University Hospitals' opening in 1967 of an eight-bed General Intensive Care Unit for both medical and surgical patients. Just a year later, the Department of Internal Medicine created its four-bed Coronary Care Unit, and a six-bed Coronary Care Unit followed at the VA. In 1975, the Department of Internal Medicine opened a new and upgraded six-bed CCU in the University Hospitals under the direction of Ernest Theilen and converted the old unit into an

Intermediate Cardiac Care Unit, recognizing a second level of technological differentiation.

Renal dialysis was another much-publicized example of medicine's new life-saving technologies. Renal dialysis also marked a new intersection of technology, medicine, and public financing of health care when Congress in 1972 extended Medicare coverage to all end-stage renal disease victims. One result of the combination of a high-technology, high-cost procedure and open-ended public financing was to make renal dialysis one of the most vigorous growth sectors in health care in the late 1960s and 1970s, sparking not just expansion in the Department of Internal Medicine's Renal Division but also making private dialysis treatment centers a major industry.

Early work in hemodialysis began at the Iowa City Veterans Administration Hospital in the late 1950s; Richard T. Smith, a Clinical Instructor in internal medicine, was a part of that effort. In 1964, a regular program in chronic hemodialysis began at the VA Hospital, those services offered to University of Iowa Hospitals and Clinics patients as well. At the same time, staff of the Department of Internal Medicine's Cardiovascular Laboratories sought to expand their own work in hemodialysis and looked forward as well to the beginning of a kidney transplant program. In 1969, the University Hospitals opened its own chronic dialysis unit under the direction of internist Richard H. Freeman, with a statewide network of affiliated dialysis centers. And in 1970, the VA began its program of home dialysis, a program soon copied at the University Hospitals.

By 1969–70, staff of the new Renal-Hypertension-Electrolyte Division handled a combined 2,350 hemodialysis and peritoneal dialysis procedures at the Veterans and University Hospitals and supervised the expanding home dialysis program. In addition, the division provided dialysis and other support services to the kidney transplant program, where kidney transplants numbered fifty each year by the mid-1970s. Underlining the procedure-oriented nature of most internal medicine subspecialties, the rapid development of dialysis and transplant programs were major factors in expansion of the Renal Division faculty. In 1971–72, the division numbered five faculty; just four years later there were eleven.

Across the Department of Internal Medicine, growth in staff numbers and expanding ward and clinic services made staff scheduling an increasingly troublesome issue. In 1962, William Bean delegated to Henry Hamilton the task of creating a formal scheduling procedure that would provide adequate staff coverage of wards and clinics—at the Veterans Administration and University Hospitals—while ensuring "that no ward will be the private preserve of an individual or a subspecialty."[62] In 1973, much the same concerns, combined with increasingly complex regulatory and reimbursement procedures, prompted formation of the department's Clinical Practice Advisory Committee charged with general oversight and coordination of the department's clinical operations and the department's four General Medical Unit Teams that assumed responsibility for specific service areas.

Increasing technological sophistication and the growth in patient service in the department placed greater responsibilities on residents as well as faculty; already in the early 1960s, there were faculty concerns over the ability of third-year residents to handle all that was expected of them. In 1971, the department for the first time designated two chief residents, each of whom spent six months at the University Hospital and six months at the Veterans Administration Hospital. In addition, each internal medicine ward had a third-year resident in charge, acting as "administrator, resident, consultant, and teacher." Other ward staff included first-year residents, interns, and rotating junior and senior clerks, all supervised by two to three senior staff.

In the 1960s, as during the Korean War, the military draft made it difficult to maintain a stable resident staff. William Bean was outspoken on that as on many other problems. "The haphazard and unfair system of drafting has been a dispiriting and disrupting influence on our whole program," Bean charged in 1964.[63] Perhaps most annoying to Bean, older residents were most susceptible to the draft, leaving a lopsided staff heavily weighted with first- and second-year residents. As the war in southeast Asia intensified in the late 1960s, the problem of "erratic and intermittent losses of residents for military service" only grew worse. "This continues to be a harassing problem," Bean lamented in 1967.[64]

By the early 1970s, the Department of Internal Medicine and the University of Iowa Hospitals also faced a rapidly changing market for hospital care. In the 1950s and 1960s, the Department of Internal Medicine had trained substantial numbers of practicing internists, and many of those had spread the new subspecialty knowledge and technologies to the larger cities of the state. At the same time, thanks to Medicare and Medicaid, Iowa's elderly and indigent patient populations had become an attractive "commodity" and offered both practicing physicians and Iowa's community and voluntary hospitals the opportunity to share directly in the flow of federal funds into the reimbursement system.

Driven by that new market calculus, many Iowa hospitals adopted marketing strategies built around enhanced patient service and aggressive advertising, competing even for many of the sophisticated procedures that had once been the sole province of the University of Iowa Hospitals. In 1968, Dean Robert Hardin warned the university's vice-president for planning that the University of Iowa Hospitals would have to keep pace in providing a more patient-centered mode of care, in particular furnishing comfortable, attractive surroundings and a variety of ancillary support services for patients and their families. "Call it 'merchandising,' or what you will," Hardin said, "the cold fact is that we no longer have an assured, captive clientele."[65] In the years that followed, market considerations played an ever larger role in the design of the University Hospitals' services and facilities.

TECHNOLOGY AND COMMUNITIES OF RESEARCH

While the role of technology in patient care and in rising health care costs quickly became a part of the popular culture in the 1960s, the impact of technology on the research enterprise was equally far-reaching. New technologies defined new physical parameters, opened new modes and new areas of measurement, and suggested new mechanisms of therapeutic intervention, and the computer revolutionized the collection and evaluation of data and the development of complex control systems.

The rapid pace of technological development in medical science tended to shrink the research communities within which concepts and languages were shared, reinforcing the tendency toward specialization and isolation, even to the point of threatening fragmentation of the subspecialties in internal medicine. Technology also defined new communities quite apart from pre-existing boundaries between specialties and subspecialties and even between the clinical and basic sciences. Interdisciplinary research and service programs, then, were a largely unanticipated outgrowth of technological development.

The Cardiovascular Division provides an example of the tendency of technology to fragment old communities and to create new ones along interdisciplinary lines. By 1963, the Cardiovascular Research Laboratories organized in the 1950s evidenced considerable subsubspecialization, embracing the Hemodynamic Laboratory directed by John Eckstein, the Arteriosclerosis and Lipid Metabolism Laboratory directed by William Connor, the Myocardial Metabolism Laboratory directed by Ernest Theilen, the Pulmonary Laboratory directed by George Bedell, the Renal and Electrolyte Laboratory directed by Walter Kirkendall, and the Clinical Pharmacology Laboratory directed by Michael Brody. In all, the Cardiovascular Research Laboratories complex was home to twelve full-time faculty and one part-time, nine full-time and two part-time fellows, nineteen full-time and four part-time laboratory technicians, and eight full-time and three part-time clerical employees.

With divisionalization in the early 1970s, the Cardiovascular Laboratories split into three autonomous divisions—renal, pulmonary, and cardiovascular. However, technology had also begun to define new interdisciplinary communities in cardiovascular research. The Specialized Center of Research in Arteriosclerosis and Thrombosis, supported by a $600,000 annual grant from the National Heart and Lung Institute, was one example. Under the direction of

William Connor, the program brought together investigators from internal medicine divisions as well as pediatrics and pathology. One of the arteriosclerosis projects of special note was the long-term assessment of coronary risk factors in children in Muscatine, Iowa.

The Regulation of the Circulation in Pathological States Program, also funded by the National Heart and Lung Institute, was a second example of an interdisciplinary community within the Department of Internal Medicine. The latter brought together a variety of clinical and basic science investigators to continue work in cardiovascular control mechanisms begun by François Abboud in the Department of Internal Medicine. Research soon branched into cellular studies, including the physiology of vascular smooth muscle and mechanisms of ion transport, and the grant renewal application in 1975 proposed a dramatic expansion of that cellular emphasis and the addition of several new researchers.

The creation of the Cardiovascular Research Center further extended the relationship between technology and interdisciplinary research. The Cardiovascular Research Center was an indirect product of the 1972 federal Heart, Lung, and Blood legislation intended by its congressional sponsors to create centers for education, research, and service combining sophisticated diagnostic and research technologies and interested investigators from related specialty areas. The University of Iowa's lengthy grant application was one of five to win final approval, but Congress appropriated sufficient funds for only one center, that at Baylor University. Undeterred, several University of Iowa researchers attained alternative funding for their proposed projects, many of them resubmitted in conjunction with either the Specialized Center for Arteriosclerosis and Thrombosis or the Regulation of the Circulation Program. In addition, alternative interdisciplinary training grants provided funding for thirteen fellowships. Despite initial disappointment, then, the Cardiovascular Center, with François Abboud as director, opened in 1974, serving as an integrating and coordinating structure for expanding programs of interdisciplinary research in the cardiovascular area.

The College of Medicine's Clinical Research Center, funded by the NIH since its opening in 1961, was closely identified with internal medicine and was the earliest of all interdisciplinary projects. The CRC had two chief purposes: to promote interdisciplinary research and to encourage scientific clinical investigation. The center was initially a cramped eight-bed facility with Robert Hodges of the Department of Internal Medicine as acting director. Subsequently, Willard Krehl joined the department and became CRC director. Expansion in the mid-1960s brought a full-time dietitian, a Ph.D. laboratory biochemist, and enlarged facilities that drew together researchers from medicine, surgery, pediatrics, and orthopaedics. In 1967, when internal medicine's William Connor replaced Krehl as director, work at the CRC involved some sixty researchers from eight departments, with Walter Kirkendall of internal medicine heading the center's protocol review committee. By 1975, the CRC was one of the College of Medicine's most active research areas, with fifty-one studies in progress involving nine departments and seven internal medicine divisions. Internal medicine studies conducted in the CRC ranged from arteriosclerosis and hypertension to anorexia nervosa.

The emergence of the Clinical Pharmacology Division was another example of the interdisciplinary potential implicit in technological innovation. In general, pharmacology blossomed with the growth of federal research funding after World War II and, to that extent, shared the pattern common to the rest of medicine. However, the growth of pharmacology was also closely linked to the postwar rise of the American pharmaceutical industry. From 1950 to 1972, drug industry investment in research and development multiplied twelve times; growth in industry sales nearly doubled the rate of growth of the gross national product.[66] Meanwhile, "wonder drugs," especially antibiotics but also diuretics and the major tranquilizers, became central elements in the popular image of medicine.

In 1962–63, the Cardiovascular Laboratories established a Clinical Pharmacology Laboratory and the Department of Internal Medicine instituted a training program in clinical pharmacology with the cooperation of Walter Kirkendall of internal medicine, Michael Brody and Lauren Woods of pharmacology, and William Wilson, who held a joint appointment in pharmacology and internal medicine. Wilson had come to the University of Iowa as a resident in internal medicine in 1953 and through his work in the Cardiovascular Laboratories had developed an interest in hypertension therapy. Wilson's part in the organization of Iowa's Clinical Pharmacology program came after a year's fellowship with Louis Lasagna at Johns Hopkins University, and he later assumed the office of program director.

Given its close association with the Cardiovascular Laboratories, the clinical pharmacology program initially emphasized clinical studies of drug therapies in cardiovascular disorders, particularly the action of diuretics in the treatment of hypertension.[67] In the early 1970s, Clinical Pharmacology became a full-fledged division of the department, and although consultations regarding poisonings and adverse drug reactions were its principal patient service missions, the division's research activity retained much of its cardiovascular focus.

The Infectious Disease Division illustrates yet another facet of the influence of technology upon subspecialty development and research interests. Because Infectious Disease, like Clinical Pharmacology, lacked the independent clinical practice dimension that most internal medicine divisions enjoyed, its growth was to a significant extent contingent upon developments, especially technological developments, in other departments and subspecialties.[68] Despite that limitation, or in illustration of it, the Infectious Disease Division, like the department's other divisions, expanded significantly in the late 1960s and early 1970s. In 1975, the division numbered one Ph.D. senior scientist, three research fellows, and three faculty, including Sam T. Donta, who had replaced Ian Smith as director. The chief factor in that modest expansion was the ability of division staff to bend their expertise and research work to clinical problems in areas such as the renal transplant program, the burn unit, and oncology where infectious disease control was a critical factor in the success of highly refined technology-based procedures.

In all, such linkages across newly recognized divisional boundaries within internal medicine and across traditional boundaries separating internal medicine from other clinical specialties and the basic science disciplines constituted one of the major innovations in the department in the late 1960s and early 1970s. A product of the evolution of modern science and technology, the multi-disciplinary cross-fertilization in medical research and patient service and the associated ad hoc organizational forms, perhaps best exemplified by the Cardiovascular Center, constructed across the College of Medicine's traditional departmental structures provided a pattern that became more accepted and more common in subsequent years.

CONCLUSION: AN END AND A BEGINNING

In 1975, James Clifton asked Dean John Eckstein of the College of Medicine to relieve him of his duties as department chair, recalling that it was never his intention "to hold this position more than a few years."[69] In his six years as chair from 1970 to 1976, Clifton left an indelible mark on the department. Most importantly, he had instituted major changes in departmental organization and administration, energized the department's second major postwar recruitment drive, and directed the department's wholehearted commitment to scientific research.

By 1975, however, the job of chair of a major department of internal medicine was far more complicated and, so many observers argued, far less desirable than had been the case even a decade earlier. As departments grew in size and complexity, and as their education, research, and service missions broadened, the turnover rate among department chairs seemed to accelerate, and fewer faculty were prepared to take on the demanding and sometimes thankless responsibilities.[70] In the past, expectations were that the chair would spend more time in teaching and research than in administration, but those days, although not so distant in time, were buried by accelerating rates of growth and change. One authority remarked that the time had come when "there are no longer any great chairmen, only great committees."[71]

The immediate future held little prospect of relief. Departments of internal medicine continued to expand through the late 1970s and into the 1980s, encompassing increasingly diverse research interests and patient service areas and necessitating increasingly complex administrative structures. Indeed, at least at the University of Iowa, the rate of growth accelerated, and funding pressures likewise increased as competition for both sponsored program grants and patient care revenues grew more intense.

The spiral of technology also accelerated. Investment by private industry in research and development increased faster from 1975 to 1980 than did government spending in that area, surpassing $2.4 billion in 1980. Especially heavy investment came in pharmaceutical technology and diagnostic- and research-related computer applications. At the same time, corporate marketing strategies became more aggressive, more sophisticated, more expensive, and—arguably at least—more successful.

Similarly, the commercialization of health care delivery continued. The combination of high-cost technology, third-party funding, and the lack of effective cost controls made many sectors of the health care market increasingly profitable. Health care enterprises—both non-profit and for-profit—became larger, and the stake of corporate business in health care increased. In Arnold Relman's memorable phrase, the era of the "medical-industrial complex" had arrived.[72]

Finally, physicians and patients alike continued to seek a meaningful balance between the technical and the interpersonal in health care, between the science and the art of medicine, between the signs elucidated by machines and the symptoms experienced by patients. While few questioned the efficacy of the expanding array of technological procedures, the human dimensions of health care delivery remained open to criticism on several counts, and patients felt, perhaps more than ever, the need of "someone who lays on the hands, does natural, touching things."[73]

Still, the mid-1970s constituted a period of promise for the University of Iowa Department of Internal Medicine. First, the department had achieved a critical mass in size and reputation that seemed to secure its place in the first rank of departments of medicine. Second, despite slower growth in federal funding of medical research and increasing efforts at controlling health care costs, extraordinary sums of money continued to pour into medical research and health care. Federal spending for health research and development in fact would rise 68 percent between 1975 and 1980, and spending on Medicare and Medicaid would increase over 110 percent in that period. That largess was not spread so evenly as in earlier years, but it promised abundant growth potential for those institutions positioned to take advantage of it.

7

The Department
and the College

1960–1975

I N medical education as in research and patient care, the 1960s and 1970s
constituted an era of increasing federal involvement. In the 1960s, rising
public expectations of medical science coupled with recurrent worries of
a shortage of health care personnel led to direct federal subsidies to medical
education in the form of construction grants, training grants, student loans, and
capitation grants. At the same time, funding agencies designated special funds
as rewards for expanding overall student enrollments, and federal legislation
was instrumental in opening medical education to women and minorities.
However, in medical education, as in many other areas, the early 1970s brought
a reduction in funding levels in many programs and slower rates of growth in
others.

Meanwhile, internal developments in medical science and practice intensified the ongoing debate over what medical education should be and what it
should accomplish. As was the case in the 1950s and before, much of that
debate had to do with the definition of a core of essential medical knowledge
and its relationship to the specialties and subspecialties. However, the worsening
problem of too much to teach in too little time led also in the 1960s to the first
concerted attempts to incorporate educational theory and models of learning into
medical education. In all, the dynamism of medicine and the debate over the
form and substance of medical education kept the medical curriculum in a
constant state of flux.

The development of medical education also reflected systemic conflicts in academic medicine. For example, many feared that the growing importance of research, as a source of institutional funding and as a measure of faculty worth, had devalued teaching. Likewise, the transformation of teaching hospitals into regional referral centers coupled with the importance of practice income in funding medical school operations also threatened to diminish the teaching function.[1] To a worrisome degree, the academic physician's roles in teaching, research, and patient care seemed to have come unhinged by the 1970s. The traditional correlation between teaching needs and faculty numbers clearly diminished, and research potential tended more and more to displace teaching needs in the evaluation of faculty candidates.

At the University of Iowa, local politics also continued to play a part in the development of medical education. By the late 1960s, the disappearance of general practitioners and particularly the decline of rural health care services in Iowa were inescapable problems. However, an unprecedented boom in the agricultural economy masked an underlying—and accelerating—economic and demographic decline of Iowa's rural communities, a decline that in fact lay behind the loss of rural health services. As a result, public debate tended to focus on rural health care issues in isolation from the larger changes in rural life, and just as was the case two decades earlier, the College of Medicine bore a heavy load of criticism for its failure to supply rural physicians.

Because of its central place in clinical instruction and in research training at undergraduate and graduate levels, internal medicine was intimately involved with the varied developments in medical education. Not only did internal medicine faculty play an important part in the ongoing reform of the undergraduate curriculum; they also contributed much to undergraduate teaching, from lectures in basic science courses and the sophomore introduction to clinical medicine to junior and senior clerkships and senior electives. At the same time, the expanding world of graduate education, including "straight" internships, residencies, and fellowships, claimed an enlarged share of faculty time, and the department also played an important, if sometimes reluctant role in the development of the family practice program.

In administration, meanwhile, the 1960s marked a culmination of the democratizing tendencies of the previous decade. Generally, the power of medical school deans in America had been in decline throughout the postwar period, in no small part because of the predominant practice—common to federal agencies, voluntary associations, and industry—of awarding research funds to individuals rather than to institutions.[2] Beyond that, two local factors were crucial to further change in governing structures in the University of Iowa College of Medicine. First, Virgil Hancher's retirement in 1964 after twenty-four years as university president fundamentally changed the political climate at the university. Second, although student unrest in the 1960s dominated newspaper headlines, faculty likewise raised political demands and brought about significant changes in the governance of the university and its component colleges and departments.

At the same time, the 1960s highlighted the growing prominence of the Department of Internal Medicine in College of Medicine affairs. Internal medicine's expanded administrative role was most immediately visible in the elevation of Robert Hardin to the deanship in 1962 and his succession by John Eckstein in 1970, but internal medicine faculty found places among the ranks of assistant and associate deans in the college as well. The relationship between internal medicine and the university at large also broadened as Robert Hardin served simultaneously as dean of the College of Medicine and as a vice-president of the university.

THE DEMOGRAPHICS OF MEDICAL EDUCATION

Despite the Department of Internal Medicine's growing commitment to scientific research and the department's rapidly expanding role in patient care, medical education remained its principal responsibility. The years from 1960 to 1975 brought important changes in the size and makeup of the medical student body at both undergraduate and graduate levels, and those changes serve as essential background for a discussion of developments in the substance and organization of medical education.

After the postwar boom in applications, American medical schools had faced stiff competition in student recruitment in the 1950s, particularly from graduate programs in the sciences.[3] However, the first half of the 1960s brought a sharp turnaround. From 1961 to 1965, the number of applicants to U.S. medical schools rose steadily, climbing from just over 14,000 to 19,000, far exceeding the growth in the size of beginning medical school classes. In 1965, the total number of applications reached its highest point since the GI bubble of 1949–1950,[4] and the upward spiral continued in the last half of the decade and spilled over into the first half of the 1970s. More than 24,000 prospective medical students filed over 134,000 applications for fall 1970 entering classes, and more than 42,000 applicants filed an average of 8.5 applications each in 1975.[5]

At the University of Iowa College of Medicine, there were just 172 applicants for the 116 openings in the beginning class of 1961. Moreover, only 184 Iowans applied for medical school admission nationwide.[6] In contrast, 1965 saw a total of 259 Iowans applying to American medical schools, 149 of whom were accepted, 107 of those at the University of Iowa. Three years later, in 1968, the college received 383 final applications, 222 from Iowa residents.

President Howard Bowen's 1965 call for a major expansion of the University of Iowa College of Medicine profoundly influenced recruitment patterns in the late 1960s and beyond. The college, Bowen charged in 1965, bore "a heavy responsibility to respond to the clear social need for more physicians," and he called for an entering class of 180 by 1975 with total enrollment of 650, plus an increase from 250 to 400 in the numbers of interns, residents, and fellows.[7] In the fall of 1970, a first-year class of 131 boosted total enrollment to 502, and the fall of 1975 brought 148 beginning students and a total enrollment of some 600.[8]

The reasons behind the surge of interest in medical school attendance were many and varied. Certainly scientific and technological advances of the 1960s transformed the image of medicine from that of a conservative, even stodgy, career to an exciting field at the cutting edge of science and technology. Certainly, too, the increase in medical school applicants reflected the movement of the baby boom generation into graduate education in general and owed something as well to the fact that medical students were relatively draftproof in a period of increasingly heavy military draft calls. Also, the opening of twenty-seven new medical schools between 1965 and 1975 meant enlarged opportunities in medical education, as did significant expansion at established schools like the University of Iowa.

Also important in the applications explosion were enlarged federal investments in medical education, including direct financial aid programs. In the late 1950s, cost was a serious deterrent to medical education. Medical students faced double the average tuition and received one quarter the average stipend income of graduate students in programs in the arts and sciences, and medical students relied far more on family resources, loans, and outside work, including a spouse's income to support their studies.[9] Also, student loan programs in medicine relied heavily on private memorials, funds from philanthropic and voluntary agencies, alumni contributions, and appropriations from school budgets.[10]

Federal programs of the 1960s, beginning with the Health Professions Educational Assistance Act of 1963, substantially changed that equation, providing direct assistance to students and to institutions as well. Construction grants, training grants, and capitation grants based on student enrollments funded new facilities and equipment as well as faculty salaries. By 1974–75, the University of Iowa College of Medicine received $1.3 million in capitation funds alone.[11]

Another factor in the rise in medical school applications was the increase in female applicants; indeed, the years from 1960 to 1975 constituted a watershed in the gender makeup of American medical education. In 1960–61, women made up just 8.4 percent of American medical students, and just nine women applied for admission to the entering class at the University of Iowa College of Medicine in the fall of 1961. As late as 1964–65, only thirty, or 7.1 percent, of the 424 medical students at the University of Iowa were women, and women made up just 6 percent of the total of medical students, interns, residents, and fellows at the College of Medicine and the University Hospitals. However, in 1975, 21 percent of first-year medical students at Iowa were women; nationwide the figure was 22 percent.[12]

Minority enrollments, although much smaller, showed a similar pattern of change. In 1970, African Americans constituted only 2.7 percent and Hispanics 0.2 percent of American medical students. Moreover, if students at Howard and Meharry Universities were excluded, African Americans were barely represented at all in American medical education. But a 1970 task force report assembled by representatives of the Association of American Medical Colleges, American Medical Association, American Hospital Association, and National Medical Association symbolized a new concern over minority enrollments,[13] and just five years later, African Americans made up 6.5 percent and Hispanics 1.4 percent of total enrollments. At the University of Iowa College of Medicine in 1974–75, the student body included nineteen African Americans, or 3 percent of total enrollments, and one American Indian.[14]

President Howard Bowen was instrumental in increasing the enrollments of women and minorities at the University of Iowa. Just a year after taking office, Bowen noted that women constituted just 35 percent of total university enrollments, 10 percentage points lower than in 1925, and that women were especially underrepresented in programs such as engineering, the sciences, business, pharmacy, and medicine. "I would suggest," Bowen said pointedly, "a review of the admissions and recruitment policy with respect to women, not only in Liberal Arts but also in the professional colleges."[15] Similarly, in 1968, Bowen suggested to Robert Hardin "the desirability of adding Negroes to the student body of the College of Medicine."[16] One product of Bowen's concerns over the enrollment of women and minorities was the College of Medicine's Educational Opportunities Program, an "affirmative action effort to identify, recruit, retain and graduate" such students.

A remarkable influx of foreign students, chiefly at the graduate level, preceded the movement of women and native-born minorities into American medical education. That phenomenon reflected the international prestige of American medical science and medical institutions, the political linkages and obligations attendant to America's superpower status, and the shortage of American-trained physicians to fill available internship and residency positions. As might be expected, the origins of foreign interns and residents tended to follow the fault lines of contemporary geopolitics and past colonial history. For example, of the nearly 9,000 foreign students in American internship and residency programs in 1963, 675 came from Iran, 343 from Cuba, and 700 from India, while all of Africa accounted for only 177.

Already in 1960–61, foreign-trained physicians constituted 17 percent of interns and residents in the state of Iowa. Nationwide in 1963, the 9,000 foreign-trained physicians filled nearly 27 percent of medical internships and 24 percent of residencies. In internal medicine, 23 percent of residents nationwide were foreign-trained physicians in 1963, and in 1964–65, foreign-trained physicians also filled 31 percent of internal medicine research and clinical fellowships. By 1975, the United States was host to over 18,000 foreign medical graduates, with the three most common places of origin—India, the Philippines, and South Korea—accounting for more than half of that total.[17]

In sum, extraordinary demographic ferment underlay the development of American medical education in the period from 1960 to 1975. The global prestige of American medical science and education and domestic political and cultural trends promoting wider access to medical education introduced unprecedented diversity among both undergraduate and graduate medical students. Moreover, the changing demographics of medical education at the University of Iowa in those years increasingly reflected that diversity.

INTERNAL MEDICINE AND THE UNDERGRADUATE CURRICULUM

During its 1960 inspection visit, the Council on Medical Education and Hospitals and Association of American Medical Colleges Liaison Committee "was generally well impressed" with the University of Iowa College of Medicine. Nonetheless, committee members were troubled by an undergraduate curriculum they described as "a ponderous one ... developed over the years by accretion." Specifically, the committee recommended increased time for elective course work and less lecture time in clinical subjects.[18]

The curriculum was admittedly an unwieldy structure. The problem lay in deciding what to do about it and in generating the political will to make major reforms. In May 1961, the College of Medicine's Curriculum Committee, chaired by Elmer DeGowin of internal medicine, reported on its somewhat drawn-out study of the undergraduate curriculum begun in the late 1950s. The committee's wide-ranging recommendations included the expansion of junior and senior clerkships and major reductions in lecture time in junior and senior classes, a proposal that would cost internal medicine half its allotted lecture hours. In December 1961, a faculty conference, which James Clifton of internal medicine helped organize, added further recommendations, including less emphasis on grades, more emphasis on self-motivated learning, and the integration both of clinical concepts into the pre-clinical years and of basic science concepts into clinical studies.[19]

Those varied recommendations led to significant revisions in the undergraduate curriculum over the next two years. Under the new regime, students spent more time in the clerkship in the junior year, where all lectures were abolished and clerks spent all their instructional time on the wards. In learning clinical medicine, went the new thinking, study properly centered on the patient rather than the classroom. As junior clerks rotated through medicine, surgery, obstetrics, and pediatrics, each hospital ward was furnished with textbooks and laboratory facilities to encourage self-study, while various department conferences substituted to some extent for the missing lectures.

Senior students, like juniors, spent their time in clerkships in the various specialties. However, seniors for the first time had the option of specialized elective courses. Internal medicine electives were an immediate success, offering an early introduction to the subspecialties in a clinical setting, with diabetes-endocrinology, cardiology, gastroenterology, allergy, and outpatient attracting considerable interest. Overall, the revamped clerkship was designed to confront seniors "with increased responsibility but less than that of an intern,"[20] and throughout both junior and senior clerkships the trend toward bedside teaching in small groups intensified.

In the 1960s, significant changes in basic science departments in American medical schools forced two important changes in undergraduate teaching strategies, both of which affected internal medicine. First, basic science departments such as anatomy, biochemistry, and physiology had become increasingly like the science departments in the liberal arts. With more and more basic science faculty holding Ph.D.'s rather than M.D.'s, their knowledge and research interests bore only indirectly upon medical practice. Moreover, the substance of those basic sciences, thus the substance of classroom presentations and laboratory experience, reflected less the needs of medical education than the independent development of increasingly specialized areas of scientific knowledge.

In 1961, as an example, the Physiology Department at the University of Iowa shifted its instructional emphasis from the organ to the cell, reflecting a larger shift in physiology research. As a result, much of the responsibility for the teaching of organ physiology fell to internal medicine staff, in the context of the introduction to clinical medicine course or the junior and senior clerkships. Similarly, in order to integrate clinical applications into basic science instruction, internal medicine faculty participated as guest lecturers in the freshman and sophomore basic science courses. The alternative—a not very attractive one— was to rely on the students to construct a coherent whole out of isolated bits and pieces of scientific knowledge.

In the fall of 1961, the Department of Internal Medicine revised its introduction to principles of medicine, a part of the introductory sophomore sequence in clinical medicine that had replaced the Coordinated Clinical Program in the early 1950s. In a new series of thirty topical lectures, organized under the title

"Mechanisms of Disease: Disease as a Breakdown in the Ecology of Man," the department offered a more comprehensive and more tightly organized survey of medicine. However, pressure from the dean's office—then occupied by Robert Hardin—led to a major reorganization of the entire introduction to clinical medicine course the following year. To the chagrin of many faculty in the college, not least department heads, the new organizational scheme eliminated the discrete blocks of student time previously assigned to the various specialties, creating instead an integrated series of clinical lectures coordinated as much as possible with the presentation of related topics in the basic science courses.

Such major changes were only a prelude to an extended curricular debate that carried through the decade. From the mid- to the late 1960s, the College of Medicine's Medical Education Committee grappled with the problem of curriculum revision. In 1965, faculty organized a series of noon faculty conferences devoted to the complicated questions of curriculum content and organization. In the fall of 1966, Dean Robert Hardin appointed several subcommittees—including an introduction to clinical subcommittee chaired by internal medicine's John Hoak—to study various aspects of the curriculum problem, an undertaking that led to an August 1967 synthesis by the full Medical Education Committee. That report in turn became the basis for a thoroughgoing restructuring of the medical curriculum.

With so much attention focused on curriculum issues, some of the fundamental premises of medical education came under scrutiny as well, at the University of Iowa and across America. For example, many educators questioned the usefulness of time-consuming laboratory sessions that had lain at the heart of scientific medical education since the turn of the century. Even in internal medicine's course in laboratory diagnosis, "the increased complexity" of diagnostic work and "the rise of a host of technicians to carry out laboratory tests" raised questions about how much knowledge of those highly technical procedures students needed, or could be expected to absorb.[21] Similar concerns extended to clinical instruction which was, in its way, a species of laboratory instruction. The authors of a 1963 study at the University of Rochester School of Medicine, for example, expressed surprise at finding much that was "haphazard and mediocre" in third- and fourth-year clinical instruction, including lack of immediate faculty supervision, lack of discussion of basic science principles on teaching rounds, and lack of encouragement of students to seek new knowledge and skills through further study of a particular problem.[22]

In general, such studies suggested that a major problem in medical education was the need to motivate students to take responsibility for their own educational progress. Familiar to all educators in all fields, that problem had become more troublesome as medical education became more demanding and as successive revisions of the curriculum placed greater responsibilities on students with no assurance that students were prepared to shoulder the additional burdens. On the contrary, there seemed abundant evidence that they were not. This called into question one of the fundamental premises of scientific medical education: the ideal of the highly motivated, self-guided student embarking upon a lifelong educational journey.

Internal medicine's Elmer DeGowin encountered both the unevenness of clinical training and the uncertainty of student motivation in his course in physical diagnosis. With several faculty involved in instruction, each of them responsible for a group of five students, DeGowin noted considerable variation in instructional methods and results. DeGowin noted also that students seemed to lack the ambition needed to fill in the gaps in their knowledge and that in general their logical skills were poorly developed, or at least poorly applied. As DeGowin saw it, students were "conditioned to study only to pass examinations," studied "only when an examination is in prospect," and then studied "only those topics likely to be subjects of examination questions."[23] In short, medical students behaved much like students everywhere.

Similar complaints surrounded the junior clerkship program. Many faculty instructors questioned the ideal of self-guided study that had led to the elimination of lectures in the clerkship and argued for the reinstitution of selected lectures. Most junior clerks, William Bean complained in the late 1960s, were "at a loss ... to know how to handle the increased responsibility they are given for their own education," refusing, for example, to "accept the responsibility for independent study."[24]

For his part, Elmer DeGowin did not doubt that medical students were a highly motivated group. His concern was that their goal was not necessarily intellectual adventure but more likely success on examinations. Moreover, as the knowledge explosion packed the curriculum, students' tendencies to focus on examinations became more pronounced and more understandable. One obvious strategy to counter what, to many faculty at least, seemed like student apathy was to stress the relevancy of subject matter, relating basic science knowledge—which students found increasingly difficult to connect with real medicine—to clinical applications.[25] Indeed, the backward and forward articulation of basic sciences and clinical practice became a major theme in medical education in the 1960s.

As the pressures on medical students and on curriculum time mounted, medical educators sought more sophisticated educational methodologies, often collaborating with educational psychologists in their search for answers to the problem of information transfer in medical education. "Information processing models" of learning designed to aid in the transfer of large bodies of knowledge were especially attractive.[26] One of the foremost exponents of such models argued that memorizing vast quantities of factual material provided medical students no clue how to organize and use the information, while the time-consuming and uneven learning-by-doing approach, as in the typical laboratory experience and in much of clinical training, was embarrassingly inefficient.[27] It was pointless, such experts counseled, to hope that student motivation would surmount those obstacles; the only solution lay in better organization of the material and in improvement of students' cognitive abilities.

Programmed instruction was perhaps the most popular variant of the information processing concept among medical educators. By breaking down a subject matter, such as etiology and control of diabetes or renal physiology and disease, into its component parts, beginning with basic concepts and progressing to specific detail, programmed instruction presented information in a logical sequence of building blocks that could be extended to any level of sophistication and that students could and would, proponents hoped, absorb at their own pace.

The literature of medical education in the 1960s was littered with proposals, reports, and studies about such instructional innovations, but the results were at best mixed. To begin with, harried instructors seldom relished the considerable investment of time and energy necessary to master the relevant principles of educational psychology and to undertake such a thoroughgoing overhaul of basic course organization and materials. Moreover, it was difficult to match such highly structured instructional approaches to the often eclectic scope of medical education. The teaching of clinical medicine, for example, was quite different from the teaching of geometry or physics. Finally, outcomes measurement was also difficult and discouragingly inconclusive in the assessment of such innovations.[28]

Educational theory, however diluted, nonetheless became a fixture in medical schools. The setting of explicit educational goals and objectives became commonplace, and many schools established student learning services to facilitate self-study. In the early 1970s, the University of Iowa College of Medicine organized an Office of Instructional Resources, directed by Henry Hamilton of internal medicine, that designed and constructed self-teaching packages—including written materials, audiotapes, and slides—and provided study space and facilities. The college also hired a full-time educational consultant to advise faculty on instructional methods. In the mid-1970s, the Department of Internal Medicine created its own specialized learning center.

In the University of Iowa College of Medicine, the decade-long focus on curriculum revision culminated in the late 1960s and early 1970s. Supported in part by a five-year grant from the Bureau of Health Professions Education and Manpower Training, the new revisions—the fruit of several years of faculty committee work—were predictably oriented toward emphases on independent study, small-group teaching, and elective course work. Predictably also, the new revisions sought to delineate a core of essential knowledge for the medical student and to integrate specialized knowledge into both basic science and clinical studies.

One of the major changes in the new curriculum was the reduction of the basic science portion of the curriculum from four semesters to three, with the second semester of the sophomore year devoted to a more intensive introduction to clinical medicine course. One of the proposals first suggested by the Medical Education Committee in 1966, the new sophomore course—in which internal medicine faculty assumed a prominent role—opened with a series of demonstrations, films, and discussions on patient-physician communication, history-taking, and physical examination, then proceeded to a general overview of medicine in a format that included small-group learning activities.

The senior elective year, begun at the University of Iowa in 1972, was another major innovation, one that also significantly increased the teaching duties of internal medicine faculty. The genesis of the elective senior year was complicated. Changes in the junior clerkship in the early 1960s had invested junior clerks with increasing responsibility in patient care and appeared, to some extent, to make the conventional senior clerkship redundant. For example, junior clerks examined new patients, took patient histories, and presented tentative diagnoses and plans for therapy to supervising staff. At the same time, the elective senior year offered a partial solution to the apparently intractable problem of representing all specialties and subspecialties in the undergraduate curriculum. Instead, the plan allowed students to choose their own concentrations. While many faculty hoped that substantial numbers of students would opt for additional work in the basic sciences, the various clinical electives attracted overwhelming interest; for example, students spent 45 percent of their elective time in internal medicine offerings.

INTERNAL MEDICINE GRADUATE PROGRAMS

Critics of the elective senior year were quick to point out that it effectively pushed the threshold of specialization from the graduate to the undergraduate years.[29] While that was true, the move toward undergraduate specialization was consistent with significant changes in graduate education between 1960 and 1975. One of the most striking of those changes was the transformation and eventual demise of the internship. During the 1950s, the number of interns in the United States had grown 106 percent, but by 1960–61, some 27 percent of internship positions were vacant. Across Iowa in 1964, just sixty-four of eighty-two available internship positions were filled, 28 percent of those by foreign graduates.[30] Moreover, by the mid-1960s, the straight internship providing training in a single specialty was rapidly displacing the traditional rotating internship in America's teaching hospitals. In 1965, just half of American internship programs, most of those in smaller community hospitals, were of the rotating kind, while 35 percent were straight internships. William Rothstein maintains that, on the whole, students and faculty preferred the rotating internship and that the straight internship was chiefly a convenience to department chairs anxious to maintain continuity in their services and to cultivate potential residents and fellows. Had more rotating internships been available, Rothstein argues, straight internships would have had few takers.[31] Yet while 21 percent of all internships were vacant in 1965, 93 percent of straight internships in internal medicine were filled.[32]

The straight internship may well have been a convenience to department administrators, but its rapid growth was at least in part an accommodation to the many pressures toward earlier specialization in medical education and toward shortening the lengthy course of graduate study. Just as important, the straight internship was consistent with traditional student preferences for a practical education, and in the 1960s, the American Board of Internal Medicine endorsed one year's straight internship and three years' general internal medicine residency as sufficient qualification for its certification examination.

At the University of Iowa in the early 1960s, the basic pattern of the rotating internship had changed little since the 1920s, as interns moved through four-month stints in internal medicine and surgery and two months each in pediatrics and obstetrics-gynecology. However, the University of Iowa Department of Internal Medicine inaugurated a straight medical internship in 1965, and by 1969–70, the department was training fifteen straight interns while participating in the training of only six rotating interns. By the mid-1970s, the internship, as a distinct training period, had disappeared altogether in the University of Iowa Department of Internal Medicine. Nationally, the demise of the internship followed a long period of criticism of the system's shortcomings, with increasing numbers of observers charging that too often the internship provided at best a marginal educational experience.[33] Besides, as was the case at the University of Iowa, the change to the elective senior year provided students an experience that in many respects seemed to supersede the straight internship.

Policy changes by two national accrediting agencies paved the way for the demise of the internship in internal medicine. In 1970, the American Medical Association decreed, first, that after 1975, only internship programs linked to residency programs would be accredited, thus eliminating many rotating programs at smaller hospitals, and, second, that specialty boards could approve residency programs that did not require an internship year. As a result of those policy changes, university-affiliated teaching hospitals trained nearly 93 percent of all residents in 1974–75, compared to just 62 percent in 1962–63,[34] and following the AMA's lead, the American Board of Internal Medicine altered the eligibility standards for its certification examination from four years' training in general internal medicine (i. e., one-year straight internship and three-year residency) to three years' training in general internal medicine or two years in general internal medicine and one year in an internal medicine subspecialty.

In the 1960s and 1970s, the residency program in the University of Iowa Department of Internal Medicine retained much of its traditional format. In 1960, first-year residents worked the wards; second-year residents worked the subspecialty services; third-year residents continued those subspecialty service assignments and also played an important role in ward teaching. In 1975, the residency program still provided that broad experience in general internal medicine; however, Richard Freeman, the department's Associate Chair for Education, had, as noted in the previous chapter, done much to upgrade the residency experience. The first year, which incorporated much of the defunct internship year, consisted of four to six months of general medicine, two to three months of subspecialty training, and two months of specialty training outside the department, while the later years continued the traditional mix of general medicine and subspecialty experience.

At the University of Iowa, the Veterans Administration Hospital was an increasingly important part of the teaching complex. By 1960, internal medicine staff at the Veterans Hospital numbered a dozen, seven of them primarily responsible for patient care and teaching. Overall, the six Veterans wards offered 215 beds for residency training and student teaching, and an integrated residency program at the University of Iowa Hospitals and Clinics and the Veterans Hospital began in 1960. By 1973–74, in the wake of the reorganization described in the previous chapter, twelve residents and some fifteen fellows in internal medicine received all or part of their training at the Veterans Administration Hospital.

The 1960s and 1970s also brought a vigorous expansion of fellowship programs, an expansion that, like the ascendancy of the residency in the 1920s and 1930s, marked an important phase in the development of medical training in America. Just as the internship had supplemented basic undergraduate medical education with general practical experience, and the residency had supplemented the internship with specialized practical experience, so the fellowship supplemented the residency with a more intense and still more highly focused experience. Thus, first the internship, then the residency, and finally the fellowship considerably lengthened the course of medical education in the twentieth century, and the fellowship became an increasingly common route to both academic positions and to private practice.

The causes behind the rise of the fellowship were essentially those behind the general expansion of departments of internal medicine in post–World War II America: the explosion of scientific knowledge and technologies on the one hand and large-scale funding from federal agencies, especially the National

Institutes of Health, and voluntary health organizations on the other. Moreover, unlike the slow growth in federal investment in undergraduate medical education prior to the mid-1960s, funding of federal graduate research training programs rose from $48,000 in 1948 to $75 million in 1963, the latter nearly ten times the funding level of undergraduate training.[35]

While the growth in internal medicine fellowship programs at the University of Iowa was explosive in the late 1960s and early 1970s, it was also uneven, skewed by patterns of available funding and historic patterns of development in the subspecialties and divisions within the department. For example, the department first received funding for cardiovascular fellowships in the 1950s. Indeed, all seven of the department's fellowships in 1960–61 were in cardiovascular fields, a result both of the established position of the National Heart Institute within the National Institutes of Health and of cardiovascular's place as the Department of Internal Medicine's oldest and best developed subspecialty interest.

By 1963, there were three separate fellowship programs in cardiovascular areas: clinical cardiology, cardiovascular research, and clinical pharmacology. The first of those, the clinical cardiology fellowship, was a two-year program supported by a training grant from the National Heart Institute. It offered broad training in electrocardiography, cardiac catheterization, and clinical work, providing an intensive exposure to cardiology appropriate to either specialized private practice or academic medicine. The cardiovascular research fellowship and the clinical pharmacology fellowship were likewise supported by the National Heart Institute, but from the first they were meant to provide training chiefly for careers in academic research. Over the long term, the Cardiovascular Laboratories and its successor units—Cardiovascular, Nephrology, and Pulmonary Divisions—maintained some of the department's most expansive fellowship programs. By 1964, twenty of the department's cardiovascular trainees already held academic positions, twelve at the University of Iowa and eight more scattered from Missouri, Minnesota, and Oregon to England, Lebanon, and Japan.

Gastroenterology, another of the department's oldest interest sections, was also an early center of fellowship training and one in which expansion came rapidly. The Gastroenterology Training Program began in 1962, funded by a grant from the National Institute of Arthritis and Metabolic Diseases. Directed by James Clifton and Harold Schedl, whose reputations for clinical and laboratory skills were well established, the program expanded to four fellows in 1967–68, and in 1969–70, additional funding from the Veterans Administration pushed the number of fellows to eight.

Through the 1960s, fellowship programs also developed elsewhere in the department, first in diabetes-endocrinology and hematology, then in metabolism, infectious diseases, and allergy. By the 1970s, active fellowship programs of varying sizes were the norm in all divisions and sections. Meanwhile, the system of subspecialty and interdepartmental conferences put together in the late 1940s and 1950s expanded into the 1960s in support of fellowship programs, serving often as forums for the exchange of ideas and presentation of research results.

The internal medicine fellowship programs, in part because of their research emphasis, were increasingly a meeting ground between the clinical and basic sciences, yet another instance of the interdisciplinary potential inherent in highly specialized scientific and technological areas. That interdependence was evident early on, for example, in the Gastroenterology Training Program, which incorporated a considerable emphasis in physiology, and it was true also of the cardiovascular research and clinical pharmacology programs, the latter standing with one leg in pharmacology while the former focused increasingly on cellular biology.

Overall, the many changes in undergraduate and graduate education coupled with the increasing diversity in the student body substantially broadened and intensified the teaching responsibilities of internal medicine faculty in the 1960s and early 1970s. From basic science courses and the introductory clinical medicine course to junior clerkships, senior electives, and residency and fellowship programs, internal medicine faculty spent more hours in instruction than ever before and did so in closer contact with individual students. Likewise, they gave more attention to pedagogical methods and did more soul-searching over outcomes than ever before.

THE GENERAL PRACTITIONER CONTROVERSY AGAIN

Through the 1950s and 1960s, the structure of Iowa's health care market, tracing the movement of Iowa's population and much of its economy, continued its long shift from rural to urban. Simultaneously, medical practice in Iowa continued the long trend toward specialization. As a result, by 1970 even many of Iowa's larger market centers and county seats—towns of 5,000–10,000 population—felt the pinch of diminishing health care services.[36] In retrospect, however, it is not self-evident that health care had in fact become less readily available to Iowans, even rural Iowans. First, the ten years from 1950 to 1960 had seen a revolution in Iowa's transportation system with the addition of thousands of miles of paved highways and the grading of virtually all rural roads. To rural Iowans, physicians twenty-five or even fifty miles distant in 1965 were likely as accessible as physicians five miles distant had been in 1940. Second, the spread of third-party health coverage had likewise contributed to the revolution in the accessibility of health care. Third, the technologies that helped to make access to health care services such a vital issue were not, in any event, readily adaptable to small-town medical practice, both because of their expense and because they often required extensive networks of support services.

Nonetheless, local concerns meshed with a larger national consensus over the need for vastly expanded programs of medical education in order to supply the anticipated demand for physicians in the 1970s and beyond.[37] President Bowen's plan for expansion of enrollments at the University of Iowa College of Medicine was a product of that consensus. But as Dean Robert Hardin sagely noted in 1968, past enrollment expansions had not increased the physician population of Iowa. Moreover, the rural states of the Midwest—e.g., Iowa, Nebraska, Kansas—where the physician shortage was deemed most acute already led the nation in the rate at which their residents entered medical school.[38] As had been true at least since the early twentieth century, Iowa residents commonly left the state after graduation from medical school and few returned. Of the 139 Iowans in internship programs in 1974, for example, just 19 were located in Iowa; of the 605 Iowans in residencies in 1974, just 178 held positions in Iowa. Meanwhile, a total of ninety-two internships and residencies in Iowa were held by foreign-trained physicians, and a good many positions were vacant.[39]

However, rightly or wrongly, medical education and the University of Iowa College of Medicine once again became targets of criticism. As John Eckstein commented, the litany of complaints against academic medicine was a long and venerable one: academic physicians were suspected of restricting enrollments in order to boost physicians' incomes; they were accused of an Ivory Tower syndrome manifesting itself as an insensitivity to the health needs of the public; and they were charged with promoting overspecialization. In short, it was widely supposed "that the [medical] educational system is at the heart of today's problems, both for what it has done, and what it has failed to do."[40] More colloquially and more to the point, one Iowan inquired of President Bowen why the people of Iowa should "continue to support a medical college that has no interest in them."[41]

The University of Iowa's Department of Family Practice was one product of the health care debate, established in 1970 by the Iowa legislature along with associated residency programs at satellite locations throughout the state. The Department of Internal Medicine's response to the family practice program was mixed. On the one hand, as might be expected, internists were generally skeptical of a new specialty that appeared to make direct claims on a part of internal medicine's established turf. On the other hand, department personnel in fact played key roles in the project. In particular, internal medicine's Paul Seebohm chaired a special steering committee that worked with the legislature in designing the statewide system and subsequently chaired the Family Practice Education Advisory Board.

By itself, the family practice ideal was only a partial solution to the perceived problems in health care delivery in Iowa. That was so in part at least because public debate conflated the disappearance of rural practitioners with the disappearance of general practitioners, two related yet distinct problems. Although Iowa's traditional rural physicians had indeed been, for the most part, general practitioners, both specialists and general practitioners in Iowa in the late 1960s were increasingly unlikely to practice in rural areas. Moreover, the new family practice program's effectiveness would, in the end, hinge upon its ability to stop the net out-migration of Iowa physicians, most obviously by attracting new graduates of the University of Iowa College of Medicine to graduate training programs in Iowa and, hopefully, to medical practice within the state.

THE QUESTION OF FACULTY PARTICIPATION—PART I

Prior to the 1960s, there had been two great watersheds in the governance of the College of Medicine. The first came during the tenure of Lee Wallace Dean from 1915 to 1927. Dean had inherited a loose collegial administrative structure dating to the nineteenth century, a structure suited to an era of non-resident, entrepreneurial faculty. With solid backing from presidents Thomas Macbride and Walter Jessup, Dean had forged a tightly centralized administration in which he ruled the college with the advice and consent of his department heads, each of whom in turn ruled his own domain more or less as he saw fit. The second watershed came in the early 1950s, during the four-year interregnum that followed the death of Dean Mayo Soley. The resulting power vacuum had brought long held faculty grievances into the open and led to grudging change in the governance of the college. Most immediately, as we have seen, President Virgil Hancher had appointed a temporary executive committee to govern the college, and that committee continued to function, in however perfunctory a way, through the 1950s and 1960s, providing a tentative opening to wider faculty participation in the governance of the college.

The 1960s brought a third watershed to the College of Medicine when faculty demanded a democratic overhaul of the administrative apparatus. Because of the *ad hoc* nature of the changes instituted in the early 1950s, faculty participation in college affairs survived at the sufferance of the dean and university administration, and, during Dean Norman Nelson's tenure, faculty votes on policy issues were rare. Furthermore, Nelson's critics charged that the elected Executive Committee had become a listening committee, barely distinguishable in outlook from the Medical Council made up of department heads. By the early 1960s, faculty sentiment overwhelmingly favored a written constitution for the college, one that would clarify authority relations and procedures and formalize faculty rights.

Among those spearheading the campaign for the "Manual of Procedure," as it was known, was Raymond Sheets of internal medicine. In early 1961, Sheets was at the center of an informal group known as the Committee of Twenty, a group that at different times included a half dozen of Sheets' internal medicine colleagues. Sheets and his collaborators grounded their demands for a permanent faculty voice in College of Medicine affairs in a scathing estimation of past and present College of Medicine deans. From the time of Lee Wallace Dean, they charged, "this college has made its way without much help from the front office." In particular, many shared Raymond Sheets' characterization of Norman Nelson's regime as "weak" and "unimaginative," unable or unwilling to respond to the dramatic changes in medical science and medical education in the 1950s and the promise of even more dramatic changes in coming years. "The College is floundering," Sheets maintained in 1961, and Dean Nelson's health problems only magnified his natural limitations. The fact that Robert Hardin had stood in as acting dean when Nelson took several months sick leave in late 1960 and early 1961 and that President Hancher had subsequently seen fit to shift the dean's responsibility for student recruitment, staff affairs, and curriculum to Hardin underscored Sheets' complaints.

Sheets and the Committee of Twenty charged further that the College of Medicine as a whole placed too much emphasis on patient service and too little emphasis on scientific research. Of course, to some extent that complaint reflected the strains of a transitional period in the history of the college; after all, as late as 1960 both tradition and public expectations put patient service well ahead of scholarship. However, committee members argued that the problem ran much deeper. The distribution of power within the college, they charged, was seriously distorted by the fact that several smaller clinical departments with strong service orientations effectively controlled the Medical Council made up of department heads, and the Council, especially in light of the precarious state of Dean Nelson's health and what many saw as his innate indecisiveness, seemed the real center of power in the college.

The struggle over college governance left William Bean, as head of internal medicine, in an awkward position. Throughout his career, Bean professed little interest in institutional politics; at the same time, however, his reputation for scholarship made him something of an outcast among his fellow department heads on the service-oriented Medical Council. Raymond Sheets and his supporters saw Bean as a potential ally in the corridors of power and pushed Bean to take a more active role in the reform effort. Sheets hoped to use the Committee of Twenty to bring enough pressure "from the left," as he put it, to make William Bean look like a moderate to his Medical Council colleagues.

It was not William Bean, however, but the Council on Medical Education and Association of American Medical Colleges Liaison Committee report of 1960 that was the lever forcing faculty grievances into the open. In addition to its criticisms of the curriculum, that report also criticized the subordination of scientific research to patient service in the college. For several months, Dean Nelson's administration kept the report under wraps, assuring the faculty that all was fine, or, in any event, that any weaknesses were already being addressed. The Committee of Twenty's first success was to win distribution of the report to the faculty and to call a faculty meeting to discuss the report's conclusions and recommendations.

That February 1961 faculty meeting laid bare the divisions within the college, and it and subsequent meetings provided a forum for dissenting faculty to pursue their reform agenda. At a March meeting, internal medicine's James Clifton proposed to the dean the formation of a committee to investigate forms of governance at other medical colleges and to assemble a proposed manual of procedure for the college. Thus was born the Committee on Administrative Structure, elected by the faculty and including Raymond Sheets among its members. The committee labored through fifty-three meetings in the space of a year and a half before finishing its detailed proposals in January 1963.[42]

In the meantime, Norman Nelson resigned as dean effective June 30, 1962, and, at the suggestion of Lewis January and Henry Hamilton of internal medicine, President Virgil Hancher had designated the Committee on Administrative Structure to serve simultaneously as the deanship search committee. Committee surveys of faculty opinion revealed a clear majority in favor of a clinician-dean, a not very surprising result in view of tradition and the size of clinical departments in the college. More than a third of respondents named Robert Hardin as a desirable candidate because of his highly visible role in administration during the last years of Nelson's tenure. Hardin's internal medicine colleagues William Bean, Willis Fowler, and Lewis January received significant support as well. Overall, faculty responses expressed a clear conviction that a reorganization of the College of Medicine's administrative structure was "sorely needed" and should be part of the transition to new leadership.

The Committee on Administrative Structure, in its capacity as the deanship selection committee, completed its work in short order. Members explored an extensive list of outside candidates for the deanship, and in June and July 1962, three of those visited the campus. Robert Hardin, too, was invited for a "campus visit." Well regarded by colleagues and well known nationally, Hardin possessed considerable administrative talent and ambition, and when the committee subsequently recommended him for the deanship, many saw the choice as a welcome change from the uncertainties and timid leadership of Norman Nelson's last years in office.[43]

It was Robert Hardin's misfortune that he came to the deanship with the potentially explosive Manual of Procedure issue hanging over his head. Hardin initially devoted his attention to other problems in the college, notably the relatively small size of the college's faculty, low faculty salaries, and the lack of teaching space, especially in basic science areas. Hardin also addressed the curricular weaknesses noted by the Liaison Committee Report, opposing the block time format in the early phases of clinical instruction, engineering the previously described overhaul of the sophomore introduction to clinical medicine course to create a more integrated program, and eventually overseeing the extensive curricular revisions of the late 1960s.[44]

Meanwhile, the proposed Manual of Procedure remained in limbo. The major changes recommended in the manual, Hardin noted, might properly take years to implement; in any event, he was preoccupied with what were to him more pressing issues. Hardin did not deliver his official comments on the manual until six months after the formal committee report in January 1963, and his response revealed a firm preference for the old style of governance. Most importantly, while the Committee on Administrative Structure had recommended a six-member Executive Committee with representation evenly divided between clinical and basic science areas, Hardin preferred a five-member committee with its members chosen on an at-large basis. Reformers feared, not without reason, that because of the voting strength of hide-bound clinical departments, the latter scheme would not significantly affect the existing distribution of power within the college.

FACULTY PARTICIPATION—PART II

Howard Bowen's arrival as University of Iowa president in the fall of 1964 tipped the political balance in the College of Medicine against Robert Hardin on the Manual of Procedure issue. Bowen, who was an economist by training and came to the university after several years as president of Grinnell College, set as his goal the rejuvenation of what many believed had become a complacent university. To accomplish that, Bowen undertook an extensive faculty recruitment program, encouraged faculty research, implemented an expansion and reorganization of the university administration, and championed wider faculty participation in university affairs.

Robert Hardin was sympathetic to much of President Bowen's program, including the desirability of enlarging and improving faculty and facilities in the health sciences. However, Hardin differed with Bowen on two critical points. First, Bowen was sympathetic to a fundamental redistribution of authority in the

College of Medicine; Hardin, as a disciple of Virgil Hancher, was not. Second, Bowen's administrative style was, in Stow Persons' characterization, "aloof,"[45] while Hardin preferred a more hands-on approach to administration. The fact that Robert Hardin had been among the candidates to succeed Virgil Hancher as president of the university and that he believed the Board of Regents' decision had come down to a choice between him and Howard Bowen further complicated relations between the two men.

By 1967, faculty discontent over Hardin's stonewalling of the Manual of Procedure, combined with the democratic tone of President Howard Bowen's administration and the contentious political environment on and off the campus, brought the governance issue to a boil once again. In the summer of 1967, after at least a year's gestation, President Bowen unveiled a significant reorganization of the health sciences campus and the dean's office of the College of Medicine. At the heart of Bowen's plan was a new office, Vice-President for Medical Affairs, to whom the executive of the College of Medicine and the director of the University Hospitals would report. As dean of the College of Medicine, Robert Hardin was Bowen's choice to fill the new post. At the same time, Bowen's plan created a new executive associate dean to take charge of day-to-day operations of the College of Medicine. In effect, Robert Hardin had been booted upstairs, or so it appeared.

In part, Bowen intended his reorganization to address the long-standing frictions between the College of Medicine and the University Hospitals. The relationship of teaching hospitals and medical schools in general had long been recognized as "a tender and complicated subject."[46] In 1950, President Virgil Hancher, reacting to an earlier wave of faculty complaints, had conceded the hospitals' ambiguous position as a "laboratory" of the college and a "service institution" to the state,[47] and during deanship searches in both the early 1950s and early 1960s, the medical faculty expressed the conviction that the new dean should have authority over the hospitals. Howard Bowen was sympathetic to that claim, recognizing the "primary purpose" of the hospitals as "laboratory facilities for instruction and research."[48]

In any event, the delegation of authority that Bowen instituted in the College of Medicine clearly fitted his personal style of leadership. Just as clearly, Bowen's preferences were not Robert Hardin's. Nonetheless, Bowen pushed ahead, shifting Hardin to the new vice-presidency and appointing Daniel Stone as the new executive associate dean of the College of Medicine. Like Hardin, Stone was a professor of internal medicine; in fact, Hardin, because of his interest in diabetes research, had been instrumental in bringing Stone to the University of Iowa. Thus, Stone had both Bowen and Hardin to thank for his position as chief executive officer of the College of Medicine.

From Bowen's perspective, Stone's appointment promised the smoothest possible working relationship between the dean and his chief executive in the

College of Medicine, and Robert Hardin may even have harbored similar hopes. However, such optimism was doomed to disappointment. Bowen's plan to free the dean from the day-to-day tedium of administration in order to focus on the big picture resulted in hopelessly muddled lines of communication and authority between Hardin and Stone, among Hardin, Stone, and the university administration, and among Hardin, Stone, and the College of Medicine faculty. The new arrangement also left Stone in control of the dean's office and exiled Hardin to Westlawn, the old nurses' dormitory. Meetings between Hardin and Stone failed to resolve the difficulties, and the two men became increasingly estranged.

President Bowen's summer 1967 reorganization was only the first step in a thoroughgoing overhaul of the College of Medicine administration, and, with Bowen's backing, the medical faculty in July 1967 passed a resolution to create a Committee on Faculty Participation. Chaired by Raymond Sheets, the committee's charge was to compile a Manual of Procedure for the college by November. Drawing heavily upon Sheets' earlier experience with the Committee on Administrative Structure, the new committee submitted its working draft to the university's central administration in October 1967 and presented its final draft to the faculty on November 30. Of the 295 eligible voters in the College of Medicine, 219 cast their ballots in early December, giving the Manual of Procedure 81 percent approval. William Bean later commented to President Bowen that he never doubted that "a truly secret ballot ... where everyone could vote without his boss knowing what he said" would show solid support behind the manual.[49]

However, the new Manual of Procedure, coming so close on the heels of President Bowen's summer administrative reorganization, was a bitter pill for Robert Hardin. The Manual of Procedure's expressed intent was "to foster an active, informed faculty," a faculty prepared to play a major role in procedural and policy issues in the college,[50] but Hardin argued during a November meeting with Raymond Sheets and his committee that few faculty were well enough informed on salient issues facing medical education generally and the University of Iowa College of Medicine specifically to handle the burdens that the manual would thrust upon them. Meanwhile, various department chairs, resentful of the dilution of their authority in the college, voiced similar opposition to the committee's plan.

Nonetheless, faced with the overwhelming faculty vote in December, Robert Hardin reluctantly sent the Manual of Procedure to President Bowen with his recommendation that Bowen approve the document as written, and on January 15, 1968, Bowen gave it his imprimatur.[51] One of Raymond Sheets' internal medicine colleagues welcomed the Manual of Procedure as the "most progressive step that I have seen in this institution for the some 20 years I have been here," and many others agreed.[52] In its final form the manual was of immense symbolic and practical importance. Extending and codifying the process of reform begun in the early 1950s, the manual protected the faculty's right to make policy recommendations to the dean through an elected executive committee empowered to choose its own officers. The manual also assured a distribution of power on the committee between basic science and clinical departments and guaranteed executive committee representation for assistant and associate professors. Finally, the manual set in place a mechanism for periodic departmental reviews.

For Robert Hardin, the upheavals of 1967 and 1968 were trying and painful. Not only did most of Hardin's internal medicine colleagues—many of whom otherwise liked and respected him and welcomed his return to the department in the late 1970s—oppose his position on the Manual of Procedure; the few entrenched opponents of reform elsewhere in the College of Medicine also castigated Hardin for bowing to the reformers' demands. When Howard Bowen resigned as university president in 1969, and the Board of Regents selected his chief lieutenant Willard L. Boyd to succeed him, Hardin resigned both as dean of the College of Medicine and as vice-president for medical affairs. Boyd then appointed Hardin his vice-president for health affairs, a more ambiguously defined advisory post.

Ironically, Robert Hardin had brought to the deanship much of the vigor and decisiveness that many had found wanting in his predecessor, and his tenure was, in many respects, strikingly successful. In particular, Hardin took a close interest in the modernization of the curriculum, the planning of several important construction projects on the health sciences campus, the genesis of the Iowa Regional Medical Program, the aggressive expansion in faculty numbers and salaries in the Department of Internal Medicine and elsewhere in the college, and the upgrading of facilities and programs at the Veterans Administration Hospital. Moreover, Hardin's stand on the Manual of Procedure, although not in keeping with the temper of the times, was not without merit. As he pointed out in the fall of 1967, a necessary corollary to decentralization and democratization in the College of Medicine was faculty members' willingness over the long term to accept the responsibilities vested in them. In the absence of such a commitment, Hardin warned, the college might well return to the combination of aimless drift and control by small interest groups that the Committee of Twenty had criticized. Through the 1970s and 1980s, as the college grew larger and more heterogeneous and as the political climate of the college, the university, and the nation at large became more complacent, the full participation of an active, informed faculty in fact became a matter of concern once again.

THE PASSING OF THE TORCH: JOHN ECKSTEIN

Robert Hardin's resignation of the deanship and his vice-presidency in 1969 marked the end of President Bowen's experiment in divided administration in the College of Medicine as well as his attempt to use his vice president for medical affairs to smooth relations between the college and the University Hospitals. Hardin's resignation also brought William O. Rieke—Professor in the Department of Anatomy and chair of the newly elected executive committee—to the position of dean *pro tem* in September 1969.

One of Rieke's first acts was to circulate a letter apprising faculty of the deanship's consolidation, pointedly noting that Robert Hardin's new role as vice-president for health affairs was strictly one of advisor to the president's provost. Daniel Stone—his functions as executive associate dean effectively superseded—then offered Rieke his resignation.[53] Rieke also announced a restructuring of the internal administration of the college, including the naming of four associate deans: academic affairs, student affairs, Veterans Hospital affairs, and community medicine. From internal medicine, Daniel Stone became associate dean of academic affairs and John Eckstein became associate dean of Veterans Hospital affairs, a position for which Stone, while still chief executive officer in the college, had recommended Eckstein in January.

As head of the executive committee, William Rieke also became chair of the deanship selection committee formed in the spring of 1969 when Robert Hardin gave notice of his resignation. President Howard Bowen told committee members, including James Clifton of internal medicine, that while he expected a search conducted in a "very judicious, careful manner," he also hoped to see a new dean installed by the start of the fall semester, a date that would mark the end of his tenure in office.[54]

Following much the same procedure as in 1962, the selection committee began by soliciting faculty input on several issues, including the organization of the dean's office, overall goals of the College of Medicine, desirable qualifications in a new dean, and suggestions of possible candidates. Also as in 1962, the committee gave close scrutiny to a number of candidates, both inside and outside the college. The strongest of the candidates were Robert Van Citters, then Professor of Physiology and Associate Dean at the University of Washington, and John Eckstein of the Department of Internal Medicine, whose candidacy rested upon his administrative work, particularly his work with the Veterans Administration Hospital, and his national reputation as a research scientist. Van Citters visited the campus in November 1969 to meet with the selection committee and the medical faculty; early the following month Eckstein also made a "campus visit."

Both Van Citters and Eckstein had detractors. Some disapproved of Van Citters because he was not a clinician. In the long history of the College of

Medicine, only one non-clinician, Ewen MacEwen, had served as permanent dean, and few faculty held fond memories of MacEwen's tenure. There were also rumblings that Van Citters was too ready to embrace untested innovations in medical education and to bow to political pressures for expanded enrollments. At the same time, a handful of older clinical representatives on the selection committee opposed Eckstein's candidacy, perhaps reluctant to have a former student as dean and intimidated, too, by his scientific reputation and research orientation. However, Eckstein did have strong support on the committee from basic science representatives for whom research was the *sine qua non* of academic life. In addition, John Eckstein enjoyed wide support among his peers in internal medicine and in the college generally; both William Bean and Walter Kirkendall, for example, wrote warm letters of endorsement of his candidacy.[55]

In December 1969, the selection committee unanimously recommended that President Boyd offer the deanship to Van Citters. However, he had also been negotiating for the deanship at the University of Washington, and when the Iowa offer became public, it prompted a similar offer from Washington, which Van Citters accepted. By year's end, then, the deanship selection process was effectively deadlocked, one faction of the selection committee steadfastly opposed to John Eckstein, who remained, nonetheless, the committee's only real candidate.

From a historical perspective, such an impasse was no great surprise. In the past, after all, the search for a new dean had commonly been a prolonged, politically charged affair, a time of much soul-searching and debate over the past, present, and future of the College of Medicine. The constitutional revisions of 1968 had not significantly diminished the dean's fundamental importance in directing development of the college, and most appreciated that the scope and pace of change in academic medicine during the late 1960s and 1970s made this choice of a new dean one of the most critical in the college's history.

With the deanship search at an impasse, William Rieke unexpectedly announced his desire to be named permanent dean. But Rieke's candidacy sparked immediate controversy among many selection committee members who saw his entry into the race as a blatant conflict of interest. In early January 1970, Rieke responded to his critics by circulating to committee members a four-page letter withdrawing his name from consideration and stating his intention to continue as chair of the selection committee in accordance with President Willard Boyd's wish that the original committee continue its work.[56] Committee members then turned their attentions to John Eckstein, and, in April 1970, after extensive discussions concerning, among other issues, the organization and funding of the dean's office, the committee unanimously recommended John Eckstein for the deanship, an office that he would hold for the next twenty-one years.

CONCLUSION

A colleague later remembered that John Eckstein's assumption of the deanship on June 1, 1970, rescued the College of Medicine from "troubled times."[57] Certainly, it marked the end of a tumultuous decade, both for the Department of Internal Medicine and for the college. Just as certainly, Eckstein's ascent to the deanship was a triumph for the forces of reform and modernization in the College of Medicine, an event capping twenty years of rapid growth accompanied at times by intense conflict.

In all, the two decades from 1950 to 1970 held many similarities to that earlier "golden age" from 1910 to 1930. Both periods saw fundamental administrative change in the College of Medicine, change that led in both cases to the dean's downfall; both periods also saw a heightened emphasis on medical research in the college and fundamental changes in the nature, content, and scale of medical education; and in both periods the Department of Internal Medicine itself and many individual internal medicine faculty were central actors in the drama of reform and modernization. For the Department of Internal Medicine, the years from 1960 to 1975 were especially important, as the department expanded and defined its role in the College of Medicine, broadened its participation in and commitment to the world of medical science, and multiplied and strengthened its connections with the physicians of Iowa.

The list of contributors to those developments was a long one, but Raymond Sheets deserves special mention. While Sheets did not achieve the scientific reputation of his friend and collaborator Henry Hamilton, his remarkable talent for institutional politics was a key to the adoption of the Manual of Procedure in 1968, and the importance of that document went far beyond simple questions of governance. Raymond Sheets knew full well that radical change in the College of Medicine's traditional power structure was essential to foster a more scientific orientation among his sometimes reluctant colleagues and to fit his department and the college as a whole for their roles in the increasingly competitive world of academic medicine.

It is also fitting to grant special mention to William Bean. Admittedly, Bean was to some extent a reluctant reformer, in part because of his essential conservatism and in part because of his disdain for political affairs. Nonetheless, Bean's humanism, his erudition, and his standing as an apostle of the scientific attitude that triumphed in American medicine in the 1960s made him a radical symbol throughout his years as head of the Department of Internal Medicine, a stance that sparked a mixture of respect, suspicion, and fear among his fellow department heads. While William Bean's retirement as head of internal medicine in 1970 marked the end of one era, his influence over the span of twenty years had helped to usher in a new and promising future.

8

The Challenge of Excellence

1975–1990

ROM 1945 to 1975, the transformation of the University of Iowa Department of Internal Medicine closely followed experience in American academic medicine at large. Both at a national level and at the University of Iowa, the expansion of research funding, especially from federal sources, had made academic medical research a major enterprise; indeed, medical research was one of America's premier postwar growth industries. Patient care had also become a major industry, thanks to public funding of health care for the poor and elderly, an expanded array of patient services, and technological and scientific advances that attracted a more diverse patient population. Finally, academic physicians' teaching responsibilities had expanded rapidly with surging undergraduate enrollments, greater attention to individual and small group instruction, and the proliferation of more specialized and more rigorous graduate training programs.

Those first three postwar decades had not been without problems, but the problems had chiefly to do with accommodating institutions and attitudes to the pressures of rapid growth and change. In contrast, while change remained a major theme in the years from 1975 to 1990, some aspects of that later period also bore an unsettling resemblance to the lean times of the depression and World War II, as American medicine, particularly academic medicine, staggered under the cumulative effects of a slow relative decline in the American economy. In Iowa in particular, a stubborn agricultural recession in the 1980s amplified the effect, severely straining budgets of the state and of local governments, cramping appropriations for the University of Iowa, and prompting repeated reversions of university funds to the state treasury. Between

1971 and 1991, the proportion of all university revenues derived from state appropriations fell from 34.2 to 24.9 percent, as earnings from sales and services, chiefly from the University of Iowa Hospitals and Clinics, rose from 11.4 to 36.3 percent of total university revenues.[1]

Despite the general economic downturn, health care costs continued to rise at an alarming pace through the 1980s, both in Iowa and across the nation. By 1989, Americans' total health care expenditures climbed to 600 billion dollars, up from seventy-five billion dollars in 1970, and health care expenditures consumed nearly 12 percent of the gross national product. Meanwhile, Medicare expenditures rose from 7.1 billion dollars in 1970 to 35.7 billion in 1980 and to 81.2 billion dollars in 1989, and federal Medicaid costs rose from 5.2 to 49.4 billion dollars in those two decades. In the 1980s, the average physician's income also rose 73 percent, a rate well above the growth in average household income.[2] Even though Iowans' per capita health care expenditures lagged slightly behind national averages, they, too, more than doubled in the 1980s, a 9 percent annual rate of increase, and by 1990, the cost of the average hospital stay in Iowa surpassed $5,000.[3]

The stubborn inflation throughout the health care sector intensified the cost management efforts begun in the early 1970s. And since hospital care and physicians' services together claimed some 60 percent of health care expenditures, federal and state legislatures and regulatory agencies—abetted by private insurers and large employers—produced a changing alphabet soup of regulatory acronyms, from HSA, PPS, and DRG's to MVPS and RBRVS.[4] The common thread joining such regulatory initiatives was the desire of legislators, regulators, insurers, and employers alike to inject quality assurance and accountability into the health care system, particularly into the physician's decision-making process and into the allocation of health care resources.

For their part, clinicians—accustomed to approaching health care from the perspective of individual patients rather than aggregate costs—often resented the added administrative burdens as well as the intrusion of third parties into the physician-patient relationship. Nonetheless, "cost-effectiveness," "outcomes management," and "clinical guidelines" were inevitable additions to the lexicon of health care during the 1980s,[5] and the Association of American Medical Colleges, the American Medical Association, and the American Hospital Association endorsed the incorporation of cost-management strategies into the medical curriculum and into continuing education programs as well.[6]

Medical research also came under scrutiny in the late 1970s and 1980s, and here, too, there were questions of quality and accountability. While the rate of return from medical research had been debated in the press, in congressional hearings, and elsewhere since the 1960s, the questions raised in the 1980s struck directly at the credibility and integrity of the research enterprise. One of the most striking examples was the debate over ethnic and gender bias in medical research and its implications for the quality of care accorded minorities and women, a debate that shifted from the margins to the mainstream of medical scientific dialogue. In 1985, the U.S. Public Health Service Task Force on Women's Health Issues issued a path-breaking report; in 1990, responding to mounting political pressures, the National Institutes of Health established an Office of Minority Programs and an Office of Research on Women's Health to insure fuller representation of minorities and women in clinical research; and in 1991, the American Medical Association's Council on Ethical and Judicial Affairs issued a report reiterating many of the critical women's health issues.[7]

At a more general level, some critics complained of a deterioration in the quality of published studies in the medical literature, citing flawed methodologies, inadequate controls, the proliferation of cross-sectional as opposed to longitudinal studies and clinical trials, and an increasing tendency to use the same data in several published papers.[8] At the same time, the exponential growth in specialty journals provided an expanding market for publication. To some at least, it appeared that the demand for publishable material combined with academic medicine's publish or perish ethos—critical to promotion, research funding, and professional recognition—tempted researchers to publish as much as possible as quickly as possible. In response to a handful of well-publicized scandals, the *Journal of the American Medical Association* implemented stringent new requirements for authors in October 1989.[9]

Quality and accountability figured also in the troubling relationship between the pharmaceutical industry and academic medicine. As early as 1961, one observer excoriated the "unwholesome entanglement of doctors with the makers and sellers of drugs,"[10] and that issue only intensified as the Kefauver Amendments of 1962 required more rigorous testing of drugs and as industry sales and profits skyrocketed in the 1960s and 1970s. With hundreds of millions of dollars at stake in the development and marketing of drugs, the industry was critically dependent upon the goodwill of physicians, especially academic physicians, and used a variety of devices to cultivate their cooperation. In response, the American Medical Association and the American College of Physicians issued new guidelines in the 1980s governing industry sponsored meetings, gifts and hospitality, and the conduct of clinical trials.[11]

In view of the above, it is little wonder that the authors of a 1978 article labeled the academic medical center a "stressed institution." Certainly that was true, as the authors pointed out, in terms of the apparent change from symbiosis to confrontation in the relationship between academic medical centers and the federal government.[12] Likewise, it was true in terms of faltering public trust in medicine in general and in academic medicine in particular—what Eric Cassell has called the "demystification of physicians and medicine."[13] Stress was visible also in terms of academic physicians' increasing difficulty in balancing the needs and demands of diverse constituencies.[14] Finally, academic health centers faced increasing competition in the marketing of health care services. Many observers argued in the 1980s that complex changes in the structures of health care delivery combined with increasingly intrusive regulatory mechanisms and changing consumer attitudes on health care issues had significantly undermined the academic health center's leadership position in American medicine.[15] In retrospect, perhaps little of that was unique to the 1980s; indeed, such observations tended only to underscore two central axioms from medical history. The first was Roy Porter's useful warning that "medicine has always been, to a large degree, a buyers' market." The second, a reminder from Paul Starr, was that Americans' long fixation with health "has not always produced faith in doctors."[16] Both are old lessons that American medicine had, perhaps understandably, forgotten in the flush of post–World War II growth and discovery.

While the University of Iowa Department of Internal Medicine was not immune to any of the above pressures, it nonetheless maintained an impressive rate of growth through the 1980s, a record that seemed in many respects to contradict the atmosphere of gloom said to envelop much of academic medicine. From 1975 to 1990, the internal medicine faculty increased by half; the department's patient service load—still an increasingly important source of departmental funding—held to a steady pattern of growth; the department's research budget rose nearly 400 percent; and the department also substantially enhanced its standing in the larger medical scientific community as several faculty members rose to positions of national leadership in a variety of professional organizations.

FRANÇOIS ABBOUD: AN AMERICAN SUCCESS STORY

Just as William Bean's philosophical bent had left its mark on the department in the 1950s and 1960s and James Clifton's organizational vision had shaped the department for much of the 1970s, the Department of Internal Medicine bore François M. Abboud's imprint in the 1980s. Not only was Abboud's a quintessentially American success story, one that intersected many salient trends in postwar academic medicine; his personal odyssey also illustrates the remarkable range of factors involved in the making of a modern academic career. Moreover, Abboud's story exemplifies the experiences and contributions of the foreign medical graduates who came to the United States in increasing numbers in the postwar years.[17]

François Abboud was born in Cairo, Egypt, in 1931. His father was of Palestinian and Greek descent, his mother a Lebanese Maronite Christian.

Abboud's parents placed special value on schooling, not least as a means of self-improvement, and both were closely involved with education. Abboud's mother directed Saint Theresa's, a private Christian school for girls, and his father for many years taught college English and later in life earned a journalism degree and became an editor for *Al Ahram*.

François Abboud attended one of Cairo's many Christian schools for boys, schools conducted by French religious orders and patronized by Egyptian elites—Muslim and non-Muslim alike—in the 1930s and 1940s. In 1948, Abboud moved on to university, first to the University of Cairo, where he completed the premedical scientific curriculum, and then to Ains Chams University, where he graduated in medicine in 1955. Reflecting the continuing British influence in Egypt, the medical faculty at Ains Chams in those years was still chiefly British; instruction and texts were in English; and the most ambitious and capable Egyptian medical graduates often undertook graduate work in England.

England was not in François Abboud's future, however, largely because of a Manitowoc, Wisconsin, schoolteacher named Agnese Dunne. Dunne, who was in Egypt as a Fulbright Fellow, chanced upon St. Theresa's in 1953, met François Abboud, and very soon developed a proprietary interest in his career and urged him to pursue graduate work in the United States. Taking matters into her own hands, Dunne sent Abboud's academic records to Marquette University, where they eventually reached the chief of medicine at Milwaukee County Hospital, the teaching hospital affiliated with what is known now as the Medical College of Wisconsin. To his surprise, François Abboud received an offer of a residency at County Hospital, and in June 1955, not yet having completed his internship, Abboud and his wife of two weeks left for the United States.

Agnese Dunne was not the only chance influence on Abboud's career. On the one hand, swelling Arab nationalism and anti-western sentiment in Egypt had significantly narrowed the opportunities open to a westernized Christian minority in the 1950s; that was one factor in François Abboud's decision to come to America. On the other hand, foreign physicians were not always well received in America and in the best of circumstances faced trying cultural adjustments, problems often more acute for their spouses. For the Abbouds, the move from cosmopolitan Cairo to the American Midwest was a difficult one, but the outbreak of the Suez War disrupted their plan to return to Egypt in 1956. Barely two years later, the Abbouds exchanged their temporary visas for permanent resident status.

Abboud's professional aims were also extremely fluid in those early years. His initial goal in coming to Milwaukee was a residency in pediatrics, which he planned to use as a steppingstone to a rural practice in Egypt. Instead, he opted for a residency in internal medicine, the latter a considerably larger and, so Abboud was advised, more rigorous program at County Hospital. It was only in the third year of his residency that Abboud decided to specialize in cardiology. The bulk of his subspecialty training, then, much of it in cardiac catheterization, came also at Milwaukee County Hospital during the two fellowship years that followed (1958–1960).

A Wisconsin Heart Association research grant supported François Abboud's fellowship training, but here, too, chance played an important part in shaping his career. Possessing limited research experience, Abboud had stumbled upon his research topic—arterial elasticity in essential hypertension—during a weekend spent poring over past issues of *Circulation,* where he found a 1957 study of arterial elasticity that drew his attention both for its subject matter and for its flawed methodology.[18] At that moment, although he did not yet know it, François Abboud had found not only a research topic; he had also found a career.

Abboud's two-year fellowship at Milwaukee County Hospital, crowded as it was with clinical responsibilities, afforded disappointingly little time for research. His next objective, then, was a place in a more research-oriented environment, and because of his developing interest in cardiology, Abboud thought first of Columbia University and Andre Cournand, the Nobel Prize winner. Abboud went to New York in the fall of 1959, talked with Cournand, and was accepted to Cournand's program for the following year. However, a Milwaukee cardiologist, Francis Rosenbaum, counseled Abboud not to go to Columbia, warning him that he might be overlooked among Cournand's corps of students. Instead, Rosenbaum offered to introduce Abboud to several acquaintances at the American Heart Association meeting in Philadelphia in November, and there Abboud might find other prospects.

In Philadelphia, one of Rosenbaum's and Abboud's contacts was the University of Iowa's John Eckstein. Abboud and Eckstein discovered their mutual interest in the physiology of hypertension, and Eckstein invited Abboud to visit Iowa City before making a commitment to Columbia. Arriving in late autumn, Abboud experienced Iowa City at its worst, chilled by both a cold rain and the sadly dilapidated Hotel Jefferson. Even worse, he found the facilities at the College of Medicine, where research was still an enterprise of uncertain status, lacking as well. Nonetheless, he was impressed with the warmth and personal interest displayed by several of his would-be internal medicine colleagues, especially Ernest Theilen, Walter Kirkendall, and William Connor.

Based on his mixed impressions during that brief visit, Abboud made a one-year commitment to the University of Iowa, planning then to return to Milwaukee to join the faculty at the Medical College of Wisconsin. However, that one-year commitment soon stretched to four and then five years, during which time Abboud moved from instructor to assistant professor while working happily and, at least in his retelling, in relative anonymity probing the mechanisms of arterial pressure regulation. Others, it should be noted, contend that François Abboud's devotion to his work and the echoes of his occasionally spirited debates with John Eckstein could hardly have gone unnoticed; on the contrary, they are solidly entrenched in departmental lore.

In 1961, Abboud published two important papers based on his earlier research at Milwaukee. The first of those demonstrated that arterial elasticity varied in inverse proportion to age, and the second argued that the majority of subjects with essential hypertension in fact exhibited arterial elasticities within the normal range for their age groups.[19] Building on that early work, Abboud subsequently collaborated with John Eckstein on a series of published studies on the general problem of blood pressure regulation, a partnership that lasted until Eckstein became dean in 1970.

With the formal divisionalization of the Department of Internal Medicine under department chair James Clifton, François Abboud became head of the new Division of Cardiovascular Diseases. Clifton saw that the new cardiovascular division would be the largest and most important of the department's subspecialty divisions; thus, its vitality was a key to the future of the entire department. On the basis of seniority and reputation, Lewis January was the most obvious choice to head the new division, but January had no interest in administrative duties and declined to be considered. Walter Kirkendall, then head of the Cardiovascular Laboratories, was a second obvious choice. However, Kirkendall's expertise lay in renal physiology rather than cardiology, and he, too, declined.

From the outset, François Abboud may well have been Clifton's first choice as division head. Although younger than the others, Abboud enjoyed a background in cardiology, an enviable record as a researcher, and abundant ambition. In addition, neither January, Kirkendall, nor Clifton wanted to risk losing Abboud to another institution. January and Kirkendall, then, concurred with Clifton in naming Abboud head of Cardiovascular Diseases.

As division head, one of François Abboud's most important assets was his appreciation of the value of a programmatic approach to medical research, one built upon collective rather than individual research initiatives and one emphasizing linkages across divisional and departmental lines. As research funds became relatively more scarce, he argued, only state-of-the-art research projects would be funded. For internists in particular, the growing significance of molecular biology in medical research mandated close cooperation with colleagues in basic science areas, and Abboud himself held a joint appointment in the Departments of Physiology and Biophysics. Internists, Abboud warned, could not sell second-rate basic research to funding agencies.

To support the new research agenda, Abboud saw the need for new organizational forms that he called "horizontal" structures impressed upon existing departments and divisions, or "vertical" structures. He conceded that the latter structures would survive because of their deep historical roots and their administrative convenience, but they were not well suited to the needs of the modern academic health center in either research or patient service areas. The Cardiovascular Center, which Abboud did much to establish and subsequently directed, was an example of the new institutional forms, bringing together researchers from a variety of disciplines in a coordinated research endeavor. For Abboud, the Cardiovascular Center represented the shape of the future.[20]

By its nature, interdisciplinary research heightened the degree of integration and interdependence among the various departments within the College of Medicine, helping to overcome a long tradition of competitive interdepartmental relationships. François Abboud argued, for example, that the rise of molecular biology had increased the department's dependence on certain of the basic science areas; thus, the Department of Internal Medicine had a vested interest in upgrading the basic science departments, some of which—in the view of Liaison Committee visitors—had slipped significantly in the 1950s and 1960s.

By the 1970s, many in the department saw François Abboud as an almost certain bet to become department head, if not at Iowa then elsewhere. Nonetheless, when James Clifton announced his intention in 1975 to step down from the department chair and Abboud put himself in contention for the position, his was, by most estimates, a dark horse candidacy. John Thompson, whom Clifton had recruited in the late 1960s as his vice-chair in charge of Veterans Affairs, was perhaps the odds-on favorite because of his wide-ranging service to the department. The selection committee also considered outside candidates. Whatever the odds, François Abboud viewed the position of department chair as an opportunity to apply his vision across the Department of Internal Medicine, and the detailed plans for departmental development that he presented during his interview with the selection committee propelled him to the top of the candidate list. In 1976, Abboud succeeded James Clifton as chair of the Department of Internal Medicine.

François Abboud's was arguably the most forceful personality to occupy the department chair since Campbell Howard, a gift that Abboud used to reinforce the sense of urgency and purpose that James Clifton had injected into the Department of Internal Medicine in the late 1960s and early 1970s. Abboud's particular concern was to solidify the department's position as a major research center. While he preferred to view the department's patient service mission in terms of clinical opportunities rather than clinical responsibilities, Abboud, like many of his colleagues, worried that fiscal and political factors had forced his department and the college at large to invest excessive time and energy in patient service at the expense of research. The college, Abboud warned, had been at least a decade late in embracing scientific research and had been scrambling since the 1960s to catch up with the competition.

Like many of his colleagues in academic medicine, François Abboud was skeptical of the trend toward applied research. Instead, Abboud emphasized the symbiotic relationship between basic research and practical applications. After all, he argued, most questions raised in clinical practice can be answered only in the laboratory. Often those answers come from basic research that may at first appear to be unrelated.[21] Moreover, Abboud maintained that, just as had been true in the past, uncovering causes and cures through basic research was the answer both to the spiraling cost of half-way health care technologies, such as coronary bypass surgery and kidney transplants, and to resultant schemes for the rationing of scarce health care resources.[22]

Abboud carried the same enthusiasm and conviction to his work in the broader community of medical science. During the 1970s and 1980s, he held a variety of national committee assignments with, for example, the American Heart Association, the American Physiological Society, and the National Heart, Lung, and Blood Institute, and he was president of the American Federation for Clinical Research. He was editor-in-chief of *Circulation Research* from 1981 to 1986 and president of the Central Society for Clinical Research in 1986. In 1987, he began a six-year term on the board of governors of the American Board of Internal Medicine. In 1990, he was president of both the American Heart Association and the Association of American Physicians and shared the CIBA International Prize for Hypertension Research with his longtime colleague and friend, Michael J. Brody.

By 1990, François Abboud's career had taken him a long way indeed from the Christian Brothers' School in Cairo. It had also taken him in unforeseen directions. In both respects, Abboud's personal history closely paralleled the history of the Department of Internal Medicine. However, Abboud was not yet convinced that his department's status as a major research center was secure, and a *U.S. News and World Report* survey lauding the University of Iowa College of Medicine as one of America's up-and-coming medical schools was as much cause for worry as for celebration. For the long term, Abboud argued, an established research reputation was essential to the department's ability to recruit quality faculty, to provide quality teaching and patient care, and to attract quality students to its graduate programs.

FACULTY EXPANSION: TENURE TRACK AND ASSOCIATES

Several factors drove continued expansion of internal medicine faculty ranks through the 1980s. Most important were the department's increasing teaching obligations, especially in expanding graduate areas; the department's patient care obligations pursuant to the University of Iowa Hospitals and Clinics' tertiary care mandate; the crucial place of practice income in maintaining departmental operations; and the department's extraordinary success in attracting research funding.[23]

In 1975, the last year of James Clifton's tenure as chair, the department numbered eighty-eight tenure-track faculty, including four women. A decade later, in 1985–86, the department comprised 103 tenure-track faculty, including forty professors, thirty-one associate professors, and thirty-two assistant professors. In the latter year, department staff also included three instructors, nineteen associates, fifteen clinical associate professors, and thirteen clinical lecturers. In 1989–90, mirroring the 15 percent growth in full-time internal medicine faculty nationwide since 1985,[24] the department numbered 134 tenure-track faculty, including joint appointments, plus thirty-four associates and sixteen associate and assistant research scientists. All told, the department showed an increase of 52.3 percent in tenure-track faculty in the fifteen years from 1975–1990, while the aggregate increase for all clinical departments in the college of medicine was 67.8 percent.

At the end of the 1980s, nine internal medicine faculty held primary appointments in other areas, ranging from preventive medicine to religion. At the same time, sixteen M.D. and Ph.D. staff held secondary appointments in related fields. For example, four faculty from the Division of Cardiovascular Diseases held secondary appointments in physiology and biophysics, radiology, pharmacology, and electrical and computer engineering; three faculty from the Division of Rheumatology held appointments in microbiology, pathology, and orthopedic surgery; and three faculty from the Division of General Internal Medicine held appointments in surgery, biochemistry, and family practice.

By the mid-1980s, the department had created a three-track system of associate appointments designed to address different needs and goals, in part a response to the increasingly competitive market for promising faculty candidates. The first of those associate tracks, the full-time clinical appointments, provided candidates one to three years of additional clinical experience prior to private practice. The second, the basic research training track, generally provided candidates two years of additional research training prior to an academic career. The third class of associate appointment, known as "intent to appoint to tenure track," provided candidates one to two years of protected time for additional academic experience prior to appointment as assistant professor in the department. This last afforded the department a means to hold potential faculty candidates without triggering the six-year tenure clock.

Overall, three departmental committees held responsibility for evaluating faculty performance and recommending promotions. One committee dealt with ranks of assistant professor and below, one with associate professors, and one with clinical appointments. The committees' promotion recommendations were based on several considerations, including patient care, teaching, research funding, publications, national recognition, "esprit de corps," and administrative responsibilities.[25] In 1990, the department and the College of Medicine also instituted a system of performance reviews for full professors.

Across America, women's representation among internal medicine faculty, and their rate of promotion continued to lag in the 1980s. Despite the rapid growth in female medical school enrollments in the late 1960s and 1970s, women in the late 1980s accounted for just 16 percent of all faculty with the M.D. degree in American medical schools. Only 7 percent of those had reached the rank of professor, and only 16 percent had reached the rank of associate professor.[26] At the University of Iowa in 1985–86, the roster of 103 tenured and tenure-track faculty in internal medicine included five women—one full professor, two associate professors, and two assistant professors; in addition, there were but three women among the department's associates. Moreover, women were least likely to be found in the older, more established subspecialities such as pulmonary diseases, where there were no women at all, or cardiovascular diseases, where there were just two female associates and one female assistant research scientist.

At the end of the 1980s and even more so in the early 1990s, the outlook for women's representation brightened considerably, in part because of a concerted effort to recruit more women to the department and in part because the substantial numbers of women who had first enrolled in medical schools in the early 1970s had, by the late 1980s, completed the ten to twelve years of training requisite to a career in academic medicine. In the fall of 1989, the University of Iowa Department of Internal Medicine included one woman at the rank of professor, four at the rank of associate professor, and seven at the rank of assistant professor—more than double the numbers of 1985–86. Just as important, nine of the department's thirty-three associates (27 percent) in 1989–90 were women. By the fall of 1992, the department showed twenty-two women among its tenure-track faculty of 164, an increase from 9 percent to 13.4 percent in just three years. Moreover, the latter figure placed the department in the forefront of affirmative action efforts in the College of Medicine. In the fall of 1992, for example, the Department of Anatomy numbered just three women among its eighteen faculty, Preventive Medicine just four of twenty-nine, and Obstetrics-Gynecology and Pediatrics just four of eighteen and eleven of sixty-five respectively.

The results of the Department of Internal Medicine's efforts to recruit women to faculty positions during the 1980s and early 1990s compared favorably to results across the many colleges and departments of the university. While the percentage of women in tenure-track positions in the university, standing at just over 19 percent by 1991, was 50 percent higher than in internal medicine, the percentage of women in internal medicine nearly doubled in the last half of the 1980s and rose another 50 percent by 1992, while the university as a whole saw an increase only from 16.3 percent in 1982 to 19.5 percent in 1991.[27]

The place of Ph.D. research scientists in the department was another salient issue of the 1980s. As the emphasis in medical research shifted toward molecular biology, more and more Ph.D. scientists found employment in departments of medicine. However, at the University of Iowa, the appointment of Ph.D.'s to the tenure track contravened traditional expectations of faculty teaching, research, and patient service, and it was not until February 1981 that the department established its first guidelines for the appointment of Ph.D.'s to the tenure track. Those guidelines required a secondary appointment in a basic science department in order to sidestep the issue of patient service and to fulfill the university's teaching requirement for tenure-track appointments. In January 1987, the department also created the position of Adjunct Assistant Professor—a five-year non-tenure track appointment to clarify further the ambiguous status of Ph.D.'s.

The guidelines of 1981 and 1987 proved inadequate to deal with the problem. By the end of the 1980s, the department had appointed just two Ph.D.'s to the tenure track, while many departments of medicine around the country were aggressively recruiting Ph.D.'s for research faculty positions. The department then eliminated its secondary appointment requirement for tenure-track Ph.D. scientists in March 1989. The new guidelines required that Ph.D. tenure-track candidates present outstanding scientific qualifications, sufficient to develop an independent research program and attract external funding, and in lieu of a secondary appointment in a basic science department required only that the candidate possess the qualifications for such an appointment. However, that change did not resolve questions surrounding fulfillment of the university's teaching requirement for tenure-track appointments; nor did it address requirements for subsequent promotion. Into the 1990s, the department's Committee on Appointment of Ph.D.'s continued its work on those problems as well as wrestling with the question of a desirable mix of Ph.D.'s and M.D.'s among faculty ranks.[28]

In all, the department's rising national reputation generally aided staff recruitment efforts through the 1980s, and the department was notably successful both in attracting new faculty in areas of existing strength and in bolstering weaker areas. By the end of the 1980s, fully 75 percent of current faculty members had been appointed since 1970, some 80 percent of those in the 1980s alone. In addition, as described earlier, the number of women in faculty positions and among the ranks of the department's associates showed promising growth, and the regularization of tenure-track appointments for Ph.D.'s afforded yet another career path for women in internal medicine.

THE FUNDING OF ACADEMIC MEDICINE

The flow of money from federal agencies, industry, and voluntary health organizations, augmented by funds generated from patient service, drove the postwar expansion of academic medical centers. Through the 1960s, federal funding of an expanding array of research, training, and construction programs was the most visible, the most often remarked upon, and arguably the most important component in that mix. However, as we have also seen, the prospects for unlimited growth in federal funding dimmed in the early 1970s. In fact, in the twenty years from the late 1950s to the late 1970s, federal research funds fell from 23 percent to 18 percent of total expenditures at American medical schools, and through the next decade fell to just 15 percent of medical school expenditures.[29] Likewise, during the 1980s, Veterans Administration/Veterans Affairs research funding actually declined on a constant dollar basis.[30] Those developments in turn heightened the emphasis on alternative funding sources. By the end of the 1980s, for example, service income accounted for over 38 percent of total revenues at American medical schools (38.2 percent at the University of Iowa), while all federal categorical funds accounted for just 24 percent of revenues.[31]

Teaching hospitals felt similar funding pressures. Moreover, by the 1970s, public teaching hospitals in particular had become so large that meaningful state support had become problematic. As a result, the period from the late 1960s to the late 1970s brought a marked shift among non-federal teaching hospitals away from federal and state grants toward debt financing of new construction. Between 1969 and 1977, the proportion of teaching hospitals' construction costs covered by federal grants fell from 13 percent to 1 percent, and support for construction from state and local governments fell from 24 percent to just 7 percent. In the same period, debt financing rose from 20 percent to 67 percent of construction costs.[32]

The University of Iowa Hospitals and Clinics was a case in point. Between 1968 and 1990, most of that time under the aggressive leadership of John Colloton, the University of Iowa Hospitals and Clinics invested more than $250 million in new construction, 96 percent of that total financed from present and future hospital earnings. In addition, a number of related construction projects also went forward with little or no federal or state contribution. For example, when the Cardiovascular Center moved to new quarters on the fifth and sixth floors of the Medical Research Center in 1982, the College of Medicine used $2.2 million in trust funds, individual and corporate contributions, and private bequests to cover the costs of construction.

State support for faculty salaries in the Department of Internal Medicine also declined, especially so in the 1980s. In 1984–85, state appropriations made up 34 percent of department salaries, but by 1989–90, reflecting in part the state budget woes of the 1980s, state support had fallen to 24 percent of total salaries. At the same time, from the mid- to the late 1980s, the percentage of total faculty salaries derived from research grants fell slightly, from 31 percent in 1985–86 to 29.4 percent in 1989–90. As a result, the department's Medical Service Fund shouldered an increasing share of the salary burden: 20 percent in 1985–86 and 33 percent in 1989–90. From 1986 to 1990, Medical Service Fund income rose from $6.7 million to $13.6 million, and practice income—70 percent of that coming from Medicare, Medicaid, and commercial insurance—provided more than 30 percent of the department's overall budget.[33]

As the department's dependence on practice income increased, cost-containment initiatives made it more and more difficult to maintain the expected rate of return from patient service. That was especially true of Medicare and Medicaid programs, which had been designed in the 1960s around the prevailing cottage industry myth in which patients, acting as independent agents, sought the services of equally independent, fee-for-service health care providers. By the 1980s, the fit between myth and reality seemed particularly bad at teaching hospitals with their distinctive patient populations and educational responsibilities. Standard reimbursement formulas and reduced overhead allowances raised serious budgetary problems that led to closer scrutiny of billing practices and procedures in the Department of Internal Medicine and throughout the College of Medicine and the University of Iowa Hospitals and Clinics. At the end of the 1980s, declining balances in departmental trust funds led Dean John Eckstein to warn of the need for further cost reductions and income increases.[34]

Federal research grants and contracts and sponsored research were a second major element in the Department of Internal Medicine budget, accounting for more than 40 percent of departmental revenues. Research funding grew from $5.5 million in 1975 to $16.7 million in 1985–86 and to $26.7 million in 1989–90, the latter figure representing some one-third of all grant funds coming to the College of Medicine and more than a quarter of all research grants received by the university as a whole. From 1985–86 to 1989–90, the department's National Institutes of Health support alone rose 70 percent. Despite cutbacks in Veterans Affairs research funding in the 1980s, the department drew $1.7 million in research funding from the VA in 1985–86 and $2.4 million in 1989–90, although the latter figure was down significantly from the peak of $2.8 million two years previously.

Despite its success in attracting research funding, the department felt the effects of the increasingly competitive funding race, as the growth in total research funding in the United States lagged considerably behind the growth in numbers of medical researchers and the inflation in research costs. Department faculty felt increasing pressure to obtain grants for research projects, and the College of Medicine provided seed grants to finance new research initiatives that might subsequently qualify for external support. Department faculty were also notably successful in obtaining career research support such as the NIH Research Career Development Awards, Research Scientist Development Awards, Clinical Investigator Awards, and Physician-Scientist Awards. Overall, in 1985–86, department faculty submitted 342 external grant applications, of which 224 were funded, for a success rate of 65 percent. By 1988–89, the number of applications had risen 30 percent to 443, but just 229 of those were funded, dropping the success rate to 52 percent.

In the late 1980s, a few major program grants claimed an increasing share of research funding. In 1986, for example, the Cardiovascular Center's oldest ongoing research initiatives, the Regulation of the Circulation in Pathological States program and the Specialized Center of Research in Lipids, Atherosclerosis and Thrombosis, received five-year grant renewals, totaling eight million dollars and eleven million dollars respectively. In the same year, the center received a five-year award of $7.5 million for a Specialized Center of Research in Occupational and Immunologic Lung Disease. By 1990, nearly one-third of all National Institutes of Health funds coming to the College of Medicine as a whole flowed to the Cardiovascular Center's ten major research programs, and in its first twenty years of existence, the center had drawn nearly $129 million in research support.[35]

The Department of Internal Medicine's increasing dependence on grants, contracts, and practice income highlighted the funding problems facing academic medicine in the 1980s, injecting additional uncertainty into the budgeting process and also multiplying the amount of faculty time invested in revenue-raising activities. Both patient service and research were obviously labor-intensive revenue sources, both also involving considerable unseen overhead. The administration of clinical services, for example, was increasingly time-consuming, while a major program grant proposal consumed hundreds of hours of time in preparation. To many observers, the unceasing quest for funding in modern academic medicine called to mind a treadmill on which one moves faster and faster to stay in the same place.

THE NEW SPECIALIZATION IN RESEARCH AND PATIENT SERVICE

There was more than a little irony in the fact that patient service and research became the Department of Internal Medicine's chief pillars of support, accounting for more than 70 percent of revenues in the late 1970s and 1980s. Research and patient service had been increasingly uneasy bedfellows throughout much of the post–World War II era; indeed, the proper balance in that relationship was one of the issues behind the faculty unrest at the University of Iowa College of Medicine in the 1960s. Yet the mission of the medical school as defined in the early twentieth century made scientific research and patient care necessary companions, and at the University of Iowa and a good many other schools practice income ultimately became a critical element in medical school financing. While research and patient service, then, might be to some extent competing imperatives, they were also inextricably linked.

The 1980s brought a significant shift in that sometimes troubled relationship. In a general way, as knowledge and technologies in academic medicine became more highly specialized in the 1970s and 1980s, practice specializations came more and more to mirror research specializations. In addition, the University of Iowa Hospitals and Clinics' transition to a tertiary care mission fundamentally changed the nature of the patient population and patient service in the 1970s and 1980s, increasing the focus on specialized services and further narrowing the gulf between patient service and scientific research. Meanwhile, the proliferation of what François Abboud called "horizontal structures" built on specialized areas of science and technology drew representatives from multiple departments and disciplines to create new communities of interest around critical intersections of service and research. In some of the most highly specialized and most technology dependent areas, new technologies functioned simultaneously as research tools and as tools for diagnosis and therapy.

In 1985–86, the department tallied 6,609 patient admissions at the University of Iowa Hospitals and Clinics; by 1989–90, admissions totaled 7,784, despite the fact that the number of patient beds assigned to the Department declined slightly from ninety-seven to ninety in general medicine and from 108 to 107 in subspecialty areas. In the same period, medical service admissions to the Veterans Administration/Veterans Affairs Hospital slipped from 3,386 to 3,182, as the VA tightened patient eligibility restrictions. Census figures from general medicine outpatient clinics at the UIHC and VA showed a similar pattern, with the university count rising from 11,505 to 13,288 and the VA count declining from 22,493 to 19,698. Meanwhile, patient visits at the department's subspecialty clinics climbed abruptly at the UIHC, from 36,956 in 1985–86 to 48,888 in 1989–90, and at the VA, from 7,912 to 9,292. The fastest growing subspecialty areas at the UIHC in the late 1980s were hematology–oncology (7,257 patient visits in 1985–86 and 8,730 in 1989–90), cardiology (5,940 and 6,888), gastroenterology (3,490 and 6,703), and pulmonary (2,508 and 3,682). Endocrine–diabetes (5,173 and 5,439) and rheumatology (5,120 and 5,707) also drew especially large numbers of patients but showed significantly slower growth rates.

Through the 1970s and 1980s, the Division of Cardiovascular Diseases, headed by Allyn L. Mark, remained the department's largest division and one of the most fruitful intersections of specialized technologies, interdisciplinary research and patient service. The division maintained perhaps the department's broadest array of technology-based research and patient service facilities, including the Cardiovascular Intensive Care Unit and Cardiac Physiology Unit, the twenty-nine bed Medical Cardiology Unit, the Cardiovascular Clinic and Diagnostic Laboratories, Invasive and Noninvasive Cardiac Electrophysiology Laboratories, and the Cardiovascular Center and its constituent parts. Mechanisms of circulatory control, blood pressure regulation, and arteriosclerosis were continued foci of basic research in the division through the 1970s and 1980s, including pioneering work in the direct recording of sympathetic nerve activity in humans (microneurography) and fundamental investigations of cerebral blood flow, the central nervous system integration of cardiac reflexes, and the sympathetic and parasympathetic regulation of the heart. Developments in cardiac imaging techniques to assess cardiac anatomy and function and coronary blood flow—developments owing much to Richard Kerber and Melvin Marcus—were among the more striking examples of the confluence of technology, research, and service.[36] In 1990, the Specialized Center of Research in Ischemic Heart Disease, originally headed by Marcus, received a five-year funding renewal in support of some three dozen faculty from eight different departments. General research in arteriosclerosis initiated by William Connor and Mark Armstrong in the 1960s continued as well, as did the division's connection with the Specialized Center of Research in Lipids, Atherosclerosis and Thrombosis, where faculty from other departments and divisions joined in the study of lipid absorption and metabolism.

In the Division of Gastroenterology-Hepatology, directed by James Christensen from 1972 to 1986 and subsequently by Joel Weinstock, rapidly expanding clinical services included endoscopic and biopsy procedures, secretory function tests, and treatment of the broad variety of gastrointestinal and liver diseases in inpatient, outpatient, and consultation services. Endoscopic procedures remained a major focus of clinical research, influenced by the steady refinement of fiber-optic technologies first introduced in the late 1960s, while basic research interests spanned digestion and absorption, intestinal motility and inflammation, gallstone formation, and biliary pathology. Establishment of the James A. Clifton Center for Digestive Diseases added another major interdisciplinary focus to the Department of Internal Medicine, incorporating staff from surgery, radiology, pathology, and pediatrics as well as internal medicine. Meanwhile, Douglas LaBrecque, who joined the division in 1977, significantly enhanced the division's expertise in hepatology and was an important actor in the UIHC liver transplant program, begun in 1984.

The Division of Hematology–Oncology, directed by John Hoak from 1972 to 1984 and subsequently by C. Patrick Burns, was a third major intersection of technology, specialized interdisciplinary research, and expanding patient service. For example, the Bone Marrow Transplant Program, begun at the UIHC in 1980, drew heavily upon basic research in hemopoietic mechanisms and immunology and upon the expertise of staff in general internal medicine, infectious diseases, radiology, surgery, and pathology as well as hematology–oncology. By 1988–89, under Roger Gingerich's direction, the program had expanded from two beds to ten and the number of transplant procedures had increased to nearly 100 per year, and Gingerich also initiated the use of a monoclonal antibody purge of bone marrow to remove lymphoma cells. In other areas, the division's inpatient units and its outpatient clinics offered an enlarged battery of services for the diagnosis and treatment of lymphomas, leukemia, blood diseases, and solid tumors, and several staff were involved with the Cancer Center, an interdisciplinary operation directed by Richard DeGowin since its inception in 1978. The division also became one of twenty Cancer and Leukemia Group B centers in 1986, performing studies of experimental cancer therapies.

Representing one of the Department's oldest subspecialties, the Division of Endocrinology-Metabolism, directed by Daryl Granner and then Robert Bar, became a significant center of research in the 1970s as the patient load doubled at the division's three specialty clinics. Diabetes mellitus remained a principal focus of division research, and a Diabetes-Endrocrinology Research Center funded by the National Institutes of Health opened in 1979, bringing together staff from biochemistry, physiology-biophysics, pharmacology, and anatomy in the study of insulin, insulin-like growth factors, and steroid hormones. The Diabetes–Endocrine Unit at the UIHC opened in 1982, providing a thirteen-bed inpatient unit for the treatment of diabetes mellitus patients. The division also maintained its close association with the multidisciplinary Clinical Research Center, directed by Barry Sherman from 1977 to 1985 and Janet Schlechte from 1987, both of them endocrinology–metabolism staff.

The Department's formal emphasis in rheumatology began only in the mid-1970s, with John Thompson and M. Paul Strottmann principally responsible for organizing and maintaining the new Rheumatology Division, a division that—after a slow start—expanded rapidly in the following decade under the direction of Robert Ashman. By 1988–89, the division numbered eight tenured and tenure-track faculty plus three associates and three fellows. With additional faculty came a broadened research agenda, especially basic research into the molecular mechanisms of inflammatory and autoimmune diseases. In 1982, the National Arthritis Foundation designated the division a Clinical Arthritis Research Center, and by the end of the decade externally funded research reached $1.5 million.

In the Division of Pulmonary Diseases, directed by George Bedell and—from 1981—by Gary Hunninghake, both clinical responsibilities and faculty research interests concentrated on the pathogenesis and treatment of occupational and interstitial lung diseases, pulmonary function, and exercise testing. Hunninghake also directed the Cardiovascular Center's Specialized Center of

Research in Occupational and Immunologic Lung Diseases. In the 1980s, the division created an important new research focus in cystic fibrosis. Michael Welsh, who became one of the university's two Howard Hughes Institute Investigators in 1989, directed the Cystic Fibrosis Research Center funded in 1986 with a five-year grant from the National Institutes of Health, and Welsh's work with gene therapy for cystic fibrosis earned national headlines in the early 1990s.

Other internal medicine subspecialties showed a similar pattern of development. In the Division of Allergy–Immunology, spun off from rheumatology in 1978 and directed by Hal Richerson through the 1980s, an expanding catalog of diagnostic and therapeutic tools spurred patient service, chiefly in the outpatient clinics first organized by Paul Seebohm in the 1950s, and also brought division staff into a close working relationship with other specialties. In the 1970s and 1980s, the immunologic system—e.g., adult immunodeficiency syndromes, the complement system, and cell-mediated immune responses—lay at the center of much of the basic research in allergy–immunology, research with significant interdisciplinary ramifications. The Asthma and Allergic Diseases Center, funded by the National Institute of Allergy and Infectious Diseases, was a collaborative enterprise of the Department of Microbiology, the Division of Pulmonary Diseases, and the Division of Allergy–Immunology. Allergy–immunology staff participated also in the Cardiovascular Center's Specialized Center of Research in Occupational and Immunologic Lung Disease.

In the Division of Nephrology, where John Stokes replaced Philip Steinmetz as director in 1982, division staff maintained a major clinical research emphasis in blood pressure regulation, an area pioneered by Walter Kirkendall in the 1950s and 1960s, and also studied issues related to renal transplantation and dialysis. Basic research centered in areas such as renal physiology and cell biology, neural control of renal function, and the pathophysiology of glomerulonephritis, work that overlapped Cardiovascular Center projects in the Regulation of the Circulation in Pathological States and the Specialized Center of Research in Hypertension. Begun in the 1960s and expanded under the impress of the Medicare funding commitment of the early 1970s, renal dialysis programs, directed by Richard Freeman and—from 1987—by William Lawton, were a rapidly expanding patient service area. The greatest growth came in outpatient areas, particularly the home dialysis programs initiated at the VA Hospital in the 1970s and at the UIHC in 1986. The division's kidney transplant team, headed by Lawrence Hunsicker, was a second major patient service and research innovation.

The Division of Infectious Diseases, directed by Sam Donta and—from 1983—by Robert Clark, expanded its personnel and its clinical and basic research interests in disease agents and their interactions with host defenses, with special emphasis on neutrophil structure and function and other immuno-logic studies. In 1990, the division received a five-year Program Project Grant for Phagocyte Biology. In 1986, Charles Helms, who held a joint appointment in General Internal Medicine, assumed direction of the University of Iowa component of the Midwest AIDS Training and Education Center and in 1990 was appointed to the AIDS Advisory Committee of the Health Resources and Services Administration. The Division of Infectious Diseases also continued to build on its close interdivisional and interdepartmental involvement with infectious disease control in immunocompromised patients in the bone marrow, kidney, pancreas, heart, and liver transplant programs as well as the hematol-ogy–oncology service, burn unit, and medical and surgical intensive care units.

The Division of General Internal Medicine, Clinical Epidemiology, and Health Services Research was a product of the early 1970s interest in primary care. Under John Thompson's direction in the late 1970s, the division was ini-tially service oriented, organized chiefly around outpatient services, including satellite residency programs at the Veterans Administration Hospital and Iowa Methodist Hospital, both in Des Moines. During the 1970s, the division added programs in emergency and geriatric medicine and in the 1980s established a medical psychiatry unit in cooperation with the Department of Psychiatry. Meanwhile, federal regulations led to the creation of a program in hospital epidemiology at the UIHC in 1976, from which grew a Division of Clinical Epidemiology organized in 1986 under the direction of Richard Wenzel. A 1989 reorganization that embodied much of the original concept of general medicine merged the Division of General Medicine, then headed by David Skorton, and the Division of Clinical Epidemiology into the current Division of General Internal Medicine, Clinical Epidemiology, and Health Services Research, directed by Wenzel. Accordingly, faculty clinical and research interests covered a broad territory, from hospital epidemiology and quality of care issues to coronary risk factors, geriatrics and cardiac imaging.

Finally, the Division of Clinical Pharmacology—under the direction of John Ambre to 1978, Reynold Spector to 1987, Ross Feldman to 1990, and then Howard Knapp—remained the smallest of the department's divisions from 1975 into the 1990s. The division's chief missions remained instruction of medical students, residents, and fellows, and maintenance of the clinical pharmacology consulting service, including consultations with the Poison Control Center. For the most part, the division continued its traditional research focus on cardiovas-cular pharmacology, and, until his death in 1990, Michael Brody of the Department of Pharmacology maintained his long and productive association with the division and also directed the Cardiovascular Center's Specialized Center of Research in Hypertension.

Across the divisions of the Department of Internal Medicine, then, the late 1970s and 1980s saw major growth in basic research, especially interdisciplinary research. At the same time, the research interests of individual faculty were often closely related to clinical interests and to practical clinical problems, a development that tended to blur the accepted distinction between basic and applied research. Moreover, technological innovation, ranging from fiber optics and lasers to computerization and electron microscopy, was an important element in the growth of both research and patient service.

THE DEPARTMENT AND COMMUNITIES OF MEDICAL SCIENCE

In the 1950s, despite the trend toward specialization in medical research, it was still possible to talk of a single community of medical science and medical scientists, just as it was still possible, as William Bean maintained, to envision internal medicine as a single specialty. However, by the 1970s and 1980s, medical research had become, as had internal medicine, a highly specialized endeavor, a field of multiple dialogues carried on in scores of specialized societies and journals. Simultaneously, as noted previously, the increasing focus on basic research created new communities of researchers across traditional boundaries of departments and disciplines. "The cell," François Abboud commented, "has become the great unifier in academic medicine."[37]

Faculty from the University of Iowa Department of Internal Medicine played diverse roles in those evolving communities of medical science. In 1988–89, forty-nine faculty members were fellows of the American College of Physicians; fourteen had been elected to membership in the Association of American Physicians; twenty held memberships in the American Society for Clinical Investigation; and seventy-two were members of the Central Society for Clinical Research. Overall, internal medicine faculty held memberships in more than sixty professional organizations and institutions, ranging from long-established organizations to newer specialty societies and basic science societies.

By the mid-1970s, the list of faculty offices, honors, and publications had grown too extensive to catalog. In 1978 alone, John Eckstein was elected president of the American Heart Association; James Clifton presided at the April meeting of the American College of Physicians and was selected a master of the ACP; Lewis January likewise became a master of the ACP and also received a special citation from the American Heart Association; and Gerald DiBona became president of the American Federation for Clinical Research. In the following years, new generations of faculty rose to national prominence. Richard Freeman served as president of the National Kidney Foundation in 1980; Gary W. Hunninghake followed in the footsteps of François Abboud and Gerald Dibona as president of the American Federation for Clinical Research in

1986, the same year that Lawrence Hunsicker became president-elect of the American Society of Transplant Physicians and American Council on Transplantation; and in 1989, Allyn Mark became editor-in-chief of *Hypertension.*

Since the Fred Smith era in the 1930s, the Department of Internal Medicine had used a variety of devices to encourage the participation of advanced students and younger faculty in research communities. In the 1970s and 1980s, those devices grew more numerous and more elaborate as research played an increasingly important part in academic medicine. The most important function of fellowship programs, for example, was to nurture medical researchers, and by the 1980s, several research-oriented programs fulfilled a similar purpose for undergraduates. Meanwhile, the department's short-term associate appointments provided an advanced introduction to academic research. Departmental subsidies for travel to scientific conferences continued to expand as well, and the department inaugurated "research days" when faculty shared their research findings with colleagues and polished their presentations for national scientific meetings. In addition, the example set by senior faculty remained an important mechanism of acculturation into the varied research communities, for undergraduate and graduate students as well as for younger faculty.

The national distribution of University of Iowa M.D.'s, residents, and fellows by the 1980s was another measure of the College of Medicine's and the Department of Internal Medicine's integration into the larger world of medical science. In 1990, 334 Iowa M.D.'s and forty Iowa Ph.D.'s held faculty positions in U.S. medical schools. A tabulation by the College of Medicine traced those Iowa graduates to every state with a medical school except Hawaii, Maine, Mississippi, New Hampshire, and Rhode Island.[38] The Department of Internal Medicine's Alumni Group Advisory Committee, formed in September 1984, sought to enhance those ties in several ways, as, for example, through the departmental publication *Colleague,* first issued in the fall of 1985.

While the Department of Internal Medicine's connections to the greater world of medical science diversified, so, too, did its connections to Iowa medicine. The increasing presence of the department's former students within Iowa medicine was an important factor in building those connections; by the late 1980s, more than half of Iowa's physicians were either University of Iowa graduates or had taken residencies at the University of Iowa Hospitals and Clinics. At the same time, new transportation and communications technologies and networks helped to ease long-standing problems in the interaction between academic and practicing physicians. Ironically, the pattern of centralization and specialization in rural health care services that had sparked so much controversy also facilitated interaction, and the diffusion of high technology procedures to regional medical centers—another common source of concern and controversy—likewise created new contexts for interaction among academic physicians and those in private practice.

Department faculty also maintained and extended their traditional links to practitioners through the Iowa Medical Society, through specialty consultation clinics in places such as Burlington, Muscatine, and Ottumwa, and through statewide specialty societies. Still the most prominent example of faculty outreach was Paul Seebohm who served as president of the Iowa Medical Society and the state board of health and also as a member of the Health Policy Corporation of Iowa and the Governor's Advisory Committee on Organ Transplants. In light of the fact that referrals made up some 80 percent of the patient load at the UIHC, Seebohm was especially concerned with the still sensitive issue of communication between house staff and referring physicians.[39]

While faculty interaction with physicians across the state served an informal educational function, the Department of Internal Medicine also expanded its formal continuing education programs, with John MacIndoe serving as the department's director of continuing medical education. Already in the mid-1970s, the department, in conjunction with the College of Medicine's Office of Continuing Medical Education, offered programs accredited for the American Medical Association's Physician's Recognition Award. Interest in such programs increased substantially in the wake of the Iowa legislature's passage in 1978 of a continuing education requirement for physician licensure. In the 1980s, the department's annual "Progress in Internal Medicine" conference became the centerpiece of its continuing education program, calling upon the expertise of many staff members and displaying the latest developments in science and technology to a large physician audience. In the October 1985 program, for example, some 440 participants attended 800 hours of presentations.

INTERNAL MEDICINE AND UNDERGRADUATE EDUCATION

By the end of the 1970s, the wave of expansion in medical school enrollments begun in the 1960s had crested. Fiscal constraints were in part responsible for that; however, the policy of expansionism that had governed medical education for some two decades had also come under attack. To many academic physicians, the training of more physicians no longer seemed a plausible solution to the problems in American health care. By 1989, the number of American physicians had doubled since 1960, while the population of the United States had grown just 36 percent, but the effect of that expansion in physician numbers on the public health was ambiguous. At the same time, as the authors of a 1979 article noted, innovations like the Regional Medical Program, which were meant to introduce planning and direction into a largely systemless health care system, "were given uncertain legislative mandates, little power, and insufficient funding."[40] For critics of expansionism, the most certain result of the training of more physicians was further inflation in American health care expenditures.

In any event, further expansion bumped against the hard reality of a declining pool of medical school applicants. From the peak year of 1974, the number of applicants to medical schools diminished steadily through the 1980s, dropping to 36,100 in 1980, 32,893 in 1985, and to 26,915 in 1989. From 1975 to 1989, the ratio of applicants to first-year positions plummeted from 2.8 to 1.6, the latter number matching the low point of the early 1960s. The number of medical graduates likewise slumped, falling from a peak of 16,327 in 1984 to 15,433 in 1990.[41] Most medical educators conceded that the shrinking pool of medical school applicants was an "ominous phenomenon."[42] Moreover, a marginal decline in college grade point averages and MCAT scores accompanied the decline in numbers of applicants.[43] Medicine, it seemed, had lost some of its lustre as a career choice.

Still, the trend toward demographic diversity in the medical student body continued. By 1984, nearly 32 percent of medical students nationwide were women, and 16.6 percent were minorities, one-third of them Asian.[44] By 1989–90, the proportion of women had risen to over 38 percent in entering classes, to 36 percent among the total student body, and to nearly 34 percent among graduates. In the last half of the 1980s, African American enrollments also rose by some 24 percent. However, enrollments of African American men actually fell during that period, and, by 1989, African American women medical students substantially outnumbered African American men.[45]

At the University of Iowa College of Medicine, after the vigorous enrollment growth begun in the late 1960s, entering classes stabilized at 175 in the 1980s. In some respects, those students were little different from their predecessors. In 1988–89, 87 percent were Iowa residents and 74 percent were science majors. However, the percentage of women in entering classes rose steadily from the 21 percent of 1975 to 34 percent in 1988–89. Meanwhile, the Educational Opportunities Program, in operation since the late 1960s, swelled total minority applications to near 200 by the end of the 1980s, when the College of Medicine counted forty-three African American and thirty-five Hispanic students among its student body. During the first twenty years of the Educational Opportunities Program, the College of Medicine graduated 114 African American physicians.[46]

After the ferment of the 1960s and early 1970s, centered on the revamped and expanded Introduction to Clinical Medicine course and the senior elective year, the curriculum, too, stabilized in the 1980s. From 1978, Donald Brown of internal medicine's Division of Cardiovascular Diseases directed the sophomore introduction to clinical medicine, consisting of three weeks of history and physical diagnosis, followed by fourteen weeks of presentations and patient-oriented programs in twenty-one areas of clinical medicine. Department of Internal Medicine faculty provided more than a third of total lecture hours and accounted for the large majority of program preceptors as well. For junior students, the clerkship rotation included nine weeks on internal medicine inpatient units in the University of Iowa Hospitals and Clinics and the Veterans Administration Hospital, and in 1989–90 the College of Medicine's Medical Education Committee recommended even more clinical time for junior clerks. Senior electives in internal medicine consisted of four-week rotations on inpatient and outpatient subspecialty services; in all, fifty-six such rotations were available in twelve general areas, including off-campus medical centers in Des Moines and LaCrosse, Wisconsin. Meanwhile, the Medical Education-Community Orientation program placed students in community hospitals for periods of eight to ten weeks between the first and second years. Another innovation was the Human Dimensions in Medicine program, a course for freshman students focused on physician-patient communication and cultural values in health care.

Undergraduates also had available a greater array of specialized programs of study, all of them calling upon internal medicine faculty as directors and student sponsors. The Medical Scientist Training Program was the most comprehensive of the new instructional programs. Designed to prepare students for careers in academic medicine, the program joined the undergraduate curriculum with graduate research training and led to the combined M.D.-Ph.D. in six to seven years. A second program, the Physician Scientist Program, linked basic science departments and clinical specialties in the program areas of the National Institute of Diabetes, Digestive, and Kidney Diseases and combined one to two years of specialized study and research during the undergraduate years with graduate research training designed to fit students for an academic career. A third program innovation, the American Heart Association Student Research Fellowship, engaged student participants in a one- or two-year research program in cardiology during the undergraduate years. During the 1988–89 year, the department sponsored a total of twelve students, including two women, in the Medical Scientist Training Program, Physician Scientist Program, and American Heart Association Student Research Fellowship.

The College of Medicine also offered its own Medical Student Research Fellowship Program meant to interest freshmen in research and to acquaint them with the career possibilities in academic medicine. Award recipients received a stipend for twelve weeks, usually in the summer, for participation in supervised research. Finally, the Department of Internal Medicine offered its honors program, coordinated by the senior clerkship committee. Offering senior students a taste of academic medicine through a coordinated program of senior electives and at least three months of supervised research, the honors program enrolled twenty-one students in 1988–89. In 1988–89, internal medicine faculty supervised a total of thirty-one students, including six women, in the Medical Student Research Fellowship and the department's own Senior Honors programs.

The variety of specialized undergraduate programs available by the 1980s posed alternatives to lock-step, mass production medical education and, by identifying and encouraging the expression of student interests, addressed a long-standing cause of student apathy. With their focus on research training, such programs also tended to lessen even further the distinction between undergraduate and graduate training. Moreover, they likely played a part in a vigorous rebound in applications for admission at the University of Iowa College of Medicine, as final applications rose more than 40 percent from 1989–90 to 1990–91.[47]

INTERNAL MEDICINE FELLOWSHIP AND RESIDENCY PROGRAMS

In the late 1970s and 1980s, the responsibilities of internal medicine faculty in the general area of graduate education continued the pattern of expansion begun in the mid-1960s. Growth in fellowship programs outpaced growth in residency programs, and, by the 1980s, proliferating fellowship programs came increasingly to reflect the growth of specialized, interdisciplinary research, symbolizing—indeed defining—the subspecialization that had overtaken internal medicine.

In 1975, the department counted forty-eight fellows. By 1985–86, the roster of fellows had grown to sixty-six, twenty-seven of whom were first-year. As was true in earlier periods, the Cardiovascular Division led the way with a total of eighteen first-, second-, and third-year fellows; Hematology–Oncology followed with a total of eleven. Of the twenty-eight fellowship graduates in that year, eleven entered private practice, just one in Iowa, and seventeen took academic positions at midwestern universities, fifteen of those at the University of Iowa. In 1989–90, enrollment in the department's varied fellowship programs grew to ninety-five, twenty-one in the Division of Cardiovascular Diseases; thirteen in the Division of Pulmonary Diseases; twelve in Gastroenterol-ogy–Hepatology; eleven in Hematology–Oncology; and ten in Infectious Diseases. General Internal Medicine, Nephrology, Endocrinology, Clinical Epidemiology, and Allergy–Immunology claimed from four to eight fellows each. Also, of the forty-one fellowship graduates in 1990, seventeen entered private practice—five of those in Iowa—and twelve joined the faculty at the University of Iowa.

In the 1980s, interdisciplinary research became a major theme in fellowship programs, a trend exemplified in the Cardiovascular Center with its ten major program areas bringing together faculty representatives from more than twenty departments. By 1990, four training areas funded by the National Institutes of Health constituted the center's major fellowship programs: the Cardiovascular Interdisciplinary Training Program dating from 1975, the Hemostasis and Thrombosis Training Program initiated in 1978, the Research Training Program in Pediatric Cardiology, also begun in 1978; and the newest, the Interdisciplinary Pulmonary Training Program. By the end of the 1980s, more than 200 fellows had passed through the oldest and largest of those programs, the Interdisciplinary Training Program; in all, the fellowship programs supported some 500 trainees between 1975 and 1990.

In the aggregate, the pattern of growth in fellowship programs in the University of Iowa Department of Internal Medicine approximated national trends which saw the total of internal medicine fellows rise from 5,885 in 1976–77 to 7,475 in 1987–88. The average program grew more than 22 percent in size in that eleven-year period, due chiefly to expansion of third-year offerings, and by far the largest fellowship programs were in cardiovascular areas. Likewise, cardiovascular programs showed the highest rate of growth—40 percent—during the period.[48]

From the mid-1970s to the end of the 1980s, the gender makeup of the population of internal medicine fellows changed slowly but steadily. In 1976–77, women held just 6 percent of all internal medicine fellowships nationwide.[49] However, by 1985–86, 27 percent of fellows in hematology, oncology, and combined hematology–oncology programs were women, and women also had made significant inroads in fellowship programs in cardiology (10 percent), gastroenterology (11 percent), and pulmonary diseases (13 percent).[50] At the University of Iowa, six of twenty-seven first-year internal medicine fellows in 1985–86 were women; at the end of the decade, women constituted 20 percent of the department's total of ninety fellows.

Foreign medical graduates held 26 percent of internal medicine fellowships in the United States in 1976–77,[51] a source of some concern but perhaps more so outside the medical profession than inside. Historically, foreign medical graduates had proved a capable and ambitious group; in the early 1980s, for example, they advanced from residency positions to fellowships at a 74 percent rate compared to the 40 percent rate for U.S. citizens graduated from foreign medical schools. Nonetheless, a provision of the Health Professions Educational Assistance Act of 1976, meant to restrict the opportunities for foreign medical graduates, required that they pass parts one and two of the national board examination and demonstrate proficiency in written and spoken English before taking American fellowship positions. The immediate result was a 25 percent drop between 1976 and 1981 in foreign fellows. Ironically, an influx of United

States citizens graduated from foreign medical schools, especially Caribbean schools, replaced the missing foreign medical graduates. Whether or not that exchange was, on balance, a good one is open to question. In any event, the mid-1980s saw a resurgence in the numbers of foreign fellows, a trend that continued in the last half of the decade. In contrast, the proportion of foreign medical graduates in internal medicine fellowship programs at the University of Iowa remained relatively stable throughout the period between 1975 and 1990 and, at 5 to 10 percent, fell well below national averages.

As already noted, the late 1970s and 1980s brought smaller growth in internal medicine residency programs. Nationwide in 1976–77, there were 15,185 residents in internal medicine; in 1988–89, there were 20,000. Internal medicine accounted for just 7 percent of all American residency programs in the latter year, but internal medicine residents made up 22 percent of the total resident population, although some 20 to 25 percent of those switched to another specialty after the first year. The percentage of female residents in internal medicine rose from 12 percent in 1976–77 to 22 percent in 1981–82 and to 26 percent in 1988–89. In 1988–89, 30 percent of first-year internal medicine residents were women compared to the average of 28 percent for all specialties.[52]

The presence of foreign medical graduates in internal medicine residency programs, as in fellowship programs, became a national issue in the 1970s. Foreign medical graduates accounted for 10 percent of first-year internal medicine residents in 1976–77, while an additional 4 percent of residents were U.S. citizens graduated from foreign medical schools. In 1985–86, the percentage of U.S. graduates of foreign medical schools, again chiefly in the Caribbean region, had risen to 10 percent. By 1988–89, all graduates of foreign medical schools, including both U.S. and non-U.S. citizens, made up 24 percent of the internal medicine resident population, 16 percent foreign medical graduates and 8 percent U.S. graduates of foreign medical schools.[53]

In most respects, residency programs in the University of Iowa Department of Internal Medicine followed national trends. First, the number of internal medicine residents continued the local growth trend begun in the late 1960s, swelling from sixty-eight in 1975–76 to 103 in 1989–90. Second, women held twenty-one of those 103 residency positions in 1989–90, when ten of the twenty-six first-year residents, or nearly 40 percent, were women. By 1992–93, women held nearly 34 percent of department fellowship positions. However, experience at the University of Iowa diverged significantly from national trends with regard to foreign medical graduates in residency positions. Despite receiving 400 or more applications each year from foreign medical graduates, the department's resident staff included just nine foreign medical graduates in 1989-90, six of those from the American University of Beirut.

From a national perspective, it appears that the expansion of internal medicine residency programs in the 1980s was accompanied by a significant decline in interest in internal medicine on the part of graduates—male and female—of American medical schools. Students complained that internal medicine was more stressful and less satisfying than other specialties,[54] and, as a result, internal medicine's success in the National Residency Matching Program fell. In 1978, just 13 percent of internal medicine residency positions were unmatched, by far the lowest percentage of any specialty, but during the next ten years the rate rose as high as 20 percent and was at or below 13 percent just three times. Additionally, each year as many as 30 percent of internal medicine residents held positions arranged outside the national match.[55] Just as troubling was a study of American Board of Internal Medicine examinations that showed a decline in scores on common items over a six-year period from 1983 to 1988. While the study's authors were wary of attaching too much significance to their findings, the board nonetheless revised its examinations in order to facilitate such long-term comparisons.[56]

The downturn in medical student interest in internal medicine led the University of Iowa Department of Internal Medicine to intensify its efforts to identify and recruit suitable residency candidates. By the end of the 1980s, the Department of Internal Medicine's House Staff Recruitment and Selection Committee screened over 700 applications per year, selecting 220-250 candidates for interviews, and the department's Housestaff Advisory Committee and Housestaff Evaluation Committee, with authority over administration of residency programs and evaluation of residents' performance, faced greater responsibilities as well.

While internal medicine residency training at the University of Iowa became decidedly more rigorous during the 1970s and 1980s, the basic structure of the residency program changed little over time. As was the case throughout most of the postwar era, residents first gained experience in general medicine then began rotations through subspecialty areas, with increasing responsibility in the second and third years. A variety of departmental seminars, conferences, and visiting scholars continued to augment the training of both residents and fellows. In addition, a Flexible Residency Program adopted in the 1980s allowed residents to interrupt their training for up to three years in order to engage in research related to internal medicine. Of the thirty graduating residents in June 1989, three entered private practice, one of those in Iowa, while sixteen joined fellowship programs, twelve of those at the University of Iowa.

Overall, graduate education in the Department of Internal Medicine during the 1970s and 1980s continued the general post-World War II theme of programmatic expansion and increasing intensity of instruction. Internal medicine faculty spent more time with students in an educational enterprise that grew ever more rationalized, ever more specialized, and ever more demanding for teachers and students alike. However, recent experience in graduate education differed significantly from earlier patterns in two crucial respects. First, residents and fellows became a more diverse group, most notably as women came to occupy one-quarter to one-third of available places. Second, fellowship programs grew much more rapidly than did residency programs, thus shifting the focus of graduate education even further toward scientific research and the training of academic researchers.

THE GENERAL PRACTITIONER: A MEASURE OF SUCCESS

As noted in an earlier chapter, the late 1960s and early 1970s saw a renewed emphasis at the University of Iowa and nationwide on the training of primary care physicians. At the heart of primary care, its proponents argued, lay a reconsideration of the equilibrium between science and art in medicine. For example, third-year medical students at Johns Hopkins University learned in the early 1970s that the clinician's "prime function is to manage a sick person with the purpose of alleviating most effectively the total impact of the illness upon that person." Note that the image was not one of the physician confronting disease with the aid of science and technology; rather the image was that of the physician interacting with the patient. Communication, Johns Hopkins students were taught, was the key to the successful management of the sick person.[57] By the 1980s, the Liaison Committee on Medical Education of the AMA and AAMC had adopted much the same language, counseling that medical students should learn to address "the total medical needs of their patients and the effect of social and cultural circumstances on their health."[58]

Within internal medicine, the focus on primary care was important in the birth of a new subspecialty, general internal medicine. The central premise of general internal medicine, with its emphasis on primary care for adult patients, was to "return comprehensive prevention, diagnosis, and treatment of adult illness to internal medicine's center stage." In short, the argument went, the "emergence of general internal medicine" would return internal medicine to "the patient and the practice of medicine." The new subspecialty also promised to open untapped areas of fundable research to the academic clinician, research rooted in sociology, psychology, economics, epidemiology, and the humanities.[59] As more than one observer noted, however, general internal medicine did not "flower exuberantly" through the 1970s.[60] General internal medicine divisions multiplied rapidly, but most of those programs, like the one at the University of Iowa, remained comparatively small, and few placed a high priority on the training of primary care residents.[61] Moreover, there were few fellowship programs to train young physicians for general internal medicine faculty positions, while external research funding failed to materialize as hoped.

In the 1980s, much of the early enthusiasm for general internal medicine reappeared behind primary care internal medicine, a new subspecialty of uncertain future distinguished by its proponents from both traditional internal medicine, with its supposed emphasis on technology and hospital care, and family practice, with its claims embracing pediatrics and obstetrics-gynecology.[62] In the early 1990s, however, the University of Iowa Department of Internal Medicine's attempt to establish a primary care internal medicine emphasis failed, in François Abboud's recounting, because of a dearth of suitable faculty candidates.

In part, the difficulties in establishing a primary care specialty in internal medicine reflected the success of family practice in preempting much of the field. At the University of Iowa, despite its initial grudging response to the family practice concept, the Department of Internal Medicine lent increasing support to the family practice program in the late 1970s and 1980s, and, by the end of the 1980s, local general internists recruited by the department to serve as clinical faculty shouldered the lion's share of responsibility for the training of family practice residents at satellite clinics around the state. Moreover, the family practice program had a significant impact on Iowa medicine. In 1970, only eight of 110 University of Iowa College of Medicine graduates remained in the state for their first graduate training year, while sixty-eight of 166 did so in 1977, with forty-eight of those entering residencies in family practice, internal medicine, or pediatrics.[63] Furthermore, in the years from 1974 to 1991, 22 percent of all University of Iowa College of Medicine graduates entered family practice residencies, twice the national rate, and 59 percent of the graduates of the statewide family practice residency program entered practice in Iowa, nearly half in towns of 10,000 or fewer in population.[64]

Still, the rise of family practice in the 1970s and 1980s did not lay to rest Iowa's rural health care debate. According to a 1989 *Des Moines Register* study, the physician population in Iowa grew by 19 percent in the 1980s, but the total number of family practice physicians in the state in fact fell by 5 percent.[65] At the same time, many of Iowa's rural hospitals, despite their psychological and economic importance to local communities, suffered a slow strangulation due to the continuing decline in rural populations, tighter federal and state regulations, rural-urban differentials in Medicare reimbursement formulas, and increasingly efficient transportation systems. In just six years, from 1980 to 1986, rural hospital admissions in Iowa dropped 36 percent, and in 1989, eight of Iowa's counties had no hospitals.[66]

By the 1980s, then, the College of Medicine and the Department of Internal Medicine in particular had done much to address the long-standing complaints about Iowa's declining primary care resources, but the unyielding realities of demographics and economics combined with the centralizing tendencies inherent in much of medical technology imposed very real constraints on the maintenance of rural health care services. In addition, returns from the National Residency Matching Program from 1986 to 1991 showed a worrisome general decline in student interest in primary care specialties, as matches fell 25 percent in internal medicine and 18 percent in family practice.[67] With the advent of the 1990s, the acknowledged difficulties in maintaining rural health care services in Iowa injected new life into a very old debate over the organization and delivery of rural health care services, much of that, as before, centered on the role and responsibility of the University of Iowa College of Medicine.[68]

THE JOHN ECKSTEIN ERA AT THE COLLEGE OF MEDICINE

From 1970 to 1991, internal medicine's John Eckstein served as dean of the University of Iowa College of Medicine, his twenty-one year tenure the longest in the college's history and arguably the most successful as well. Much like Lee Wallace Dean's tenure, John Eckstein's years as dean constituted a period of extraordinary expansion in the College of Medicine. As noted in the previous chapter, the early 1970s saw a major growth in undergraduate enrollments, and throughout the 1970s and 1980s, the College of Medicine's graduate programs, including residencies and fellowships, grew steadily. Likewise, faculty numbers grew exponentially, not just in the Department of Internal Medicine but across the board in the College of Medicine. Moreover, the building program set in motion in the late 1960s continued in the Eckstein years, bringing enlarged facilities for research—both basic science and clinical—and for patient service, including a major addition to the Oakdale campus and the human biology building later renamed in Eckstein's honor.

Although it may not have been explicit in 1970, the selection of John Eckstein—a man firmly committed to scientific research—as dean of the College of Medicine was a triumph for the forces of reform represented by Raymond Sheets and the "Committee of Twenty" in the 1960s. Indeed, in many accounts, Eckstein's greatest accomplishment was to put the University of Iowa College of Medicine on a course that, by the 1990s, brought national recognition for research achievement to selected faculty and departments, an outcome made all the more remarkable by the college's laggardly position as a research institution in the 1950s and 1960s and the increasingly competitive scramble for research funding in the 1970s and 1980s.

The aggressive expansion of the College of Medicine during John Eckstein's administration was of course accompanied by—and in fundamental ways dependent upon—a parallel expansion of the University of Iowa Hospitals and Clinics. By the late 1980s, the UIHC, under the capable direction of John Colloton, had become a sprawling and dynamic complex, symbolic of its role as Iowa's tertiary care facility and symbolic also of a growing body of expertise in scientific research and patient service, expertise recognized both locally and—to an increasing degree—nationally as well. During that prolonged period of symbiotic growth, the relationship between the dean and the hospitals director was far less troubled than had been the case at many times in the past. Likewise, it was perhaps less troubled than the rapid pace of expansion might have led one to expect.

Nonetheless, the potential for friction, born chiefly of the close interdependence of the two institutions, was an ever-present reality, virtually as old as the University Hospital itself, and that potential had grown roughly in proportion to the expansion of the hospitals and clinics' fiscal base, especially during the post-1965 Medicare era. President Howard Bowen's late 1960s solution, which had both the chief executive officer of the College of Medicine and the director of the University Hospitals reporting to a university vice-president, had collapsed in short order, as had its forerunner under Virgil Hancher in the late 1940s, undermined, some said, by officials in both the college and the hospitals and by Robert Hardin's own frustrations. Under John Eckstein and John Colloton, then, the relationship between the college and the hospitals reverted more or less to the status quo ante, a not altogether satisfactory arrangement with few mechanisms—apart from good will—to foster the needed inter-institutional cooperation. By the late 1980s, rumor and speculation abounded regarding the extent and nature of the rift between the dean and the hospitals and clinics director, and university president Hunter Rawlings was drawn in as mediator in that relationship. Rawlings' position was a familiar but seldom happy one for university presidents, one that Rawlings appeared to accept only reluctantly, knowing that neither side would likely welcome a solution imposed by presidential fiat.

After eight months of study, the University of Iowa Review Committee for the College of Medicine issued a report—the Bonfield Report, named for law professor Arthur Bonfield—in the spring of 1991, a report that included a review of relations between the College of Medicine and the University of Iowa Hospitals and Clinics.[69] Among the review committee's recommendations were several aimed to ease the tensions between the college and the hospitals and clinics, including formally codifying their relationship, implementing mechanisms to resolve disputes, and resurrecting the organizational scheme in which both the dean and the director reported to a vice-president. Pursuant to that report, President Rawlings introduced two major administrative innovations: first, the appointment of a UIHC chief of staff to report both to the dean and to the hospital director and, second, in an echo from the late 1960s, the creation of a vice-president for health sciences to oversee all the health sciences colleges and the UIHC.

When John Eckstein announced his retirement from the deanship in 1991, his only public explanation was the laconic comment, "I've been doing it for over 20 years."[70] In that same year, John Colloton also announced his resignation, effective in 1993, when he would take a newly created position as vice-president for statewide health services. Behind Eckstein's and Colloton's resignations lay two decades of extraordinary growth in the College of Medicine and the University of Iowa Hospitals and Clinics. During those years, John Eckstein had successfully held conflicting egos and departmental interests in a semblance of consensus, balanced the various outside constituencies—local, state, and national—with their own agendas and their own vested interests in the college and its operations, and, at least for much of the period, achieved a *modus vivendi* with the director of the university's complex of hospitals and clinics. For Eckstein's many supporters, his record of accomplishment, like John Colloton's, stood by itself.

CONCLUSION

By any measure, the University of Iowa Department of Internal Medicine made significant strides in the years from 1975 to 1990, many of those in areas of traditional strength. For example, the department's growing contributions to patient care and undergraduate and graduate teaching as well as its service to wider communities of medical science and the public continued very old trends. On the whole, too, François Abboud's ambitions for the department were not unlike those of Campbell Howard sixty years earlier. Likewise, much as was the case in the 1920s, the department's expansion in the past two decades was supported by growth throughout a complex institutional matrix, including not only the College of Medicine and the University of Iowa Hospitals and Clinics but also institutions as geographically remote as the National Institutes of Health and the Department of Veterans Affairs.

At the same time, the 1970s and 1980s brought much that was new. For example, the halting trend toward gender balance among internal medicine faculty was a striking departure from the past as was the explosive growth in the department's research efforts and accompanying growth in research-oriented fellowship programs. The same was true of internal medicine's increasing involvement with other departments in interdisciplinary research enterprises.

Similarly, although patient care was a long-established part of the department's mission, the addition of new facilities, new technologies, new faculty, and new patient populations translated quickly into new patient service areas, from laser angioplasty and catheter ablation to organ transplants and fiber-optic rhinoscopy.

In retrospect, it is clear that the late 1960s and 1970s had in fact marked an important turning point in the department's history. In the 1950s, William Bean had been content, indeed delighted, to have his faculty engage in research of any kind, but the second great postwar wave of faculty expansion that began in the late 1960s saw new faculty recruits selected specifically with an eye toward their research potential. Moreover, new faculty were increasingly selected on the basis of their fit within specific research programs, as the department moved toward a much more closely managed approach to medical research, even in areas of so-called basic research.

The department's enthusiastic embrace of research in the 1970s and 1980s and its emergence as a center for highly specialized patient care did at times exacerbate some old problems—for example, balancing competing demands on facilities and on faculty time. The new emphasis on research seemed also to create new problems—for example, Ph.D. promotion policies. However, there were benefits as well, both in the growth of knowledge and technological capabilities and in the expansion of patient services.

One of the most striking consequences of the department's transition in the 1970s was the appearance of a significant generational divide. By the 1980s, much of what had become traditional about the department was traceable to William Bean's leadership and the personnel and institutional changes of the immediate post–World War II period. During the 1980s, however, death claimed several key figures from that era, while several others moved to emeritus status. Meanwhile, much of what was new about the department in the 1980s owed its origins, directly or indirectly, to the years of James Clifton's and François Abboud's leadership. For example, faculty recruited from the late 1960s through the 1980s clearly dominated the department's research agenda. Moreover, by the early 1990s, some 80 percent of current internal medicine faculty had been recruited during François Abboud's fifteen-year tenure as department chair.

Overall, the late 1970s and 1980s, perhaps more so than earlier periods in the department's history, mixed old and new, continuity and discontinuity. While it was clear to most at least that the key to the department's future lay in research, whether in now traditional lines of scientific research or in the newer areas of health services research, all agreed, too, that the blend of old and new in the 1980s was a principal source of the department's strength. To some at least, the most important challenge for the future lay in maintaining that balance. For example, how large can the department grow and still maintain the cohesiveness and common sense of purpose that have always been a source of its strength? Can the department accommodate those faculty whose chief interests and contributions lie in teaching or patient care rather than in laboratory research? Clearly, the preservation and adaptation of the best of traditional practices while continuing to incorporate new ideas and new directions will not be a simple task.

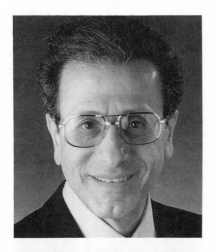

FRANÇOIS M. ABBOUD, M.D.,
President: American Federation for Clinical
Research, 1971; Central Society for Clinical
Research, 1985; Association of American
Physicians, 1990; American Heart Association,
1990. *Photographs courtesy of the Department
of Internal Medicine, University of Iowa Hospitals and Clinics.*

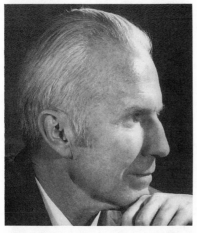

WILLIAM B. BEAN, M.D.,
President: Central Society for Clinical Research, 1950; American Society for Clinical
Nutrition, 1962; American Osler Society,
1971; American Clinical & Climatological Association, 1977.

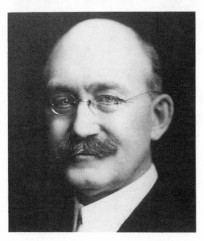

WALTER L. BIERRING, M.D.,
President: Alpha Omega Alpha, 1924-54;
American Medical Society, 1933-35; American Board of Internal Medicine, 1936-39;
American Board of Preventive Medicine,
1947-56.

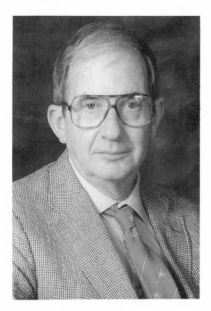

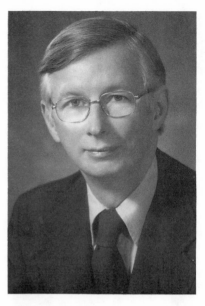

JAMES CHRISTENSEN, M.D.,
President: American Motility Society, 1982-84.

JAMES A. CLIFTON, M.D.,
President: American Gastroenterology Association, 1970; American College of Physicians, 1977. Chairman of American Board of Internal Medicine, 1980.

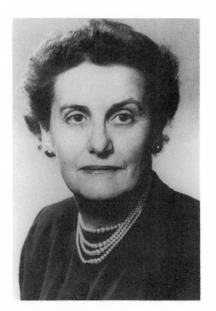

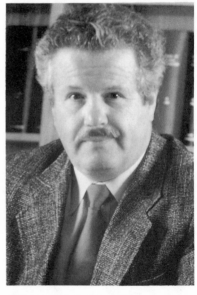

KATE DAUM, Ph.D.,
President: American Dietetic Association, 1932.

GERALD G. DiBONA, M.D.,
President: American Federation for Clinical Research, 1978.

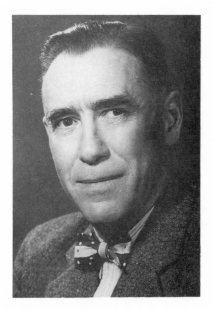

WILLIS M. FOWLER, M.D.,
President: Central Society for Clinical Research, 1949.

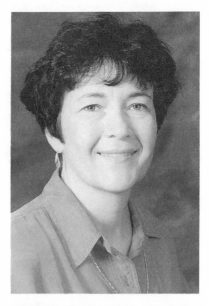

NANCY S. GOEKEN, Ph.D.,
President: American Society of Transplant Physicians, 1986; American Society for Histocompatibility and Immunogenetics, 1989.

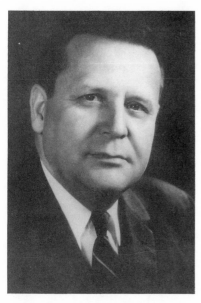

ROBERT C. HARDIN, M.D.,
President: American Diabetes Association, 1969.

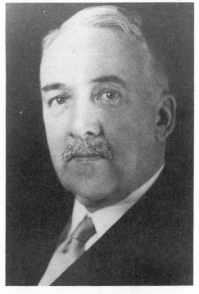

CAMPBELL P. HOWARD, M.D.,
President: Association of American Physicians, 1929.

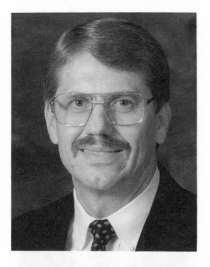

GARY W. HUNNINGHAKE, M.D.,
President: American Federation for Clinical
Research, 1986; American Thoracic Society,
1994.

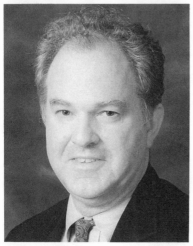

LAWRENCE G. HUNSICKER, M.D.,
President: American Society of Transplant
Physicians, 1987; American Thoracic Society,
1987.

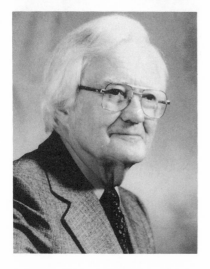

LEWIS E. JANUARY, M.D.,
President: American Heart Association, 1966.
Vice-President of International Cardiology
Federation, 1970-78.

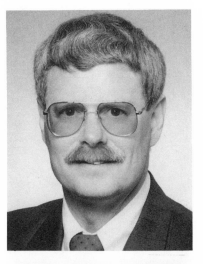

ROGER G. KATHOL, M.D.,
President: Association of Medicine and Psychiatry, 1992; Academy of Clinical Psychiatry, 1992.

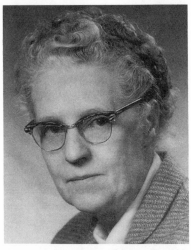

MARGARET A. OHLSON, Ph.D.,
President: American Dietetic Association, 1951.

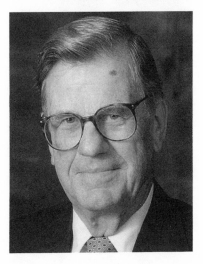

PAUL M. SEEBOHM, M.D.,
President: American Academy of Allergy, 1966.

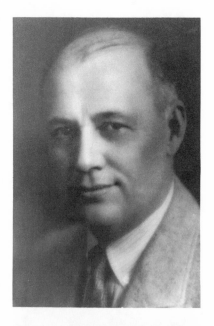

FRED M. SMITH, M.D.,
President: Central Society for Clinical
Research, 1936.

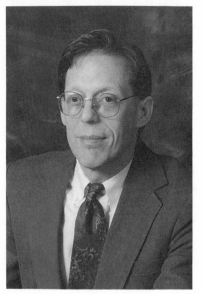

RICHARD P. WENZEL, M.D., M.Sc.,
President: Society of Hospital Epidemiology
of America, 1985.

EPILOGUE

ISTORIANS are commonly reticent on the subject of the lessons of history. Like researchers in the physical sciences, historians commonly prefer to see their work as a species of pure science, its relevance, if any, to contemporary problems and issues no more than an accident. Moreover, historians often argue that since historical knowledge is normally bounded by complex circumstances born of time and place, history seldom repeats itself in any meaningful sense. Thus, the lessons of history are not so clear as the uninitiated might think.

However, caveats and disclaimers aside, historians do in fact speculate about the lessons of history and on occasion do so with considerable passion. Moreover, whatever their philosophical objections to notions of "relevancy" in their work, historians agree at a minimum that good history provides both stimulus and guidelines for sober reflection on what is possible and even probable in the future and what is not, a process which may carry significant implications for public and private policy decisions. So it is here.

SCIENCE, TECHNOLOGY, AND THE INDUSTRIALIZATION OF MEDICINE

This history of the University of Iowa Department of Internal Medicine—with its chief focus on local issues, local institutions, and local personalities—is a chapter in the rise of scientific medicine in modern America. Rightly enough, progress and celebration figure prominently in that story. At another level, however, this local history is a chapter in the industrialization of

American medicine and American health care. That aspect of this story—marked by the development of a mass market for health care goods and services, the concentration of capital and attendant decline of artisan production in the health care marketplace, the increasing emphasis on technology and associated specialization in medicine, and the erosion of the physician-patient relationship by both technology and the cash nexus—is, in its way, a far more complicated and far more troubled one.

One of the hallmarks of the past century has been the movement, albeit irregular, toward a mass market for professional health care, a mass market that in turn spawned an array of major industries, including the health insurance industry, the pharmaceutical industry, the hospital management industry, and a variety of ancillary service industries. At the same time, the provision of health care goods and services became increasingly capital intensive, particularly so in the decades since World War II, and business management techniques and administrative structures as well as the profit motive found wider application throughout the health care marketplace, including in private medical practice, voluntary hospitals, and academic health centers. For better or worse, as one observer noted as early as 1959, American medicine adopted "more and more ... the behavior of the marketplace."[1]

Many factors lay behind that process of industrialization in American health care, including rising per capita incomes in American society, the promotional activities of organized medicine, broad changes in cultural attitudes toward health care practices, and sporadic innovations in government policy. None of those factors, however, was as important as the extraordinary pace of advance in medical science and technology, without which the modern health care marketplace would be inconceivable. Since the late nineteenth century, the public's increasing acceptance of the authority of science and technology in general and of medical science and technology in particular was the foundation upon which physicians based both their claims to professional jurisdiction and their demands upon social resources in funding the constantly evolving institutional structures of the modern health care system.

Medical science and technology were also central factors in the commercial development of health care, as the fruits of scientific research and the creation, marketing, and employment of health-related technologies as well as health care services became major revenue sources in the health care economy. At the same time, the expanding scope of scientific research and technological innovation fed the trend toward specialization and subspecialization in medical research and in clinical practice, while the closely linked scientific and technological revolutions in medicine diminished the human dimensions of the physician-patient encounter, with machines displacing both the patient's narrative and the physician's senses in diagnosis and prognosis of disease.

Science and technology, in league with political and economic currents, also enormously amplified the physician's role as gatekeeper to the health care system, defining and regulating access to the sick role in American society. Recently, Charles Rosenberg has introduced the concept of the framing of disease to describe the increasingly elaborate process by which diseases are identified scientifically and their legal and social dimensions defined. Clearly, academic physicians have played an important part in the development of that framing process, their work providing increasingly sophisticated means—for example, immunologic or genetic tests—to categorize individuals by specific diseases and disease markers. Contemporary discussion surrounding the definition of AIDS highlights both the complexity and the central importance of the disease-framing process, while ambitious new research initiatives such as the Human Genome Project promise a major expansion of the problem.[2] In October 1992, the University of Iowa College of Medicine received a $15 million grant from the National Center for Human Genome Research, making the university one of nine centers for research on the Human Genome Project.

The impact of science and technology on the health care marketplace has surely exceeded anything imagined by turn-of-the-century boosters of scientific medicine. On many occasions, and increasingly so in recent decades, the enhanced scientific and technological capabilities of twentieth-century American medicine have sparked conflict, controversy, and resistance from within the medical community and the health care industry, as well as from agencies of state and federal governments and from consumers of health care goods and services. Indeed, there is no little irony in the fact that the cumulative successes of scientific medicine have made health care policy the subject of intense political interest. As one author recently suggested, the essence of academic medicine in particular—that is, scientific research, high technology patient care, and the training of young physicians in both those areas—is inherently political. The benefits generated by academic medicine, the distribution of those benefits, the social costs, and the likely impact on various sectors of the health care industry are necessarily issues of broad interest.[3]

Still, even the most vocal critics of change during the past century, whether inside or outside the health care system, have seldom questioned the basic premises of scientific medicine. Nearly all have accepted as an article of faith that the contributions of medical science and technology to health care are inescapable and that more science and technology will make health care even more effective.[4] What has been most often in dispute are the ramifications—direct and indirect, real and imagined—of scientific and technological change, with conflict centering on the distribution of the benefits of science and technology, not excluding questions surrounding the distribution of power and profits within the health care system.

A POST-INDUSTRIAL MEDICINE?

Largely because of its striking successes, then, American medicine has become the center of intense debate. By the 1970s, a disappointed and increasingly skeptical public joined disgruntled legislators, insurers, and employers in a chorus of complaints focused chiefly on the availability and quality of medical services and spiraling health care costs. The much discussed and often excoriated political and cultural clout of organized medicine, it seemed, had evaporated virtually overnight, and the harsh criticism, coming as it did on the heels of two decades of unprecedented scientific advance and institutional growth, puzzled and angered much of the medical community.

On the whole, physicians were not insensitive to the criticisms raised by outside critics. Within some physician circles at least there was considerable self-criticism, including criticism of academic medicine and medical education. To be sure, a critique of excessive specialization and technological alienation in health care was an explicit part of the ideological foundations of the new primary care specialties that emerged in the late 1960s and 1970s. Also, some more experienced physicians whose memories stretched back before the frantic post–World War II era were well aware of the extent to which the various sectors of the health care system had changed—not, in their view, always for the better.

For various reasons, then, many observers both inside and outside medicine conceded by the end of the 1980s that the industrial model of health care, whatever its past successes, displayed serious deficiencies. Moreover, virtually everyone agreed that the regulatory experiments of the 1970s had been largely ineffective in dealing with the deep-seated problems in health care, and many maintained that the widely touted free market solutions of the 1980s that proposed to let the profit motive drive health care policy had only made matters worse. The latter, some critics charged, only encouraged the wasteful duplication of services in the name of market competition and the introduction of more expensive, but largely untested, procedures and technologies while leaving mounting numbers of Americans outside the health care system altogether. In addition, such critics found the connections between business imperatives—productivity, market shares, profit margins—and desirable patient outcomes uncertain at best.

Nonetheless, agreement that the health care system was badly in need of fixing did not lead to a consensus on precisely what to fix or how to fix it, in no small part because of the sheer complexity of the system itself and the diversity of interests and perspectives contained within it. That lack of consensus reflects the fragmentation of the "managerial function" in the health care system,[5] a function dominated by academic medicine as recently as the 1950s but since contested by a variety of other institutions, including the health insurance industry and agencies of government. In the words of one prominent academic physician, "academic medicine no longer dominates the practice of medicine."[6] That is so because of widespread disillusionment within the medical community as well as among the public with big medicine represented in the academic medical centers and because the transformation of big medicine into big business created powerful competitors for leadership. As many observers have noted, there is much irony in organized medicine's flight from big brother and the specter of socialized medicine into the beckoning and sometimes stifling embrace of big business.

By the advent of the 1990s, academic medicine was caught in an apparent paradox, its authority to order the health care system in decline even as the impact of medical science and technology upon American social institutions and values accelerated. Also by the 1990s, however, there was a growing sense that the perception of urgency surrounding health care issues provided academic medicine the opportunity to reassert the physician's position of moral authority in society and to reassert as well the leadership role of academic medicine within the health care system. Both objectives, so some argued, could be approached by bringing the intellectual resources of academic medicine to bear on the social and economic dimensions of health care, including the social and economic impacts of medical science and technology.

The growing interest in medical ethics—or, more broadly, bioethics— during the past two decades is one example of the willingness in academic medicine to seize new leadership opportunities and to expand medicine's mandate in new directions. In 1960, the heading "Ethics, Medical" in *Index Medicus* covered only a half page and included scarcely more than sixty entries; in contrast, in 1990, the same heading filled nearly six pages and ran well over 600 entries. In fact, prior to the 1960s, there was little to talk about in medical ethics, and the scope of ethical debate was generally limited by the widespread presumption that a combination of economic development and scientific advance promised to eliminate most, if not all, ethical problems from health care. At the time, the chief focus in medical ethics lay in defining the physician's responsibility as a self-governing professional and director of the health care team; issues such as the confidentiality of patient records and when and how to tell bad news to patients dominated ethical discussion. By the late 1960s and even more so in the 1970s, several factors—including the example and the language of the civil rights movement, rising cost containment pressures in health care, medicine's rapidly expanding technological capabilities, and disturbing perceptions of ethical misconduct among physicians—dramatically altered the ethical dialogue.[7] The resulting ferment called into question the authoritarian nature of existing codes of medical ethics, recast the physician-patient relationship along more egalitarian lines, and addressed a growing array of conflict of interest as well as technology- and cost-based issues in health care.

The new medical ethicists' agenda is complex. First, they have sought to create a new ethical structure to buttress the physician's moral authority by setting standards for the practice of medicine extending beyond personal values, common public ethical standards, and minimal requirements established in law,[8] with the intent of marking off a "societal space in which a profession of scientific healers can work."[9] That goal is complicated by what Edmund Pellegrino calls the "plurality of sets of ethical commitments" in contemporary health care, perhaps the most compelling of which are the often conflicting pull of humanitarian ideals and technological imperatives on the one hand and cost containment pressures on the other. Pellegrino also notes that those new ethical standards must incorporate physicians' social responsibilities as members of a privileged corporate group, taking a more active interest, for example, in assuring access to health care and in policing the medical profession.[10]

A second problem for the new generation of medical ethicists has been the implementation of new ethical precepts and perspectives within the medical profession. At many medical schools, like the University of Iowa, the new focus on medical ethics has led to the introduction of a humanist component to the curriculum, including broad emphases on the humanities and social sciences as well as on specific ethical problems in medicine and the teaching of "clinical etiquette."[11] Unlike earlier calls for the addition of a humanist dimension to medical education, the current effort is designed to inculcate a set of cognitive and affective skills rather than to make the physician a gentleman or lady. In line with that goal, the Medical College Admissions Test in 1991 added emphases in the humanities and social sciences and in critical thinking and communication skills.

Critics of such reforms have argued that students are in fact less influenced by the curriculum than by the environment—social, institutional, personal—in which they are taught. Therefore, the inclusion of social sciences, humanities, and ethics in the medical curriculum may or may not make young physicians more effective at the bedside. Reform advocates respond that such innovations are not aimed solely at bedside performance but will, at the very least, provide students a broader, more sophisticated perspective on the role of medical practice in contemporary society and on the meaning of illness, particularly in different cultural settings and population groups.[12] The response from students, who already face a daunting curriculum crowded with technical information and whose demands for a practical education are one of the constants of the history of medical education, remains to be seen.

In internal medicine, meanwhile, the aims and concerns of health services research complement and in many respects overlap the aims and concerns of the new medical ethics. Like medical ethics, health services research is designed to merge medical science and technology with cultural and economic concerns in health care, in effect addressing some of the most basic and most difficult questions confronting modern medicine. Moreover, Robert Petersdorf and others maintain that health services research is crucial to the future of medicine. The University of Iowa's François Abboud, while proud of his department's strength in cellular and molecular biology, is also acutely aware of the need for a strong base in health services research.[13] Because the tattered prestige of science is no longer sufficient to shield medical practice from outside scrutiny, more and more observers, like Petersdorf and Abboud, argue that physicians must take the initiative in the study of critical issues in medicine—issues such as clinical decision-making, patient outcomes, quality assurance, and patient satisfaction—or risk losing control of the practice of medicine to government agencies, the health insurance industry, and a growing roster of other economic and political interests.[14] Indeed, in 1985, the United States Congress established a bipartisan Biomedical Ethics Board made up of six senators and six representatives and a companion Biomedical Ethics Advisory Committee, both bodies charged with addressing "the ethical, social, and legal implications of advances in biomedical research and technology."

Health services researchers, like the new generation of medical ethicists, face difficult and sensitive problems. For the short term, a major concern is the shortage of faculty and research funding in the field, despite the establishment of the National Center for Health Services Research—now the Agency for Health Care Policy and Research—in the late 1960s. For the long term, a more formidable problem may well be the potentially divisive nature of health services research itself, work that inevitably focuses on some of the most highly charged intersections—now and for the foreseeable future—of politics and medicine. While the study of patient outcomes and the evaluation of new technologies, as examples, are areas of intense interest to government agencies, to various other third parties in health care, and to practicing physicians, the ramifications of such studies for interested parties—not least internal medicine—will not in all cases be happy ones. Such studies will challenge internal medicine, like other specialties and providers, to offer a more rigorous justification of its claims upon health care resources.

Specifically, health services research may have significant impact on the research agenda in internal medicine. Since the inception of large-scale research funding from voluntary agencies and the federal government in the wake of World War II, a complicated network of political factors—what might be called the "politics of disease"—have influenced the distribution of research funding among and within the medical specialties quite apart from—and, so some critics argue, in conflict with—rational scientific considerations. One outcome of health services research, then, might be significant shifts in research funding patterns, such as a shift in resources toward disease prevention and away from acute conditions and even away from some aspects of research associated with chronic disease states, areas in which internal medicine has historically been heavily invested.

Health services research and the new dialogue in medical ethics, then, are positioned to play major roles in an emerging post-industrial health care system. Each in its own way addresses a set of deceptively simple questions: What has medical science accomplished and for whom; what ought to be the goals of medical science; and how would those goals be attained in a workable health care system? Until the 1960s, it hardly seemed necessary to ask such questions; both the questions and their answers were subsumed in the dominant vision of medical progress. The fruits of scientific medicine were, it seemed, certain and of universal benefit. However, with what one historian has called "an end to triumphalism" in science,[15] the past and future of medical science have become areas of contention, as competing interest groups offer divergent answers to the questions posed above.

Perhaps in that diversity lies the opportunity for academic health centers to reclaim a leadership role by proposing ways to match health care institutions and resources to the needs of diverse populations. Academic health centers in fact filled that adaptive role with extraordinary success in the first half of the twentieth century, implementing a thoroughgoing vision of scientific health care through the creative agency of medical research and through substantial changes in medical education, in medical practice, and in the organizational and institutional matrix of health care delivery. The University of Iowa Department of Internal Medicine was prominent in that effort at the local level and over the years became increasingly prominent at the national level also. The creation of a post-industrial health care system—one in which nurse practitioners, pharmacists, and other health care professionals, including practicing physicians, demand expanded roles and in which on-line databases and computerized information transfer play a central part—will demand a similar commitment of energies and resources.

THE DEPARTMENT OF INTERNAL MEDICINE: PAST, PRESENT, AND FUTURE

For a century and more, the University of Iowa Department of Internal Medicine, the College of Medicine, and the University of Iowa Hospitals and Clinics, have stood as local symbols of the American faith in and expectations of scientific medicine. In turn, the history of the department and those companion institutions has mirrored—with due allowance for the distortions introduced by local conditions—the complex and dramatic forces at work in the great and much-discussed transformation of American medicine.

Viewed from a local perspective, that transformation was an extended and uneven process, an irregular series of transformations or turning points. In the twentieth century alone, the defining moments in the history of the University of Iowa Department of Internal Medicine were many, from Abraham Flexner's denunciation of the College of Medicine and the subsequent recruitment of Campbell Howard to head the Department of Internal Medicine, through Flexner's part in securing financing for the new medical campus in the 1920s and the crushing blow from the depression of the 1930s, to the remarkable post–World War II expansion spurred in part by federal funding of medical research, training, and patient care. Given the pressures currently at work in health care, the 1990s may well mark another such defining moment.

For all that, the Department of Internal Medicine has maintained much of its distinctiveness. Part of that reflects the nature of Iowa itself, a state that retains, often self-consciously, much of its rural character and one that bears admitted resemblance to many of the stereotypes commonly attached to it. Similarly, despite its many cultural amenities, Iowa City, the home of the University of Iowa, retains much of its small-town flavor. The Department of Internal Medicine's traditional emphasis on humaneness, informality, and personal interaction—particularly among faculty and students—is firmly rooted in those rural, small-town traditions of Iowa. Moreover, with no other medical schools nearby and with the relative proximity of the university's liberal arts and health sciences campuses, department faculty have been, by and large, more closely integrated into the university community than might be the case at a medical center in, say, Chicago or New York City.

Another constant in the history of the Department of Internal Medicine has been its prominent role in Iowa medicine, a role that has sometimes been troubled but one in which internal medicine faculty have invested considerable effort. Over the years, the department has provided undergraduate and graduate training to a growing proportion of Iowa physicians, spread the latest in medical science and technology to the far corners of the state through continuing education efforts, and, since the second decade of the twentieth century, served the specialized health care needs of ever larger numbers of Iowa's citizens.

Through a good part of its history, the department's original contributions to medical science were modest; its role was not unlike that of developing countries in today's world economy, dependent upon knowledge, technologies, trained personnel, and capital contributed from elsewhere. It was not until the 1960s that the department, like the College of Medicine as a whole, developed a significant research emphasis and not until the 1970s that research was firmly acknowledged as a central part of the department's mission. Thus, François Abboud's observation that his department and the College of Medicine have been engaged in a game of catchup in establishing a research orientation is not far off the mark. Yet the Department of Internal Medicine's up-and-coming status from the 1950s into the 1970s was in many respects a comfortable one. Now, however, thanks to the extraordinary exertions of the past three decades, the department looks toward its future from an acknowledged position of national leadership, and perhaps the chief question for the future is whether it can combine that newfound prominence in scientific research with its traditional strengths in the human dimensions of medicine.

NOTES

INTRODUCTION

1. Arthur L. Bloomfield, "Origin of the Term 'Internal Medicine,'" *Journal of the American Medical Association* 169 (1959), p. 1628; Paul B. Beeson and Russell C. Maulitz, "The Inner History of Internal Medicine," in Maulitz and Diana Long, eds., *Grand Rounds: One Hundred Years of Internal Medicine* (Philadelphia: University of Pennsylvania Press, 1988), pp. 16–17; Walter L. Bierring, *A History of the Department of Internal Medicine, State University of Iowa College of Medicine, 1870–1958* (Iowa City: State University of Iowa, 1958), p. 45.

2. Edward C. Atwater, "Internal Medicine," in Ronald L. Numbers, ed., *The Education of American Physicians: Historical Essays* (Berkeley: University of California Press, 1980), p. 144.

3. The Maulitz and Beeson volume, *Grand Rounds*, is an excellent introduction to various aspects of the history of internal medicine. A broader discussion of recent medical historiography has to start with such works as Paul Starr, *The Social Transformation of American Medicine: The Rise of a Sovereign Profession and the Making of a Vast Industry* (New York: Basic Books, 1982); Charles Rosenberg, *The Care of Strangers: The Rise of America's Hospital System* (New York: Basic Books, 1987); Kenneth E. Ludmerer, *Learning to Heal: The Development of American Medical Education* (New York: Basic Books, 1985); John Harley Warner, *The Therapeutic Perspective: Medical Practice, Knowledge, and Identity in America, 1820–1885* (Cambridge, Mass.: Harvard University Press, 1986).

4. See A. McGehee Harvey, Gert H. Brieger, Susan L. Abrams, and Victor McKusick, *A Model of Its Kind: A Centennial History of Medicine at Johns Hopkins* (Baltimore: Johns Hopkins University Press, 1989).

5. See Stow Persons, "The Flexner Investigation of the University of Iowa Medical School," *Annals of Iowa* 48 (Summer/Fall 1986), pp. 274–291; Lee Anderson and Lewis January, "Walter L. Bierring and the 'Flexner Revolution' at the University of Iowa College of Medicine," *The Pharos* 55 (Winter 1992), pp. 9–12.

6. See William B. Bean, "An Appreciation: Walter L. Bierring, M.D.," *Geriatrics* 16 (July 1961), pp. 355–359; Lee Forrest Hill, "In Memoriam: Walter Lawrence Bierring, M.D., M.A.C.P., M.R.C.P., Edin.," *Journal of the Iowa Medical Society* 51 (September 1961), pp. 612–613.

7. Robert H. Ebert, "Medical Education at the Peak of the Era of Experimental Medicine," *Daedalus* 115 (Spring 1986), p. 58; Caroline Bedell Thomas, "American Medicine in the Twentieth Century: Some Personal Insights," *Transactions and Studies of the College of Physicians of Philadelphia*, ser. 5 1 (December 1979), p. 251.

8. Ebert, "Medical Education at the Peak of the Era of Experimental Medicine," p. 55.

9. See Anne E. Crowley, Sylvia I. Etzel, Edward S. Petersen, "Undergraduate Medical Education," *Journal of the American Medical Association* 254 (September 27, 1985), pp. 1568–1569.

10. Genevieve Miller, "In Praise of Amateurs: Medical History in America Before Garrison," *Bulletin of the History of Medicine* 47 (1973), pp. 586–615.

11. Ronald L. Numbers, "The History of American Medicine: A Field in Ferment," *Reviews in American History* 10 (December 1982), p. 245.

12. See Susan Reverby and David Rosner, "Beyond the Great Doctors," in Reverby and Rosner, eds., *Health Care in America: Essays in Social History* (Philadelphia: Temple University Press, 1979), pp. 3–16; George Rosen, "Toward a Historical Sociology of Medicine: The Endeavor of Henry Sigerist," *Bulletin of the History of Medicine* 32 (November–December 1958), pp. 500–516.

13. See, for example, Richard H. Shryock, "The Interplay of Social and Internal Factors in the History of Modern Medicine," *Scientific Monthly* 76 (1953), pp. 221–230.

14. The medicalization of American society stood at the center of much of the debate. A good review of medicalization arguments is Renee C. Fox, "The Medicalization and Demedicalization of American Society," *Daedalus* 106 (1977), pp. 3–22; see, also, Daniel Fox, "The Decline of Historicism: The Case of Compulsory Health Insurance in the United States," *Bulletin of the History of Medicine* 57 (Winter 1983), pp. 596–610.

15. For a discussion of potential grounds of rapprochement among medical historians, see S. E. D. Shortt, "Clinical Practice and the Social History of Medicine: A Theoretical Accord," *Bulletin of the History of Medicine* 55 (1981), pp. 533–542.

16. Ludmerer, *Learning to Heal*, p. 137.

17. Genevieve Miller, "Medical History," in Ronald L. Numbers, ed., *The Education of American Physicians: Historical Essays* (Berkeley: University of California Press, 1980), pp. 290–308.

18. For early discussion of the issue, see Z. J. Lipowski, "Psychosocial Aspects of Disease," *Annals of Internal Medicine* 71 (December 1969), pp. 1197–1206; Horacio Fabrega, "The Need for an Ethnomedical Science," *Science* 189 (September 19, 1975), pp. 969–975; George L. Engel, "The Need for A New Medical Model: A Challenge for Biomedicine," *Science* 196 (April 1977), pp. 129–136.

19. Lester S. King, *Medical Thinking: A Historical Preface* (Princeton: Princeton University Press, 1982), pp. 73–89.

20. Eric J. Cassell, "The Changing Concept of the Ideal Physician," *Daedalus* 115 (Spring 1986), p. 189.

21. Edmund Pellegrino, "The Sociocultural Impact of Twentieth-Century Therapeutics," in Maurice J. Vogel and Charles E. Rosenberg, eds., *The Therapeutic Revolution: Essays in the Social History of American Medicine* (Philadelphia: University of Pennsylvania Press, 1979), p. 246.

22. William Bean, "The Scholar in Clinical Medicine," *Archives of Internal Medicine* 111 (January 1963), pp. 1–3.

23. See, for example, Roger J. Bulger, "The Modern Context for a Healing Profession," in Bulger, ed., *In Search of the Modern Hippocrates* (Iowa City: University of Iowa Press, 1987), pp. 3–8; Eric Cassell, *The Healer's Art: A New Approach to the Doctor-Patient Relationship* (Cambridge, Mass.: MIT Press, 1985); Pellegrino, "The Sociocultural Impact of Twentieth-Century Therapeutics," pp. 245–266.

CHAPTER 1

1. The transformation concept of course comes from Paul Starr, *The Social Transformation of American Medicine: The Rise of a Sovereign Profession and the Making of a Vast Industry* (New York: Basic Books, 1982).

2. See, for example, Ronald L. Numbers and Judith Walzer Leavitt, eds., *Medicine Without Doctors: Home Health Care in American History* (New York: Science History Publications/USA), 1977); Lee Anderson, *Iowa Pharmacy, 1880–1905: An Experiment in Professionalism* (Iowa City, Iowa: The University of Iowa Press, 1989).

3. For early patterns of disease, see R. Carlyle Buley, "Pioneer Health and Medical Practices in the Old Northwest Prior to 1840," *The Mississippi Valley Historical Review* 20 (1933–34), pp.

497–520; Erwin H. Ackerknecht, "Diseases in the Middle West," in *Essays in the History of Medicine in Honor of David J. Davis, M.D., Ph.D.* (Chicago: University of Illinois Press, 1965), pp. 168–181.

4. William Watson, "Early Medical Practitioners," in *Historical Lectures upon Early Leaders in the Professions in the Territory of Iowa* (Iowa City, Iowa: State Historical Society of Iowa, 1894), p. 18.

5. For discussion of alternatives to orthodox medicine, see Norman Gevitz, ed., *Other Healers: Unorthodox Medicine in America* (Baltimore: Johns Hopkins University Press, 1988); Robert C. Fuller, *Alternative Medicine and American Religious Life* (New York: Oxford University Press, 1989).

6. S. B. Chase, [Presidential Address], *Transactions of the Iowa State Medical Society* 5 (1881–82), p. 10.

7. Daniel Drake, *Practical Essays on Medical Education and the Medical Profession in the United States* (Baltimore: Johns Hopkins University Press, 1952), pp. 45–59.

8. See John T. McClintock, "Medical Education in Iowa," in *One Hundred Years of Iowa Medicine* (Iowa City, Iowa: Athens Press, 1950), pp. 224–309.

9. See Kenneth Ludmerer, *Learning to Heal: The Development of American Medical Education* (New York: Basic Books, 1985), pp. 127–28; much of the discussion of William Robertson and medical reform in Iowa is adapted from Lee Anderson, "'Headlights upon Sanitary Medicine': Public Health and Medical Reform in Late Nineteenth-Century Iowa," *Journal of the History of Medicine and Allied Sciences* 46 (April 1991), pp. 178–200.

10. James B. Miner, "Medical History of Floyd County," *Journal of the Iowa Medical Society* 32 (1942), p. 441.

11. The reorganization of the larger economy and society in the late nineteenth century is the subject of a vast historiography. Representative early views are Robert Wiebe, *The Search for Order, 1877–1920* (New York: Hill and Wang, 1967); and Louis Galambos, "The Emerging Organizational Synthesis in Modern American History," *Business History Review* 44 (1970), pp. 279–290. More recent works of note are Thomas Bender, *Community and Social Change in America* (Baltimore: Johns Hopkins University Press, 1982); and Martin J. Sklar, *The Corporate Reconstruction of American Capitalism: The Market, the Law, and Politics* (New York: Cambridge University Press, 1988).

12. For the origins and meaning of the medical police concept, see George Rosen, "Cameralism and the Concept of Medical Police," *Bulletin of the History of Medicine* 27 (1953), pp. 21–41; Leona Baumgartner and Elizabeth Ramsey, "Johann Peter Frank and His 'System einer vollstandigen medicinischen Polizey,'" *Annals of Medical History* 5 (1933), pp. 525–32; 6 (1934), pp. 69–90.

13. *Transactions of the Iowa State Medical Society* 1 (1867–71), p. 59.

14. See general discussions in Charles Rosenberg, "Science and Social Values in Nineteenth-Century America: A Case Study in the Growth of Scientific Institutions," in *No Other Gods: On Science and American Social Thought* (Baltimore: Johns Hopkins University Press, 1978), pp. 135–152; Jean B. Quandt, "Religion and Social Thought: The Secularization of Post-Millennialism," *American Quarterly* 25 (1973), pp. 390–409; Burton Bledstein, *The Culture of Professionalism: The Middle Class and the Development of Higher Education in America* (New York: W.W. Norton & Co., 1976).

15. William S. Robertson, "Sanitary Science and Public Hygiene," Paper delivered before the Iowa State Medical Society on May 16, 1883, State Historical Society of Iowa Archives.

16. Stephen Smith, "On the Reciprocal Relations of an Efficient Public Health Service and the Highest Educational Qualifications of the Medical Profession," *Reports and Papers of the American Public Health Association* 2 (1874–75), p. 196.

17. *Transactions of the Iowa State Medical Society* 4 (1879–80), p. 15.

18. *Transactions of the Iowa State Medical Society* 2 (1872–76), p. 181.

19. *Transactions of the Iowa State Medical Society* 4 (1879–80), pp. 10–18.

20. John M. Toner, "Boards of Health in the United States," *Reports and Papers of the Amer-*

ican Public Health Association 1 (1873), pp. 499–500.

21. G. C. Morehead, *Fourth Biennial Report of the Board of Health of the State of Iowa* (1885–87), p. 157.

22. John Shaw Billings, "The Registration of Vital Statistics," *The American Journal of the Medical Sciences* 85 (January 1883), p. 46.

23. P. J. Farnsworth, "Relation of the State to Sanitary Science," *Transactions of the Iowa State Medical Society* 2 (1872–76), p. 172.

24. *Transactions of the Iowa State Medical Society* 4 (1879–80), p. 11.

25. Charles E. Rosenberg, "Doctors and Credentials—The Roots of Uncertainty," *Transactions and Studies of the College of Physicians of Philadelphia*, ser. 5, vol. 6 (1984), p. 297.

26. *Transactions of the Iowa State Medical Society* 4 (1879–80), pp. 27–28.

27. *Transactions of the Iowa State Medical Society* 4 (1879–80), pp. 53–55. In Iowa, there were over 300 homeopathic practitioners in the early 1880s, as compared to perhaps 150 eclectics and some 2,000 regulars: *Annual Directory of Homeopathic Physicians of Iowa, Minnesota, and Wisconsin* (Iowa City, Iowa: Iowa City Publishing Company, 1880), pp. 1–7; Charles H. Lothrop, *Medical and Surgical Directory of the State of Iowa, 1883–1884* (Clinton, Iowa: Allen Steam Printing and Binding, 1883).

28. *Iowa State Register*, February 12, 1880.

29. *Laws of Iowa, 1886*, Chapter 104.

30. See, for example, George E. MacLean's inaugural address as president of the University of Iowa, "The New University," delivered September 29, 1899; Edward Shils, "The Order of Learning in the United States: The Ascendancy of the University," in Oleson and Voss, eds., *The Organization of Knowledge in Modern America, 1860–1920* (Baltimore: Johns Hopkins University Press, 1979), pp. 19–47.

31. John P. Irish, "Some Episodes in the History of the Founding of the Medical College of the State University of Iowa," *The Iowa Journal of History and Politics* 18 (January 1920), p. 125.

32. *Transactions of the Iowa State Medical Society* 1 (1867–71), pp. 129–132.

33. Clarence Ray Aurner, *History of Education in Iowa*, Vol. VI (Iowa City, Iowa: State Historical Society of Iowa, 1916), pp. 137–38.

34. *Iowa City Republican*, January 4, 1871. See also John P. Irish, "Some Episodes in the History of the Founding of the Medical College of the State University of Iowa," *The Iowa Journal of History and Politics* 18 (January 1920), pp. 125–129.

35. *Davenport Democrat*, October 14, 1870.

36. Unidentified newspaper clipping, University of Iowa College of Medicine Papers, Folder 1, 1852–1940, State Historical Society of Iowa.

37. John B. Roberts, "The Science of Successful Surgery," *Journal of the American Medical Association* 12 (February 16, 1889), p. 217.

38. J. M. Angear, "Medicine," *Transactions of the Iowa State Medical Society* 2 (1872–76), p. 109.

39. See, for example, Russell M. Jones, "American Doctors in Paris, 1820–61: A Statistical Profile," *Journal of the History of Medicine and Allied Sciences* 25 (1970), pp. 143–157.

40. William H. Draper, "On the Relations of Scientific and Practical Medicine," *Transactions of the Association of American Physicians* 3 (1888), p. 4.

41. James B. Herrick, "Changes in Internal Medicine Since 1900," *Journal of the American Medical Association* 105 (October 26, 1935), p. 1314.

42. J. M. DaCosta, "Tendencies in Medicine," *Transactions of the Association of American Physicians* 12 (1897), p. 1.

43. See Russell C. Maulitz, "Physician Versus Bacteriologist," in *Grand Rounds*, pp. 91–107; Gerald L. Geison, "Divided We Stand: Physiologists and Clinicians in the American Context," in *The Therapeutic Revolution*, pp. 67–90; L. S. Jacyna, "The Laboratory and the Clinic: The Impact of Pathology on Surgical Diagnosis in the Glasgow Western Infirmary, 1875–1910," *Bulletin of the History of Medicine* 62 (Fall 1988), pp. 384–406.

44. See Walter Bierring, "Reveries of a Doctor: The Old Medical Building," *The Iowa Alumnus*

(February 1919).

45. Walter Bierring, *A History of the Department of Internal Medicine, State University of Iowa College of Medicine, 1870–1958* (Iowa City, Iowa: The University, 1958), pp. 22, 24.

46. See, for example, Middleton's introductory paper on thermometry delivered to the Iowa State Medical Society, "The Thermometer in Disease," *Transactions of the Iowa State Medical Society* 2 (1872–76), pp. 124–30.

47. For the influence of continental European science on American medical science, see Kenneth Ludmerer, *Learning to Heal*, pp. 22–23; Thomas Neville Bonner, "The German Model of Training Physicians in the United States, 1870–1914: How Closely Was It Followed," *Bulletin of the History of Medicine* 64 (Spring 1990), pp. 18–34; William Osler, "The Coming of Age of Internal Medicine in America," *International Clinics*, 25th series 4 (1915), pp. 1–2.

48. See Fritz K. Ringer, "The German Academic Community," in *The Organization of Knowledge in Modern America, 1860–1920*, pp. 409–29.

49. Edwin D. Kilbourne, "The Emergence of the Physician-Basic Scientist in America," *Daedalus* 115 (Spring 1986), pp. 47, 49.

50. Lawrence Littig, "The Practitioner, the Profession and the Medical Organization," *Journal of the American Medical Association* 58 (June 1, 1912), p. 1655.

51. Joseph B. Priestley, "Iowa's Osler," *Journal of the Iowa State Medical Society* 47 (August 1957), pp. 471–74; William B. Bean, "In Memoriam: Walter Lawrence Bierring," *The Pharos* (July 1961), p. 185.

52. See Walter L. Bierring, "The Story of Bacteriology at the University of Iowa," *Journal of the Iowa State Medical Society* 27 (October–November 1937), pp. 555–557, 656–659.

53. Kenneth Ludmerer, *Learning to Heal*, pp. 132–33.

54. C. S. Chase, University of Iowa College of Medicine Papers, Folder 5, State Historical Society of Iowa.

55. Walter Bierring, "The Modern Treatment of Diphtheria with Demonstration of Method of Preparation of Antitoxin," reprinted in *Journal of the Iowa State Medical Society* 25 (April 1925), p. 7.

56. See "Rules and Regulations for the Government of the University Hospital" in Walter Bierring, *A History of the Department of Internal Medicine*, pp. 36–42. For a description of the nineteenth-century hospital, including its moral universe, see Charles Rosenberg, *The Care of Strangers: The Rise of America's Hospital System* (New York: Basic Books, 1988), pp. 15–121; and Morris Vogel, *The Invention of the Modern Hospital: Boston, 1870–1930* (Chicago: University of Chicago Press, 1980), pp. 5–58.

57. C. E. Barrett, "Memorandum Concerning Medical Schools," Box 23, File 2, 1910, George E. MacLean Papers, University of Iowa Archives.

58. Nancy Knight, "'The New Light': X-Rays and Medical Futurism," in Joseph J. Corn, ed., *Imagining Tomorrow: History, Technology, and the American Future* (Cambridge, Mass.: MIT Press, 1986), pp. 67–90.

59. There are, of course, far more conspiratorial interpretations; see, for example, E. Richard Brown, *Rockefeller Medicine Men* (Berkeley: University of California Press, 1979).

60. Ludmerer, *Learning to Heal*, pp. 105–108.

61. Frank Billings, "Medical Education in the United States," *Journal of the American Medical Association* 40 (May 9, 1903), p. 1272.

62. Victor C. Vaughan, "The Functions of a University Medical School," *Journal of the American Medical Association* 54 (April 19, 1910), p. 1191.

63. See Paul Starr, *The Social Transformation of American Medicine*, pp. 114–15; Kenneth Ludmerer, *Learning to Heal*, pp. 84–89.

64. See Rosemary Stevens, *American Medicine and the Public Interest* (New Haven: Yale University Press, 1971), pp. 60–61.

65. Abraham Flexner, *An Autobiography* (New York: Simon and Schuster, 1960), p. 74.

66. Abraham Flexner, *Medical Education in the United States and Canada: A Report to the Carnegie Foundation for the Advancement of Teaching* (New York: The Foundation, 1910). For

a detailed, if skeptical, treatment of the Flexner report and its context, see Howard S. Berliner, *A System of Scientific Medicine: Philanthropic Foundations in the Flexner Era* (New York: Tavistock Publications, 1985). See also Berliner, "A Larger Perspective on the Flexner Report," *International Journal of Health Services* 5 (1975), pp. 573–92.

67. For an insightful account of Flexner's visit and its immediate consequences, see Stow Persons, "The Flexner Investigation of the University of Iowa Medical School," *Annals of Iowa* 48 (Summer/Fall 1986), pp. 274–91.

68. Flexner to George E. MacLean, April 22, 1909, MacLean Papers, University of Iowa Archives, Box 19, File 5.

69. Howard S. Berliner, *A System of Scientific Medicine*, pp. 104–05.

70. Flexner to MacLean, April 25, 1909, George E. MacLean Papers, University of Iowa Archives, Box 19, File 5.

71. File 1(a), 1920–21, Walter A. Jessup Papers, University of Iowa Archives.

72. "State University of Iowa. Medical Department," George E. MacLean Papers, University of Iowa Archives, Box 25, File 5.

73. Kenneth Ludmerer, "The Plight of Clinical Teaching in America," *Bulletin of the History of Medicine* 57 (1983), p. 219.

74. See Thomas Bonner, "German Doctors in America, 1887–1914: Their Views and Impressions of American Life and Medicine," *Journal of the History of Medicine and Allied Sciences* 14 (January 1959), pp. 1–17.

75. See Kenneth Ludmerer, *Learning to Heal*, pp. 83, 92, 113–122.

76. Edward C. Atwater, "Internal Medicine," in Ronald Numbers, ed., *The Education of American Physicians: Historical Essays* (Berkeley: University of California Press, 1980), p. 151.

77. George E. MacLean, July 7, 1909, George E. MacLean Papers, University of Iowa Archives, Box 19, File 7.

78. Chase to MacLean, July 10, 1909, George E. MacLean Papers, University of Iowa Archives, Box 19, File 6.

79. Rockwood to MacLean, July 8, 1909, George E. MacLean Papers, University of Iowa Archives, Box 19, File 6.

80. Jepson to MacLean, July 12, 1909, George E. MacLean Papers, University of Iowa Archives, Box 19, File 6.

81. Flexner to James H. Trewin of the Iowa State Board of Education, November 8, 1909, George E. MacLean Papers, University of Iowa Archives, Box 19, File 6.

82. Whitehead to Henry S. Pritchett, George E. MacLean Papers, University of Iowa Archives, Box 19, File 6.

83. See Persons, "The Flexner Investigation of the University of Iowa Medical School,", pp. 280–81. A board of education replaced the university's board of regents as of July 1, 1909, bringing the university, the agricultural college at Ames, the normal school at Cedar Falls, and the school for the blind at Vinton under a single administration.

84. Minutes of the State University of Iowa Medical Faculty, December 7, 1909, University of Iowa Archives.

85. Minutes of the Iowa State Board of Education, December 10, 1909.

86. First Biennial Report of the State Board of Education of Iowa (1909–10), pp. 10–11; Murdoch Bannister, Board of Control of State Institutions, to MacLean, July 5, 1910, George E. MacLean Papers, University of Iowa Archives, Box 23, File 2; Whitehead's Report to Henry S. Pritchett, November 7, 1909, George E. MacLean Papers, Box 19, File 6.

87. J. Trewin to A. Flexner, April 1910, George E. MacLean Papers, University of Iowa Archives, Box 27, File 2.

88. H. Pritchett to J. Trewin, George E. MacLean Papers, University of Iowa Archives, Box 27, File 2.

89. J. Pratt to G. MacLean, June 5, 1910, George E. MacLean Papers, University of Iowa Archives, Box 26, File 2.

90. J. Guthrie to G. MacLean, June 21, 1910, George E MacLean Papers, University of Iowa

Archives, Box 24, File 5.

91. J. Trewin to G. MacLean, June 20, 1910, and July 16, 1910, George E. MacLean Papers, University of Iowa Archives, Box 27, File 2 and Box 24, File 4.

92. MacLean to G. C. Moorehead, July 19, 1910, George E. MacLean Papers, University of Iowa Archives, Box 25, File 5.

93. R. Palmer Howard, *The Chief: Dr. William Osler* (New York: Science History Publications/USA, 1983), p. 54.

94. *Ibid.*, p. 55.

95. J. Guthrie to G. MacLean, July 9, 1910, George E. MacLean Papers, University of Iowa Archives, Box 24, File 5.

96. C. Howard to G. MacLean, July 19, 1910, George E. MacLean Papers, University of Iowa Archives, Box 25, File 1.

97. G. MacLean to Faculty Committee, State Board of Education, July 19, 1910, George E. MacLean Papers, University of Iowa Archives, Box 25, File 3.

98. Minutes of the State Board of Education of Iowa 2 (July 1, 1910–June 30, 1911), p. 11.

99. G. MacLean to Senator A. B. Funk, July 26, 1910, George E. MacLean Papers, University of Iowa Archives, Box 24, File 4.

100. W. Boyd to G. MacLean, July 26, 1910, George E. MacLean Papers, University of Iowa Archives, Box 23, File 3.

101. G. MacLean to C. Howard, July 28–29, 1910, George E. MacLean Papers, University of Iowa Archives, Box 25, File 1.

102. C. Howard to G. MacLean, August 3, 1910, George E. MacLean Papers, University of Iowa Archives, Box 25, File 1.

CHAPTER 2

1. Daniel Fox, *Health Policies, Health Politics: The British and American Experience, 1911–1965* (Princeton, N.J.: Princeton University Press, 1986), pp. 15–20.

2. James Ewing, "The University and the Medical Profession," *Bulletin of the New York Academy of Medicine*, ser. 2 8 (1932), p. 13.

3. Theodore Hough, "The University the Natural Home of the Medical School," *Proceedings of the Association of American Medical Colleges* 32 (1922), pp. 5–18. Hough's reference to Iowa was no coincidence. President Walter Jessup was one of the respondents to a questionnaire Hough had circulated on the issue; see Theodore Hough to W. A. Jessup, July 10, 1920, File 1(b), 1920–21; March 1, 1921, File 1(d), 1920–21, Walter A. Jessup Papers, University of Iowa Archives.

4. Medical Faculty Minutes, May 10, 1910, University of Iowa Archives.

5. "Report on Medical Education in Iowa," *Journal of the Iowa State Medical Society* 4 (July 15, 1914), p. 79.

6. Medical Faculty Minutes, May 31, 1907, University of Iowa Archives.

7. Ludmerer, *Learning to Heal*, pp. 123–38.

8. Leadership in medicine is highly contested, and academic physicians are clearly but one of the interested parties. Over time there is considerable variation in the relative influence of the various parties; see discussion in David B. Smith and Arnold D. Kaluzny, *The White Labyrinth: Understanding the Organization of Health Care* (Berkeley, Calif.: McCutchan Publishing, 1975), p. 56.

9. R. Palmer Howard, *The Chief*, p. 65.

10. C. P. Howard to L. W. Dean, May 13, 1916, Thomas H. Macbride Papers, File 6, 1916, University of Iowa Archives.

11. L. W. Dean to T. H. Macbride, April 26, 1915, Thomas H. Macbride Papers, File 6(a), 1915, University of Iowa Archives.

12. C. P. Howard, "The Etiology and Pathogenesis of Bronchiectasis," *American Journal of*

the Medical Sciences 147 (March 1914), pp. 313–332.

13. Walter Bierring, *A History,* p. 59.

14. James Young, oral interview with Richard Caplan, September 25, 1985, Department of Internal Medicine Archive.

15. Medical Faculty Minutes, January 3, 1922, University of Iowa Archives.

16. Medical Faculty Minutes, September 22, 1920, University of Iowa Archives; W. A. Jessup to L. W. Dean, May 25, 1923, Walter A. Jessup Papers, File 1(a), 1922–23, University of Iowa Archives.

17. See Rosemary Stevens, *American Medicine and the Public Interest,* pp. 116–120.

18. Medical Faculty Minutes, May 1, 1916, University of Iowa Archives. The Iowa Board of Medical Examiners made one years' hospital experience a requirement for licensure beginning in September 1918.

19. J. T. McClintock to J. G. Bowman, March 19, 1912, John G. Bowman Correspondence, Box 4, File 225, University of Iowa Archives.

20. See Paul B. Beeson, "The Natural History of Medical Subspecialties," *Annals of Internal Medicine* 93 (October 1980), pp. 624; Paul B. Beeson and Russell C. Maulitz, "The Inner History of Internal Medicine," in *Grand Rounds,* pp. 22–25.

21. *Cedar Rapids Republican,* November 23, 1913.

22. Medical Faculty Minutes, December 13, 1915, University of Iowa Archives.

23. See L. W. Dean to T. H. Macbride, January 3, 1916, and T. H. Macbride to L. W. Dean, January 5, 1916, Thomas H. Macbride Papers, File 6, 1916, University of Iowa Archives.

24. Hugh Hawkins, "University Identity: The Teaching and Research Functions," in *The Organization of Knowledge in Modern America,* pp. 285–312.

25. In addition to articles cited elsewhere, see C. P. Howard, "The Medical Aspects of Sarcoma," *Iowa Medical Journal* 20 (March 15, 1914), pp. 467–72; "The Iron Metabolism of Hemochromatosis," *Archives of Internal Medicine* 20 (December 1917), pp. 896–918; "Functional Diagnosis of Polyglandular Disease in Acromegaly and Other Disturbances of the Hypophysis," *American Journal of the Medical Sciences* 158 (December 1919), pp. 830–9; "Progressive Lenticular Degeneration Associated with Cirrhosis of the Liver," *Archives of Internal Medicine* 24 (November 15, 1919), pp. 497–508; "Metabolic Studies in Pernicious Anemia," *Archives of Internal Medicine* 32 (July 1923), pp. 1–16; with Louis Baumann, "Metabolism and Scurvy in an Adult," *Archives of Internal Medicine* 9 (1912), pp. 665–679.

26. *Transactions of the Association of American Physicians* 26 (1911), p. xv; 29 (1914), p. xii.

27. See Lawrence D. Thompson, "Early History of the Central Society for Clinical Research," *Journal of Laboratory and Clinical Research* 41 (1953), pp. 3–5; A. McGehee Harvey, *Science at the Bedside: Clinical Research in American Medicine* (Baltimore: Johns Hopkins University Press, 1981), pp. 122–23; A. McGehee Harvey, *The Interurban Clinical Club, 1905–1976: A Record of Achievement in Clinical Science* (The Club, 1978).

28. See Michael Bliss, *The Discovery of Insulin* (Chicago: University of Chicago Press, 1982).

29. Simon Flexner to C. P. Howard, June 5, 1923; Simon Flexner to W. A. Jessup, June 12, 1923; C. P. Howard to Simon Flexner, June 28, 1923, Walter A. Jessup Papers, File 1, 1922–23, University of Iowa Archives; F. M. Smith to Simon Flexner, October 7, 1924, Walter A. Jessup Papers, File 73, 1924–25, University of Iowa Archives.

30. George Rosen, *The Structure of American Medical Practice, 1875–1941* (Philadelphia: University of Pensylvania Press, 1983), p. 46.

31. Virginia Luckey, "The First Rural Public Hospital," *Journal of the Iowa State Medical Society* (March 1960), pp. 165–66.

32. State University of Iowa Hospital Report, March 4, 1912, President John G. Bowman Correspondence, Box 6, University of Iowa Archives.

33. L. W. Dean to T. H. Macbride, October 26, 1914, Thomas H. Macbride Papers, File 6, 1914, University of Iowa Archives.

34. Hospital Superintendent's Statistical Report, November 1–November 30, 1916, Walter A. Jessup Papers, File 6(a), 1916–17, University of Iowa Archives.

35. Medical Faculty Minutes, December 13, 1915, University of Iowa Archives.

36. W. A. Jessup to Norman Walker [Royal College of Physicians, Edinburgh], July 26, 1921, Walter A. Jessup Papers, File 1(f), 1921–22, University of Iowa Archives.

37. A. Flexner to J. G. Bowman, June 25, 1913, John G. Bowman Papers, Box 2, File 157, University of Iowa Archives.

38. G. Canby Robinson, "The Use of Full-Time Teachers in Clinical Medicine," *Southern Medical Journal* 15 (December 1922), pp. 1009–13.

39. *Des Moines Register and Leader,* July 14, 1914.

40. William Osler, "The Coming of Age of Internal Medicine in America," *International Clinics,* 25th series 4 (1915), p. 4.

41. Sydney R. Miller, "Contemporary Deterrents to the Progress of Clinical Medicine," *Annals of Clinical Medicine* 1 (July 1922), pp. 10–17. For full discussion of the ideological basis of the full-time plan and its implementation, see Berliner, *A System of Scientific Medicine*; Steven C. Wheatley, *The Politics of Philanthropy: Abraham Flexner and Medical Education* (Madison, Wisc.: University of Wisconsin Press, 1988), pp. 59–82. Controversy over the full-time system outlived Flexner, animating both medical historians and academic physicians; see, for example, Michael J. Lepore, M.D., *Death of the Clinician* (Springfield, Ill.: Charles C. Thomas, 1982).

42. Medical Faculty Minutes, June 28, 1915, University of Iowa Archives.

43. L. W. Dean to W. A. Jessup, October 6, 1922, Walter A. Jessup Papers, File 1(b), 1922–23, University of Iowa Archives.

44. Medical Faculty Report to W. A. Jessup, December 1922, Walter A. Jessup Papers, File 1(a), 1922–23, University of Iowa Archives.

45. C. P. Howard to W. A. Jessup, January 9, 1923, Walter A. Jessup Papers, File 1, 1922–23, University of Iowa Archives.

46. Medical Faculty Minutes, June 7, 1915, University of Iowa Archives.

47. C. P. Howard to L. W. Dean, January 6, 1915, Thomas H. Macbride Papers, File 6(a), 1915, University of Iowa Archives.

48. L. W. Dean to W. A. Jessup, April 14, 1920, Walter A. Jessup Papers, File 1(a), 1919–20, University of Iowa Archives.

49. Lawrence W. Littig, "The Practitioner, the Profession, and the Medical Organization," *Journal of the American Medical Association* 58 (June 1, 1912), p. 1656.

50. "Report on Medical Education in Iowa," *Journal of the Iowa State Medical Society* 4 (July 15, 1915), p. 81; *Des Moines Register and Leader,* May 18, 1914.

51. Arther Dean Bevan to T. H. Macbride, April 6, 1914, Thomas H. Macbride Papers, File 6, 1914, University of Iowa Archives.

52. J. H. Trewin to T. H. Macbride, June 9, 1914, Thomas H. Macbride Papers, File 47, 1914, University of Iowa Archives.

53. J. W. Kime, M.D., to T. H. Macbride, April 3, 1914, Thomas H. Macbride Papers, File 6, 1914, University of Iowa Archives.

54. T. H. Macbride to Iowa State Medical Society, May 7, 1914, Thomas H. Macbride Papers, File 6, 1914, University of Iowa Archives.

55. See, for example, Medical Faculty Minutes, October 4, 1916, University of Iowa Archives.

56. On the national level, the American Congress on Internal Medicine was designed to serve a similar post-graduate function, bringing noted medical researchers to a different medical center for a week of seminars and demonstrations.

57. Medical Faculty Minutes, April 19, 1917, University of Iowa Archives.

58. Iowa City *Press Citizen,* June 6, 1936.

59. Medical Faculty Minutes, January 15, 1924, University of Iowa Archives.

60. Stow Persons, *The University of Iowa in the Twentieth Century: An Institutional History* (Iowa City, Iowa: University of Iowa Press, 1990), p. 221.

61. See, for example, Flexner's letter to L. W. Dean, February 12, 1920, Walter A. Jessup Papers, File 1(a), 1919–20, University of Iowa Archives. Much of the description of events surrounding financing of the new complex comes from Lee Anderson, "'A Great Victory': Abra-

ham Flexner and the New Medical Campus at the University of Iowa," *Annals of Iowa* 51 (Winter 1992), pp. 231–251.

62. Stephen C. Wheatley, *The Politics of Philanthropy*, p. 86.

63. See File 1(a), 1920–21, and W. A. Jessup to Abraham Flexner, August 30, 1920, File 1(b), 1920–21; L. W. Dean to W. A. Jessup, December 11, 1920, Walter A. Jessup Papers, File 1(e), 1920–21, University of Iowa Archives.

64. Abraham Flexner, *I Remember: The Autobiography of Abraham Flexner* (New York: Simon and Schuster, 1940), pp. 292–293.

65. Abraham Flexner to Walter A. Jessup, November 27, 1922, File 1, 1922–23, Walter A. Jessup Papers, University of Iowa Archives.

66. Flexner, *I Remember*, pp. 295–296.

67. W. R. Boyd to W. A. Jessup, April 20, 1921, Walter A. Jessup Papers, File 1(c), 1920–21, University of Iowa Archives.

68. Abraham Flexner to Walter A. Jessup, May 25, 1921, File 1, 1920–21, Walter A. Jessup Papers, University of Iowa Archives.

69. W. H. Gemmill and W. R. Boyd to Abraham Flexner, May 28, 1921; Walter A. Jessup to Abraham Flexner, June 1, 1921, File 1, 1920–21, Walter A. Jessup Papers, University of Iowa Archives.

70. Abraham Flexner to Walter A. Jessup, June 7, 1921, File 1, 1920–21, Walter A. Jessup Papers, University of Iowa Archives.

71. William R. Boyd to Walter A. Jessup, May 13, 1922, File 1(f), 1921–22, Walter A. Jessup Papers, University of Iowa Archives.

72. Abraham Flexner to Walter A. Jessup, May 26, 1922, File 1(f), and June 7, 1922, File 1(c), 1921–1922, Walter A. Jessup Papers, University of Iowa Archives.

73. Henry S. Pritchett to Walter A. Jessup, October 31, 1922, and November 8, 1922, Walter A. Jessup Papers, File 1, 1922–1923, University of Iowa Archives.

74. Wheatley, *The Politics of Philanthropy*, p. 105.

75. Abraham Flexner to Walter A. Jessup, November 6, 1922, File 1, 1922–1923, Walter A. Jessup Papers, University of Iowa Archives.

76. Walter A. Jessup to Abraham Flexner, November 9, 1922, File 1, 1922–1923, Walter A. Jessup Papers, University of Iowa Archives.

77. Flexner, *I Remember*, p. 294.

78. Quoted in Wheatly, *The Politics of Philanthropy*, p. 103.

79. Flexner, *I Remember*, p. 296.

80. Quoted in Wheatley, *The Politics of Philanthropy*, p. 105.

81. Abraham Flexner to Walter A. Jessup, November 23, 1922, and Abraham Flexner to W. H. Gemmill, November 24, 1922, File 1, 1922–1923, Walter A. Jessup Papers, University of Iowa Archives.

82. George E. Vincent to Walter A. Jessup, December 7, 1922, File 1, 1922–1923, Walter A. Jessup Papers, University of Iowa Archives.

83. Flexner, *I Remember*, p. 292.

84. Copies of the press release are in the Walter A. Jessup Papers, File 1, 1922–23, University of Iowa Archives.

85. File 1, 1922–23, Walter A. Jessup Papers, University of Iowa Archives.

86. George E. MacLean to L. W. Dean, January 19, 1923, Walter A. Jessup Papers, File 1(a), 1922–23, University of Iowa Archives.

87. *Marshalltown Times-Republican*, February 18, 1923.

88. File 1, 1922–23, Walter A. Jessup Papers, University of Iowa Archives contains excerpts from dozens of Iowa newspapers.

89. *Cedar Rapids Evening Gazette*, December 27, 28, 1922.

90. Resolution of Farmers Union of Emmet County, January 10, 1923, Walter A. Jessup Papers, File 1, 1922–23, University of Iowa Archives.

91. Lee Wallace Dean to Walter A. Jessup, January 21, 1923, Walter A. Jessup Papers, File 1,

1922–23, University of Iowa Archives.

92. Tom B. Throckmorton to Walter A. Jessup, January 26, 1923; Walter A. Jessup to Tom B. Throckmorton, January 27, 1923, File 1, 1922–23, Walter A. Jessup Papers, University of Iowa Archives; *Journal of the Iowa State Medical Society* 13 (February 15, 1923), p. 61.

93. Stow Persons, *The University of Iowa in the Twentieth Century*, pp. 77–83.

94. Iowa State Budget for the Biennium Ending June 30, 1919, p. 21; Budget Report for the Biennium Beginning July 1, 1925, and Ending June 30, 1927, p. 101. The Iowa experience was consistent with the nationwide pattern of rising state support for higher education; see *Historical Statistics of the United States, Colonial Times to 1970*, Part 2 (Washington, D.C.: U.S. Government Printing Office, 1975), p. 1128.

95. See Marcel C. LaFollette, *Making Science Our Own: Public Images of Science, 1910–1955* (Chicago: University of Chicago Press, 1990).

96. See, for example, the *Des Moines Register*'s late December numbers celebrating the agricultural recovery.

97. *Journal of the Senate, 40th General Assembly, 1923*, pp. 471, 861, 966.

98. *Journal of the House, 40th General Assembly, 1923*, pp. 531, 824, 1262, 1291–96.

99. Walter A. Jessup to Abraham Flexner, March 30, 1923, Walter A. Jessup Papers, File 1, 1922–23, University of Iowa Archives.

100. *Des Moines Register*, March 31, 1923.

101. *Acts and Resolutions of the 40th General Assembly of the State of Iowa*, ch. 63, pp. 65–66.

102. Abraham Flexner to Walter A. Jessup, April 2, 1923, Walter A. Jessup Papers, File 1(a), 1922–23, University of Iowa Archives.

103. Walter L. Bierring to Walter A. Jessup, March 31, 1923, File 1(a), 1922–23, Walter A. Jessup Papers, University of Iowa Archives.

104. R. Palmer Howard, *The Chief*, p. 57.

105. William Osler to James B. Herrick, September 17, 1910, C. P. Howard File, University of Iowa Archives.

106. L. W. Dean to T. H. Macbride, February 20, 1915, Thomas H. Macbride Papers, File 6(a), 1915, University of Iowa Archives.

107. L. W. Dean to T. H. Macbride, September 19, 1915, Thomas H. Macbride Papers, File 6(b), 1915, University of Iowa Archives.

108. Dean's search, then, was necessarily short; however, G. Canby Robinson was one of the men recommended as "apt to take that position and who would do good work": Dean of Stanford School of Medicine to David Starr Jordan, Chancellor, September 10, 1915, Thomas H. Macbride Papers, File 6(b), 1915, University of Iowa Archives.

109. Howard's return was cause for a faculty dinner at the Jefferson Hotel and a reception for all medical college and nursing school personnel: Medical Faculty Minutes, January 20, 1916, and January 31, 1916, Thomas H. Macbride Papers, File 6, 1916, University of Iowa Archives.

110. R. Palmer Howard, *The Chief*, p. 76.

111. L. W. Dean to W. A. Jessup, April 8, 1920, Walter A. Jessup Papers, File 1(a), 1919–20, University of Iowa Archives.

112. C. P. Howard to L. W. Dean, March 27, 1924, Walter A. Jessup Papers, File 74, 1923–24, University of Iowa Archives.

113. C. P. Howard to L. W. Dean, May 25, 1924, Walter A. Jessup Papers, File 74, 1923–24, University of Iowa Archives.

114. L. W. Dean to W. A. Jessup, May 26, 1924, Walter A. Jessup Papers, File 74, 1923–24, University of Iowa Archives.

115. Iowa City *Press Citizen*, May 27, 1924, p. 2.

116. Norman C. Miller to C. P. Howard, June 12, 1924, Walter A. Jessup Papers, File 74, 1923–24, University of Iowa Archives.

117. W. L. Bierring to L. W. Dean, June 24, 1924, Walter A. Jessup Papers, File 74, 1923–24, University of Iowa Archives.

118. George F. Dick to W. A. Jessup, August 9, 1924, Walter A. Jessup Papers, File 73, 1924–

25, University of Iowa Archives.

119. James B. Herrick to L. W. Dean, July 20, 1924, Walter A. Jessup Papers, File 73, 1924–25, University of Iowa Archives. Many years later, Herrick spoke warmly of Fred Smith in his memoirs, *Memories of Eighty Years* (Chicago: University of Chicago Press, 1949), pp. 245–6.

120. Fred M. Smith, "The Ligation of Coronary Arteries with Electrocardiographic Study," *Archives of Internal Medicine* 22 (1918), pp. 8–27; see, also, Joel D. Howell, "Early Perceptions of the Electrocardiogram: From Arrhythmia to Infarction," *Bulletin of the History of Medicine* 58 (Spring 1984), pp. 83–98.

121. L. W. Dean to W. A. Jessup, August 9, 1924, Walter A. Jessup Papers, File 73, 1924–25, University of Iowa Archives.

122. F. J. Rohner to L. W. Dean, August 11, 1924, Walter A. Jessup Papers, File 73, 1924–25, University of Iowa Archives.

123. Internal Medicine Faculty to W. A. Jessup, August 12, 1924, Walter A. Jessup Papers, File 73, 1924–25, University of Iowa Archives.

124. W. E. Gatewood to W. A. Jessup, August 12, 1924, Walter A. Jessup Papers, File 73, 1924–25, University of Iowa Archives.

125. R. B. Gibson to W. A. Jessup, August 12, 1924, Walter A. Jessup Papers, File 73, 1924–25, University of Iowa Archives. Gibson presented Fred Smith with an ultimatum on the salary issue, but the administration turned down Smith's recommendation for a raise. Nonetheless, Gibson stayed.

126. L. W. Dean to W. A. Jessup, August 13, 1924, Walter A. Jessup Papers, File 73, 1924–25, University of Iowa Archives.

127. C. P. Howard to L. W. Dean, August 24, 1924, Walter A. Jessup Papers, File 73, 1924–25, University of Iowa Archives.

128. W. R. Boyd to W. A. Jessup, August 21, 1924, Walter A. Jessup Papers, File 73, 1924–25, University of Iowa Archives.

129. L. W. Dean to T. H. Macbride, November 23, 1914, Thomas H. Macbride Papers, File 6, 1914, University of Iowa Archives.

130. *The Daily Iowan,* May 13, 1927.

131. W. A. Jessup to Abraham Flexner, June 13, 1924; General Education Board to W. A. Jessup, June 19, 1924, Walter A. Jessup Papers, File 101A, 1923–24, University of Iowa Archives.

132. See, as examples, F. J. Rohner, C. W. Baldridge, G. H. Hansmann, "Glandular Fever (Infectious Mononucleosis)," *Archives of Internal Medicine* 38 (1926), pp. 413–48; Wesley E. Gatewood, "Syphilis of the Digestive Organs," *American Journal of the Medical Sciences* 169 (February 1925), p. 253.

133. Iowa City *Press Citizen,* May 5, 1927.

134. Iowa City *Press Citizen,* May 12, 1927.

135. Medical Faculty to W. A. Jessup, May 17, 1927, Walter A. Jessup Papers, File 73, 1926–27, University of Iowa Archives.

136. *Des Moines Sunday Register,* July 24, 1927.

137. F. M. Smith to L. W. Dean, April 22, 1927, Walter A. Jessup Papers, File 73, 1926–27, University of Iowa Archives.

138. L. W. Dean to W. A. Jessup, April 7, 1920, Walter A. Jessup Papers, File 73, 1926–27, University of Iowa Archives.

139. W. A. Jessup to F. M. Smith, May 27, 1927; F. M. Smith to W. A. Jessup, June 1, 1927, Walter A. Jessup Papers, File 73, 1926–27, University of Iowa Archives.

140. The story of Peking Union is sketched in Jeffrey W. Cody, "Building Peking Union Medical College," Research Reports from the Rockefeller Archive Center (Spring 1990), pp. 7–9.

141. F. M. Smith to W. A. Jessup, July 14, 1927, Walter A. Jessup Papers, File 73, 1927–28, University of Iowa Archives.

142. W. A. Jessup to G. Canby Robinson, June 27, 1927, Walter A. Jessup Papers, File 73, 1926–27, University of Iowa Archives.

143. F. M. Smith to W. A. Jessup, July 14, 1927; W. A. Jessup to H. M. Korns, July 20, 1927;

Horace M. Korns to W. A. Jessup, July 23, 1927, Walter A. Jessup Papers, File 73, 1927–28, University of Iowa Archives.

144. W. A. Jessup to Earle P. Scarlett, September 22, 1927, Walter A. Jessup Papers File 73, 1927–28, University of Iowa Archives.

CHAPTER 3

1. See Leland Sage, *A History of Iowa* (Ames, Iowa: Iowa State University Press, 1974); Theodore Salutos and John D. Hicks, "The Farm Strike," in Dorothy Schwieder, ed., *Patterns and Perspectives in Iowa History* (Ames, Iowa: Iowa State University Press, 1973), pp. 361–77.

2. File 73, 1929–30, W. A. Jessup Papers, University of Iowa Archives.

3. File 73, 1930–31, W. A. Jessup Papers, University of Iowa Archives; File 73, 1931–32, W. A. Jessup Papers, University of Iowa Archives.

4. File 67, 1931–32, W. A. Jessup Papers, University of Iowa Archives.

5. File 67C, 1932–33, W. A. Jessup Papers, University of Iowa Archives; File 67, 1931–32, W. A. Jessup Papers, University of Iowa Archives.

6. *Daily Iowan,* April 18, 1933.

7. *Des Moines Sunday Register,* August 7, 1932.; File 73, 1932–33, W. A. Jessup Papers, University of Iowa Archives. The latter was computed on an ascending scale, beginning with 15 percent of the first $2,000 and an additional 1 percent of each subsequent $1,000.

8. H. S. Houghton to O. J. Fay [telegram], February 11, 1933, File 73, 1932–33, W. A. Jessup Papers, University of Iowa Archives.

9. W. A. Jessup to Cliff Millen, August 4, 1931, File 67, 1931–32, W. A. Jessup Papers, University of Iowa Archives.

10. E. A. Gilmore to Iowa State Board of Education, May 21, 1935, File 73, 1935–36, E. A. Gilmore Papers, University of Iowa Archives. MacEwen's appointment had been under consideration since at least the previous summer; see H. S. Houghton to E. A. Gilmore, August 30, 1934, File 73, 1934–35, E. A. Gilmore Papers, University of Iowa Archives.

11. E. M. MacEwen to E. A. Gilmore, June 30, 1936, and July 6, 1936, File 73, 1936–37, E. A. Gilmore Papers, University of Iowa Archives.

12. File 73, 1936–37, E. A. Gilmore Papers, University of Iowa Archives.

13. File 57B, 1929–30, W. A. Jessup Papers, University of Iowa Archives.

14. File 67C, 1932–33, W. A. Jessup Papers, University of Iowa Archives.

15. W. A. Jessup to Cliff Millen, n. 13.

16. File 57B, 1930–31, W. A. Jessup Papers, University of Iowa Archives.

17. File 57B, 1929–30, W. A. Jessup Papers, University of Iowa Archives.

18. File 57B, 1929–30, and File 57B, 1930–31, W. A. Jessup Papers, University of Iowa Archives.

19. *University of Iowa Extension Bulletin,* October 28, 1933.

20. H. S. Houghton to W. A. Jessup, July 15, 1932, File 73, 1932–33, W. A. Jessup Papers, University of Iowa Archives.

21. *Journal of the American Medical Association* 105 (August 31, 1935), p. 683.

22. Abraham Flexner to W. A. Jessup, March 20, 1934; J. T. McClintock to W. A. Jessup, March 27, 1934, File 73, 1933–34, W. A. Jessup Papers, University of Iowa Archives.

23. J. T. McClintock to George T. Baker, December 7, 1933, File 73, 1933–34, W. A. Jessup Papers, University of Iowa Archives.

24. *Journal of the American Medical Association* 109 (August 28, 1937), p. 671.

25. See, for example, Arthur Dean Bevan, "The Overcrowding of the Medical Profession," *Journal of the Association of American Medical Colleges* 11 (1936), pp. 377–84.

26. Herman G. Weiskotten, *Journal of the American Medical Association* 108 (June 19, 1937), p. 2134.

27. *Bulletin of the Association of American Medical Colleges* 1 (July 1926), p. 32.

276 NOTES TO PAGES 63–68

28. See Paul Starr, *The Social Transformation of American Medicine*, pp. 261–266.

29. Rosemary Stevens, *American Medicine and the Public Interest*, pp. 186–87.

30. *Final Report of the Commission on Medical Education* (New York: The Commission, 1932), pp. 174–75.

31. E. M. MacEwen to Virgil M. Hancher, August 29, 1940, File 107, 1940–41, Virgil M. Hancher Papers, University of Iowa Archives.

32. *Journal of the American Medical Association* 108 (March 27, 1937), pp. 1026–29.

33. File 73, 1934–35, E. A. Gilmore Papers, University of Iowa Archives.

34. Lewis January, Interview, May 3, 1990; see, also, Charles F. Wooley, "Fred M. Smith (1888–1946)," *Journal of Laboratory and Clinical Medicine* 108 (December 1986), pp. 635–636.

35. See, as examples, Fred Smith, "The Coronary Circulation," *Archives of Internal Medicine* 40 (1927), pp. 281–291; Fred Smith, G. H. Miller, and V. C. Graber, "The Effect of Caffeine Sodio-Benzoate, Theobromine Sodio-Salicylate, Theophylline and Euphylline on the Coronary Flow and Cardiac Action of the Rabbit," *Journal of Clinical Investigation* 2 (December 1925), p. 157; Fred Smith, W. D. Paul, and H. W. Rathe, "Significance of the Coronary Circulation in Arteriosclerotic Heart Disease," *Transactions of the Association of American Physicians* 49 (1934), pp. 163–65; Fred Smith, "The Diet and Theophylline in the Treatment of Cardiac Failure," *Transactions of the Section on Practice of Medicine of the American Medical Association* (1928), pp. 174–81.

36. William W. Moore, *Fighting for Life: The Story of the American Heart Association, 1911–75* (Dallas, TX: American Heart Association, 1983), p. 13; Joel D. Howell, "Hearts and Minds: The Invention and Transformation of American Cardiology," in Maulitz and Long, eds., *Grand Rounds*, pp. 244–48.

37. Willis M. Fowler, *Hematology for Students and Practitioners* (New York: P. B. Hoeber, Inc., 1945; Second Edition, 1949).

38. F. M. Smith to E. M. MacEwen, October 16, 1935, File 73P, 1935–36, E. A. Gilmore Papers, University of Iowa Archives.

39. *American Medical Association Daily Bulletin* 34 (June 10, 1937), p. 1.

40. Minutes of the Iowa State Board of Education, March 7, 1929.

41. H. S. Houghton to W. A. Jessup, May 31, 1929, File 73, 1929–30, W. A. Jessup Papers, University of Iowa Archives.

42. File 73, 1932–33, W. A. Jessup Papers, University of Iowa Archives.

43. Minutes of the Finance Committee of the Iowa State Board of Education, August 6, 1928.

44. See, for example, John P. Swann, *Academic Scientists and the Pharmaceutical Industry: Cooperative Research in Twentieth-Century America* (Baltimore: Johns Hopkins University Press, 1988), pp. 118–169.

45. Harry P. Smith of the Department of Pathology won the Ward Burdick Medal of the American Society of Clinical Pathologists in 1941 for his work in blood clotting.

46. *University of Iowa Extension Bulletin*, July 15, 1934.

47. T. U. McManus to W. A. Jessup, June 18, 1930, File 73, W. A. Jessup Papers, University of Iowa Archives.

48. *Journal of the Iowa State Medical Society* 15 (July 1925), p. 414.

49. Russell Cecil, *A Textbook of Medicine, by American Authors* (Philadelphia: W. B. Saunders and Company, 1928).

50. *American Heart Journal* 1 (October 1925), p. 115.

51. H. G. Weiskotten, "Present Tendencies in Medical Practice," *Bulletin of the Association of American Medical Colleges* 2 (January 1927), pp. 34–5.

52. Rosemary Stevens, *American Medicine and the Public Interest*, p. 162.

53. Rosemary Stevens, "The Changing Idea of a Specialty," *Transactions and Studies of the College of Physicians of Philadelphia*, ser. 5 2 (1980), pp. 159–177.

54. Lewis Thomas, "On the Science and Technology of Medicine," *Daedalus* 106 (Winter 1977), pp. 35–46.

55. Paul B. Beeson, "The Natural History of Medical Subspecialties," *Annals of Internal*

Medicine 93 (1980), pp. 624–626.

56. File 57B, 1930–31, W. A. Jessup Papers, University of Iowa Archives.

57. *Journal of the American Medical Association* 109 (August 28, 1937), p. 668.

58. Rosemary Stevens, *American Medicine and the Public Interest,* pp. 121, 156.

59. *Ibid.*, pp. 167–68, 231–35; George Morris Piersol, *Gateway of Honor: The American College of Physicians, 1915–1959* (Lancaster, Pa.: The College, 1962), pp. 98, 101, 106, 117, 125, 135.

60. See Margaret W. Rossiter, *Women Scientists in America: Struggles and Strategies to 1940* (Baltimore: Johns Hopkins University Press, 1984); Regina Markell Morantz-Sanchez, *Sympathy and Science: Women Physicians in American Medicine* (New York: Oxford University Press, 1985).

61. At one level this is a simple proposition, reflected, for example, in the paucity of female subjects in medical research. At a higher level of abstraction, the study of language and metaphor in scientific rhetoric suggests the same conclusion, at least to some observers. For general discussions of gender and science, see Ruth Bleier, *Feminist Approaches to Science* (New York: Pergamon Press, 1986); Nancy Tuana, ed., *Feminism and Science* (Bloomington, Ind.: Indiana University Press, 1989).

62. Mary Roth Walsh, "Doctors Wanted: No Women Need Apply": *Sexual Barriers in the Medical Profession, 1835–1975* (New Haven: Yale University Press, 1977), p. 224.

63. Robert E. Neff to Margaret E. Nelson, September 13, 1939, File 107, 1940–41, Virgil M. Hancher Papers, University of Iowa Archives.

64. *Journal of the American Medical Association* 115 (August 31, 1940), pp. 765–7.

65. File 107, 1940–41, Virgil M. Hancher Papers, University of Iowa Archives.

66. Charles Rosenberg, *The Care of Strangers,* pp. 327–332.

67. Campbell P. Howard, "The Sphere of the Dietitian," *Journal of the American Dietetic Association* 2 (June 1926), pp. 1–5.

68. E. Neige Todhunter, "Ruth Wheeler," *Journal of the American Dietetic Association* 47 (December 1965), p. 465.

69. Albert H. Byfield to Ruth Wheeler, June 2, 1922, File 1 [Nutrition], 1921–22, Walter A. Jessup Papers, University of Iowa Archives.

70. Ruth Wheeler to A. J. Lomas, April 6, 1923, File 1, 1922–23, Walter A. Jessup Papers, University of Iowa Archives.

71. A. J. Lomas to Lee W. Dean, April 9, 1923, File 1, 1922–23, Walter A. Jessup Papers, University of Iowa Archives.

72. Ruth Wheeler to Walter A. Jessup, June 25, 1923, File 1, 1922–23, Walter A. Jessup Papers, University of Iowa Archives.

73. Lee W. Dean to Walter A. Jessup, April 25, 1923, File 1, 1922–23, Walter A. Jessup Papers, University of Iowa Archives.

74. Ruth Wardall to Lee W. Dean, January 20, 1926, File 73, 1925–26, Walter A. Jessup Papers, University of Iowa Archives.

75. Ruth Wheeler to Lee W. Dean, December 4, 1925, File 73, 1925–26, Walter A. Jessup Papers, University of Iowa Archives.

76. E. Neige Todhunter, "Kate Daum," *Journal of the American Dietetic Association* 47 (November 1965), p. 434; Nelda Ross Larson, "Dr. Kate Daum," *Journal of the American Dietetic Association* 32 (March 1956), pp. 229–230; Patricia Aleson, "Who's It Named For? Kate Daum House," *SUI Staff Magazine* 16 (January 1966), pp. 13–16.

77. State University of Iowa Medical Faculty Minutes, March 8, 1927, University of Iowa Archives.

78. "Nutrition Is No Longer the Step-Child of Medicine," Dietetics Collection, University of Iowa Hospitals.

79. "Personnel and Organization of a Hospital Dietary Department," Dietetics Collection, University of Iowa Hospitals.

80. Walsh, "The Professional Standing of the Dietitian in the Hospital," *Journal of the Amer-*

ican Dietetic Association 1 (December 1925), pp. 103–105.

81. Wilder, "The Hospital Nutrition Expert," *Journal of the American Dietetic Association* 1 (December 1925), pp. 118–127.

82. Standard histories of nutrition are chronicles of great men and their discoveries; see, for example, Elmer Verner McCollum, *A History of Nutrition: The Sequence of Ideas in Nutrition Investigations* (Boston: Houghton Mifflin Company, 1957).

83. Harold H. Williams, "Relationship of the Journal to the American Institute of Nutrition," *The American Institute of Nutrition: A History of the First 50 years, 1928–1978* (Bethesda, Md.: American Institute of Nutrition, 1978), pp. 1–2.

84. Erlene Churchill to Kate Daum, February 25, 1946; Dayna Klisurich to Kate Daum, May 26, 1943, Dietetics Collection, University of Iowa Hospital.

85. Margaret A. Ohlson and Kate Daum, "A Study of the Iron Metabolism of Normal Women," *Journal of Nutrition* 9 (January 1935), pp. 75–89.

86. See, for example, Fred M. Smith and Nelda Ross, "The Importance of Diet in the Treatment of Cardiac Failure," *Journal of the American Dietetic Association* 4 (June 1928), pp. 15–20.

87. Kate Daum to Catherine Kock, April 17, 1930; Kate Daum to Grace H. Smith, June 6, 1934, Dietetics Collection, University of Iowa Hospital.

88. Kate Daum to Mrs. Theo Stebbins, February 22, 1932, Dietetics Collection, University of Iowa Hospital.

89. See Kathleen Wolf, *A History of the Iowa Dietetic Association, 1930–1970* (The Association, 1971).

90. Paul Beeson and Russell Maulitz, "The Inner History of Internal Medicine," in *Grand Rounds*, pp. 22, 27–8.

91. *Ibid.*, p. 29.

92. Harold C. Leuth, "Economic Aspects of Future Medical Practice," *Journal of the American Medical Association* 128 (June 16, 1945), pp. 528–29.

93. *Historical Statistics of the United States, Colonial Times to 1970* (Washington, D.C.: Department of Commerce, 1975), p. 1140.

94. W. Paul Havens, Jr., ed., *Internal Medicine in World War II*, vol. 1 (Washington, D. C.: Office of the Surgeon General, Army Medical Department, 1961), p. 27. Volume one of Havens' official history details the organization and work of consultants in internal medicine; volumes two and three present a compilation of experience with specific diseases.

95. "Activities of the Medical Department in Augmentation of the Army," *War Medicine* 1 (January 1941), p. 73.

96. Roscoe G. Leland, "A Census of Physicians for Military Preparedness," *War Medicine* 1 (January 1941), pp. 95–101.

97. See "Report of the Committee on Military Preparedness," *Journal of the American Medical Association* 119 (June 20, 1942), pp. 650–3.

98. Victor Johnson, "Four Academic Years in Three Calendar Years," *Journal of the Association of American Medical Colleges* 17 (January 1942), pp. 9–15.

99. *Journal of the Association of American Medical Colleges* 17 (January 1942), pp. 48–9.

100. Ewen M. MacEwen to Virgil M. Hancher, March 6, 1942, File 108, 1941–42, Virgil M. Hancher Papers, University of Iowa Archives. Only five medical schools did not immediately undertake the accelerated program: Oklahoma, Baylor, Kansas, Howard, and Meharry: *Journal of the Association of American Medical Colleges* 17 (May 1942), p. 185.

101. Friction between the Procurement and Assignment Service and the military is obvious in official histories; see, for example, John H. McMinn and Max Levin, *Personnel in World War II* (Washington, D.C.: Office of the Surgeon General, Department of the Army, 1963), pp. 74–5, 168–73.

102. *Journal of the American Medical Association* 129 (September 1, 1945), p. 45.

103. *Journal of the American Medical Association* 129 (September 1, 1945), p. 53.

104. File 109, 1942–43, Virgil M. Hancher Papers, University of Iowa Archives.

105. E. M. MacEwen to V. M. Hancher, September 5, 1942, File 109, 1942–43, Virgil M.

Hancher Papers, University of Iowa Archives.

106. See Rosemary Stevens, *American Medicine and the Public Interest*, pp. 277–80.

107. For the story of the Army Air Forces Medical Department, see Mae Mills Link and Hubert A. Coleman, *Medical Support of the Army Air Forces in World War II*, 3 vols. (Washington, D.C.: Office of the Surgeon General, United States Air Force, 1955).

108. Lewis E. January, Interview, May 3, 1990; "Subacute Bacterial Endocarditis Treated with Penicillin," *Journal of the Iowa State Medical Society* 36 (March 1946), pp. 104–6; "Subacute Bacterial Endocarditis Treated with Penicillin," *Air Surgeon's Bulletin* 2 (1945), p. 361.

109. The official history of the blood program, compiled by one of the principals, is Douglas B. Kendrick, *Blood Program in World War II* (Washington, D.C.: Office of the Surgeon General, Army Medical Department, 1964). Kendrick's work is a valuable resource, very detailed and forcefully written; it provided much of the material in this section.

110. See Robert A. Kilduffe and Michael DeBakey, *The Blood Bank and the Technique and Therapeutics of Transfusions* (St. Louis: C. V. Mosby Co., 1942).

111. The findings were published in a series of papers by Elmer DeGowin and various collaborators: E. L. DeGowin, J. E. Harris, and E. D. Plass, "Studies in Preserved Human Blood. I. Various Factors Influencing Hemolysis"; "Studies on Preserved Blood. II. Diffusion of Potassium from the Erythrocytes During Storage"; E. L. DeGowin, R. C. Hardin, and J. E. Harris, "Studies on Preserved Human Blood. III. Toxicity of Blood with High Plasma Potassium Transfused into Human Beings"; E. L. DeGowin, R. C. Hardin, and L. W. Swanson, "Studies on Preserved Human Blood. IV. Transfusion of Cold Blood into Man," *Journal of the American Medical Association* 114 (March 9, 1940), pp. 850–55, 855–57, 858–59, 859–61; E. L. DeGowin and R. C. Hardin, "Studies on Preserved Human Blood. VI. Reactions from Transfusion," *Journal of the American Medical Association* 115 (September 14, 1940); E. L. DeGowin, "Grave Sequelae of Blood Transfusions: A Clinical Study of 13 Cases Occurring in 3500 Blood Transfusions," *Annals of Internal Medicine* 11 (April 1938), pp. 1777–91. See also, Robert C. Hardin, "A History of Blood Banking: Early Days at Iowa," Unpublished Paper presented at the dedication of the Elmer L. DeGowin Memorial Blood Center, December 11, 1981, Department of Internal Medicine Files.

112. Kendrick, *Blood Program in World War II*, p. xiv; E. L. DeGowin and R. C. Hardin, "A Plan for Collection, Transportation and Administration of Whole Blood and of Plasma in Warfare," *War Medicine* 1 (May 1941), pp. 326–341; DeGowin and Hardin continued their collaboration after the war as co-authors, with John B. Alsever, of *Blood Transfusion* (Philadelphia: W. B. Saunders, 1949).

113. Kendrick, *Blood Program in World War II*, pp. 470–71.

114. *Ibid.*, pp. 473–74, 498–99.

115. Lester Maris Dyke, *Oxford Angel: The 91st General Hospital in World War II* (Richmond, Va.: Published privately, 1966), p. 42. Dyke, then a colonel and a career medical officer, was a 1926 Iowa M.D. As a further illustration of the small world of military medicine, Dyke's chief of urology was Dr. Eddie Anderson, who, as coach of the famed University of Iowa "Iron Men" and Heisman Memorial Trophy winner Nile Kinnick, had been the American Football Coaches Association coach of the year in 1939.

116. Kendrick, *Blood Program in World War II*, p. 480.

117. *Ibid.*, pp. 559, 565.

118. See, for example, Elmer DeGowin, "Errors in Mass Blood Grouping and Methods of Minimizing Them," *War Medicine* 4 (October 1943), pp. 410–14.

119. Kendrick, *Blood Program in World War II*, p. ix.

120. E. M. MacEwen to V. M. Hancher, August 29, 1940, File 107, 1940–41, Virgil M. Hancher Papers, University of Iowa Archives.

121. E. M. MacEwen to V. M. Hancher, September 26, 1941, File 108, 1941–42, Virgil M. Hancher Papers, University of Iowa Archives.

122. E. M. MacEwen to V. M. Hancher, January 18, 1943, File 109, 1942–43, Virgil M. Hancher Papers, University of Iowa Archives.

PART II—INTRODUCTION

1. Many Americans approached the postwar years with trepidation, their attitudes and expectations tempered by the harsh realities of fifteen years of depression and war; see William Graebner, *The Age of Doubt: American Thought and Culture in the 1940s* (Boston, Mass.: Twayne Publishers, 1990).

2. For background on the federal government's limited role in scientific research prior to World War II, see A. Hunter Dupree, *Science in the Federal Government: A History of Policies and Activities* (Baltimore: Johns Hopkins University Press, 1986).

3. American Cancer Society News Release, File 1, 1949–50, Virgil M. Hancher Papers, University of Iowa Archives.

4. William Moore, *Fighting for Life: The Story of the American Heart Association, 1911–1975* (New York: The Association, 1983), pp. 56, 83

5. See A. N. Richards, "The Impact of the War on Medicine," *Science* 103 (May 10, 1946), pp. 575–578; George B. Darling, "How the National Research Council Streamlined Medical Research for War," in Morris Fishbein, ed., *Doctors at War* (New York: E.P. Dutton and Company, 1945), pp. 363–398.

6. Elizabeth Brenner Drew, "The Health Syndicate: America's Noble Conspirators," *Atlantic Monthly* (December 1967), 75–82.

7. William Rothstein, *American Medical Schools and the Practice of Medicine: A History* (New York: Oxford University Press, 1987), pp. 236–37.

8. The notion of science as enterprise, however, preceded World War II; see, for example, J. L. Heilbron and Robert W. Seidel, *Lawrence and His Laboratory: A History of the Lawrence Berkeley Laboratory,* vol. I (Berkeley: University of California Press, 1990).

9. Robert H. Ebert, "Medical Education at the Peak of the Era of Experimental Medicine," *Daedalus* 115 (Spring 1986), p. 58.

10. Robert H. Ebert, *Ibid.,* pp. 58–59.

11. For a critical discussion of the intrusion of business management into the conduct of basic science research, see Robert P. Crease and Nicholas P. Samios, "Managing the Unmanageable," *The Atlantic* 267 (January 1991), pp. 80–88. For a local view, see "Research Plan Raked: Iowa Scientists Fear Pursuit-of-Knowledge Curbs," *Des Moines Sunday Register,* September 6, 1992.

CHAPTER 4

1. V. M. Hancher to G. H. Scanlon, April 2, 1948, Medicine File, University of Iowa Archives.

2. V. M. Hancher to A. Flexner, June 21, 1950, File 115, 1949–50, Virgil M. Hancher Papers, University of Iowa Archives.

3. V. M. Hancher to G.H. Scanlon, April 2, 1948, Medicine File, University of Iowa Archives; V.M. Hancher to Faculty Committee, State Board of Education, August 5, 1951, Medicine File, University of Iowa Archives; *Des Moines Register,* October 19, 1947.

4. File 109, 1942–43; File 109J, 1943–44, Virgil M. Hancher Papers, University of Iowa Archives.

5. Stow Persons, *The University of Iowa in the Twentieth Century,* p. 227.

6. V. M. Hancher to L.W. Swanson, April 18, 1949, File 117, 1948–49, Virgil M. Hancher Papers, University of Iowa Archives.

7. V. M. Hancher to A. Flexner, June 21, 1950, File 115, 1949–50, Virgil M. Hancher Papers, University of Iowa Archives.

8. File 109, 1942–43; File 109J, 1943–44, Virgil M. Hancher Papers, University of Iowa Archives.

9. V. M. Hancher to G. H. Scanlon, File 109J, 1943–44, Virgil M. Hancher Papers, University of Iowa Archives.

10. Fred Smith's death in 1946 led to his replacement by Frank Peterson, head of surgery, and a staunch champion of private practice.

11. *Des Moines Register,* October 19, 1947.

12. *Journal of the Iowa State Medical Society* 37 (July 1947), p. 305.

13. L. J. O'Brien to V. M. Hancher, April 9, 1947, File 111, 1946–47, Virgil M. Hancher Papers, University of Iowa Archives.

14. A. W. Dakin to V. M. Hancher, April 8, 1947, File 111, 1946–47, Virgil M. Hancher Papers, University of Iowa Archives.

15. Persons, *The University of Iowa in the Twentieth Century,* pp. 233–234.

16. V. M. Hancher to L.W. Swanson, April 18, 1949, File 117, 1948–49, Virgil M. Hancher Papers, University of Iowa Archives.

17. E. M. MacEwen, n.d., File 111, 1946–47, Virgil M. Hancher Papers, University of Iowa Archives.

18. Lester M. Dyke to V. M. Hancher, July 1, 1949, File 115, 1949–50, Virgil M. Hancher Papers, University of Iowa Archives.

19. Department of Internal Medicine, *Annual Report, 1946.* The Department began compiling sketchy reports in the late 1930s; however, comprehensive annual reports appeared in the postwar period. Hereafter, all references to *Anual Report* are to those departmental documents.

20. The general account of William Bean's selection was compiled from "Memorandum Concerning the Appointment of Dr. William Bean," File 112F, 1947–48, Virgil M. Hancher Papers, University of Iowa Archives; Department of Internal Medicine, *Annual Report, 1948,* p. 13; William B. Bean, Interview, November 16, 1988; and Lewis E. January, Interview, January 15, 1991.

21. Dean Ewen MacEwen, for example, was privately critical of both Smith and Korns: E. M. MacEwen to V. M. Hancher, March 20, 1947, File 111, 1946–47, Virgil M. Hancher Papers, University of Iowa Archives.

22. A. W. Dakin to V. M. Hancher, August 18, 1947, File 112F, 1947–48, Virgil M. Hancher Papers, University of Iowa Archives.

23. V. M. Hancher to C. Jacobsen, September 8, 1947, File 112F, 1947–48, Virgil M. Hancher Papers, University of Iowa Archives.

24. Eugene Ferris subsequently became Medical Director of the American Heart Association, and Richard Vilter succeeded Blankenhorn at Cincinnati.

25. William B. Bean, Interview, November 16, 1988. See William B. Bean, "Nutrition Survey of American Troops in the Pacific," *Nutrition Reviews* 4 (September 1946), pp. 257–259; "Field Testing of Army Rations," *Journal of Applied Physiology* 1 (December 1948), pp. 448–457; "Performance in Relation to Environmental Temperature," *Bulletin of the Johns Hopkins Hospital* 76 (January 1945), pp. 25–58. See, also, Rohland H. Isker, "Research in Army Subsistence," *Journal of the American Dietetic Association* 18 (January 1942), pp. 20–22; James A. Tobey, "The Army's Nutritional Problems," *War Medicine* 2 (May 1942), pp. 437–444.

26. W. B. Bean to C. Jacobsen, March 10, 1948; C. Jacobsen to W. B. Bean, March 16, 1948, File 112F, 1947–48, Virgil M. Hancher Papers, University of Iowa Archives.

27. W. B. Bean to V. M. Hancher, March 23, 1948, File 112F, 1947–48, Virgil M. Hancher Papers, University of Iowa Archives.

28. *Annual Report, 1954–55,* p. 2.

29. William B. Bean, Interview, November 16, 1988; "A Department of Internal Medicine," *Journal of Medical Education* 29 (June 1954), p. 25–26.

30. Staff, Department of Internal Medicine, "An Appraisal of Our Present Department of Medicine," *Annual Report, 1957–58.*

31. *Annual Report, 1954–55,* p. 1.

32. William B. Bean, "A Department of Internal Medicine," p. 27.

33. W. B. Bean to F. J. L. Blasingame, February 12, 1959, File 65G, 1958–59, Virgil M. Hancher Papers, University of Iowa Archives.

34. William B. Bean, "Careers in Medicine," *Archives of Internal Medicine* 99 (June 1957),

p. 851.

35. See also Bean's comments on Kate Daum's death in the *Iowa City Press Citizen*, December 31, 1955, and his comments marking the death of June Fisher: *Annual Report, 1963–64.*

36. File 25, 1954–55, Virgil M. Hancher Papers, University of Iowa Archives.

37. *Annual Report, 1948–49*, p. 14; *Annual Report, 1954–55*, p. 63; *Annual Report, 1959–60*, p. 39.

38. *Journal of Medical Education* 34 (October 1959), p. 167.

39. *Journal of the American Medical Association* 129 (September 1, 1945), p. 55.

40. *Journal of the American Medical Association* 140 (May 14, 1949), p. 178; 159 (September 24, 1955), p. 258; 171 (October 10, 1959), p. 716.

41. *Journal of the American Medical Association* 140 (May 14, 1949), p. 181; 171 (October 10, 1959), p. 718.

42. W. B. Bean to F. J. L. Blasingame, February 12, 1959, File 65G, 1958–59; W. B. Bean to V. M. Hancher, November 30, 1959, File 65G, 1959–60, Virgil M. Hancher Papers, University of Iowa Archives.

43. William B. Bean, "A Department of Internal Medicine," p. 24.

44. *Journal of the American Medical Association* 144 (September 9, 1950), pp. 128–129.

45. *Journal of the American Medical Association* 171 (November 14, 1959), p. 1518.

46. N. B. Nelson to V. M. Hancher, November 3, 1954, File 118, 1954–55, Virgil M. Hancher Papers, University of Iowa Archives.

47. Robert C. Hardin, "The Medical Center," (Unpublished Report, 1966), p. 21.

48. *Annual Report, 1948–49*, p. 4.

49. Minutes of the Compensation Committee, Iowa Medical Service Plan, 1946–60, p. 4; also, Carlyle Jacobsen, Ewen MacEwen, Gerhard Hartman, and Dabney Kerr, "Research in Medicine," February 1, 1947, File 111, 1946–47, Virgil M. Hancher Papers, University of Iowa Archives.

50. *Annual Report, 1949–50*, p. 16; *Annual Report, 1952–53*, p. 17.

51. *Annual Report, 1952–53*, Appendix I, p. 9.

52. Womack Report, File 108, 1950–51, Virgil M. Hancher Papers, University of Iowa Archives.

53. *Annual Report, 1953–54*, pp. 2–3.

54. File 118, 1954–55, Virgil M. Hancher Papers, University of Iowa Archives.

55. File 120, 1955–56, Virgil M. Hancher Papers, University of Iowa Archives.

56. See *University of Iowa Medical Bulletin*, Winter 1957–58.

57. For a brief overview, see William B. Bean, "Recent Advances in Internal Medicine, A Review of Five Years' Progress in the Department of Medicine of the S.U.I. College of Medicine," *Journal of the Iowa State Medical Society* 44 (November 1954), pp. 497–504.

58. *Annual Report, 1947–48*; *Annual Report, 1958–59*, p. 8.

59. *Annual Report, 1951–52*, p. 11.

60. *Annual Report, 1950–51*, p. 10; *Annual Report, 1954–55*, p. 9.

61. *Annual Report, 1954–55*, p. 9.

62. See Victor Cornelius Medvei, *A History of Endocrinology* (Boston: MTP Press Limited, 1982), pp. 385–542.

63. For a description of the Metabolic Ward and its operations, see William Bean and Robert Hodges, "The Operation of a Metabolic Ward," *Nutrition Reviews* 18 (March 1960), pp. 65–67.

64. See, for example, W. D. Paul, R. L. Dryer, and J. I. Routh, "Effect of Buffering Agents on Absorption of Acetylsalicylic Acid," *Journal of the American Pharmaceutical Association* [Scientific Edition] 39 (January 1950), pp. 21–24.

65. See Glenn Gritzer and Arnold Arluke, *The Making of Rehabilitation: A Political Economy of Medical Specialization, 1890–1980* (Berkeley: University of California Press, 1985), Ch. 5, pp. 86–122.

66. W. D. Paul to H. H. Davis, September 21, 1950, File 108F, 1950–51, Virgil M. Hancher Papers, University of Iowa Archives.

67. *Annual Report, 1952–53*, p. 7.

68. *Annual Report, 1948.*

69. *Annual Report, 1954–55,* p. 13; *Annual Report, 1958–59,* p. 6.

70. E. M. MacEwen to V. M. Hancher, March 26, 1947, File 111, 1946–47, Virgil M. Hancher Papers, University of Iowa Archives.

71. *Annual Report, 1952–53,* p. 13; *Annual Report, 1959–60,* p. 6.

72. Kirkendall had, for example, published an early clinical report on chlorothiazide: "A Clinical Evaluation of Chlorothiazide," *Circulation* 19 (June 1959), pp. 933–941.

73. Joseph H. Roe to Kate Daum, May 9, 1951, Dietetics Collection, University of Iowa Hospitals.

74. See "A Report on the Recent Research in Nutrition at the State University of Iowa Hospitals," *Journal of the Iowa State Medical Society* (April 1956), pp. 199–201.

75. Those investigations appeared in the *Journal of the American Dietetic Association* between 1951 and 1955 and in *A Complete Summary of the Iowa Breakfast Studies,* published by the Cereal Institute in 1962.

76. See, for example, Lydia J. Roberts, "Beginnings of the Recommended Dietary Allowances," *Journal of the American Dietetic Association* 34 (September 1958), pp. 903–908.

77. Agnes Fay Morgan, "The Dietitian's Place in the Hospital Research Program," *Journal of the American Dietetic Association* 15 (December 1939), p. 857.

78. Martha Nelson Lewis to Kate Daum, July 12, 1945; Kate Daum to Martha Nelson Lewis, July 23, 1945, Dietetics Collection, University of Iowa Hospitals.

79. Kate Daum to Norman Nelson, August 19, 1953, Dietetics Collection, University of Iowa Hospitals.

80. *Annual Report, 1963–64,* p. 26.

81. File 115, 1949–50, Virgil M. Hancher Papers, University of Iowa Archives.

82. See, for example, *Iowa City Press Citizen,* August 14, 1947.

83. See, for example, James V. Maloney, Jr., "A Report on the Role of Economic Motivation in the Performance of Medical School Faculty," *Surgery* 68 (1970), pp. 1–15.

CHAPTER 5

1. *Historical Statistics of the United States from Colonial Times to the Present* (Washington, D.C.: Bureau of the Census, 1975), p. 76.

2. *Journal of the American Medical Association* 171 (November 14, 1959), p. 1536; John M. Stalnaker, "The Study of Applicants for Admission to United States Medical Colleges in 1953–54," *Journal of Medical Education* 29 (April 1954), pp. 13–20.

3. Mary Roth Walsh, *"Doctors Wanted: No Women Need Apply": Sexual Barriers in the Medical Profession, 1835–1975* (New Haven: Yale University Press, 1977), pp. 230–233, 245; see also, "Women in Medicine," *Journal of Medical Education* 38 (June 1963), pp. 518–519.

4. *Journal of the American Medical Association* 144 (September 9, 1950), pp. 118–119.

5. *Journal of the American Medical Association* 171 (November 14, 1959), pp. 1535, 1544.

6. See Regina Markell Morantz-Sanchez, *Sympathy and Science: Women Physicians in American Medicine* (New York: Oxford University Press, 1985), pp. 329–331.

7. "Women in Medicine," pp. 518–519.

8. *Daily Iowan,* February 13, 1989, p. 1.

9. M. Steinbrink to V. M. Hancher with note from E. M. MacEwen, March 28, 1947, File 111, 1946–47, Virgil M. Hancher Papers, University of Iowa Archives.

10. *Journal of the American Medical Association* 141 (September 3, 1949), p. 33; 171 (November 14, 1959), p. 1542.

11. File 115, 1949–50, Virgil M. Hancher Papers, University of Iowa Archives.

12. *Annual Report, 1953–54,* p. 5.

13. *New York Times,* "Medical Colleges in Vast Expansion," March 2, 1952.

14. See, for example, "Rural Health: Vanishing Country M.D.'s," *Newsweek* (March 24, 1947),

pp. 56–60.

15. See, for example, Lewis Mayers and Leonard Harrison, *The Distribution of Physicians in the United States* (New York: General Education Board, 1924).

16. M. E. Barnes to M. Soley, June 8, 1949, File 117, 1948–49, V. M. Hancher Papers, University of Iowa Archives.

17. V. M. Hancher to H. R. Gross, April 15, 1949, File 117, 1948–49, V. M. Hancher Papers, University of Iowa Archives.

18. Enrollment in several professional programs had in fact dropped precipitously during the war. For example, in pharmacy, total enrollment fell by two-thirds, from 154 to 53 between 1940 and 1945; in engineering, from 478 to 150; and in business administration, from 467 to 141. Hancher may well have supposed that the pattern in the College of Medicine was the same.

19. *Des Moines Register,* June 19, 1949.

20. "Is the Medical Profession Restricting Enrollment of Medical Students?" *Journal of the Iowa State Medical Society* 40 (February 1950), pp. 79–80.

21. Daniel J. Glomset, "The Relation of Research to the Practice of Medicine," *Journal of the Iowa State Medical Society* 36 (June 1946), pp. 231–36.

22. V. M. Hancher to A. Flexner, June 21, 1950, File 115, 1949–50, Virgil M. Hancher Papers, University of Iowa Archives.

23. Virgil M. Hancher, "The Social Responsibilities of Medicine," *Journal of the Association of American Medical Colleges* 25 (March 1950), pp. 81–89.

24. The American Medical Association had established its Section on General Practice in 1945; the American Academy of General Practice was organized in June 1947 and began publication of *GP* in April 1950.

25. E. M. MacEwen to V. M. Hancher, March 26, 1947, File 111, 1946–47, Virgil M. Hancher Papers, University of Iowa Archives.

26. C. A. Nicoll to V. M. Hancher, December 28, 1949, File 115, 1949–50, Virgil M. Hancher Papers, University of Iowa Archives.

27. "Report of the Committee on General Practice," *Journal of the Iowa State Medical Society* 42 (July 1952), pp. 337–338.

28. *Des Moines Sunday Register,* "SUI Medical Wage System Aids Research," February 10, 1952.

29. *Journal of the Iowa State Medical Society* 40 (April 1950), p. 186.

30. W. W. Morris to V. M. Hancher, August 5, 1958, File 65, 1958–59, Virgil M. Hancher Papers, University of Iowa Archives.

31. Anna E. Sevringhaus, "Distribution of Graduates of Medical Schools in the United States and Canada According to Specialties, 1900–1964," *Journal of Medical Education* 40 (August 1965), pp. 733.

32. S. F. Gibbs to *Des Moines Register,* July 22, 1958, File 65, 1958–59, Virgil M. Hancher Papers, University of Iowa Archives.

33. William Bean, "A Department of Internal Medicine," *Journal of Medical Education* 29 (June 1954), p. 13.

34. *Ibid.,* p. 12.

35. William Bean, "Convocation Comments," *Journal of the Iowa State Medical Society* 40 (January 1950), pp. 22–24; see also, "Preparing for a Medical Education and Practice," Proceedings of University of Iowa Symposium, November 9, 1951.

36. William Bean, "A Department of Internal Medicine," p. 13.

37. See James A. Greene, "Coordination of Clinical Teaching: Method and Results of an Experiment," *Journal of the Association of American Medical Colleges* 20 (May 1945), pp. 129–134.

38. William Bean, "The Rise and Fall of the Correlated Clinical Courses at Iowa," *Journal of Medical Education* 31 (February 1956), p. 98.

39. *Annual Report, 1953–54,* p. 4.

40. William B. Bean, "Delirium Cordis," *Diseases of the Chest* 26 (October 1954), p. 390.

41. Walter Bierring, *A History of the Department of Internal Medicine*, p. 98.

42. Edmund Pellegrino, "The Sociocultural Impact of Twentieth-Century Therapeutics," in Morris Vogel and Charles Rosenberg, eds., *The Therapeutic Revolution: Essays in the Social History of American Medicine* (Philadelphia: University of Pennsylvania Press, 1979), pp. 245–246.

43. William Bean, "Caritas Medici," *Archives of Internal Medicine* 92 (August 1953), pp. 153–161.

44. *Annual Report, 1951–52*, p. 9.

45. *Annual Report, 1950–51*, p. 2.

46. File 58, 1946–47, Virgil M. Hancher Papers, University of Iowa Archives.

47. *Annual Report, 1953–54*, p. 7.

48. *Annual Report, 1958–59*, p. 10.

49. *Des Moines Register*, June 30, 1950.

50. *Annual Report, 1952–53*, p. 1; *Annual Report, 1951–52*, p. 2.

51. W. B. Bean to N. B. Nelson, December 8, 1958, File 65G, 1958–59, Virgil M. Hancher Papers, University of Iowa Archives.

52. *Annual Report, 1951–52*, p. 2.

53. Robert C. Hardin, "The Teaching Value of the Veterans Hospital," *Journal of the Iowa State Medical Society* 43 (April 1953), p. 161.

54. H. H. Davis to V. M. Hancher, March 9, 1951, File 108, 1950–51, Virgil M. Hancher Papers, University of Iowa Archives.

55. Walter A. Bloedorn, "Financial Aid to Medical Education," *Journal of the Association of American Medical Colleges* 23 (November 1948), p. 358.

56. Rosemary Stevens, *American Medicine and the Public Interest*, pp. 356–357.

57. N. G. Alcock to V. M. Hancher, March 1, 1950, File 115, 1949–50, Virgil M. Hancher Papers, University of Iowa Archives.

58. V. M. Hancher to Harry M. Neas, January 29, 1951, File 108, 1950–51, Virgil M. Hancher Papers, University of Iowa Archives.

59. *Des Moines Register*, January 23, 1951.

60. *Journal of the American Medical Association* 171 (November 14, 1959), p. 1547. The American Medical Association also had its American Medical Education Fund, established in 1951, to raise money within the medical profession for the support of medical education.

61. W. B. Given to V. M. Hancher, January 10, 1958, File 65G, 1957–58, Virgil M. Hancher Papers, University of Iowa Archives.

62. See Stow Persons, *The University of Iowa in the Twentieth Century*, p. 235.

63. College of Medicine Faculty to V. M. Hancher, June 23, 1949, File 115, 1948–49, Virgil M. Hancher Papers, University of Iowa Archives.

64. V. M. Hancher to Medical Faculty, June 28, 1949, File 115, 1948–49, Virgil M. Hancher Papers, University of Iowa Archives.

65. File 115, 1949–50, Virgil M. Hancher Papers, University of Iowa Archives. For biographical information on Wearn, see Philip Handler, "Joseph Treloar Wearn," *Journal of Medical Education* 40 (November 1965), pp. 1009–1012.

66. Selection Committee Report, August 1947, File 112F, 1947–48, Virgil M. Hancher Papers, University of Iowa Archives.

67. V. M. Hancher to John M. Russell, July 12, 1950; V. M. Hancher to Major General Paul R. Hawley, July 17, 1950, File 110Z, 1952–53, Virgil M. Hancher Papers, University of Iowa Archives.

68. V. M. Hancher to C. Jacobsen, July 7, 1949, File 115, 1949–50, Virgil M. Hancher Papers, University of Iowa Archives.

69. September 27, 1949, File 115, 1949–50, Virgil M. Hancher Papers, University of Iowa Archives.

70. R. T. Tidrick to V. M. Hancher, February 28, 1950, File 115, 1949–50, Virgil M. Hancher Papers, University of Iowa Archives.

71. N. G. Alcock to V. M. Hancher, April 3, 1950, File 115 [Confidential], 1949–50, Virgil M. Hancher Papers, University of Iowa Archives.

72. W. B. Bean to V. M. Hancher, April 3, 1950, File 115 [Confidential], 1949–50, Virgil M. Hancher Papers, University of Iowa Archives.

73. M. E. Barnes to V. M. Hancher, April 3, 1950, File 115 [Confidential], 1949–50, Virgil M. Hancher Papers, University of Iowa Archives.

74. L. W. Swanson to V. M. Hancher, May 24, 1950, File 115F, 1949–50, Virgil M. Hancher Papers, University of Iowa Archives.

75. V. M. Hancher to W. B. Bean, June 22, 1950, File 115F, 1949–50, Virgil M. Hancher Papers, University of Iowa Archives.

76. V. M. Hancher to Faculty Committee, State Board of Education, August 8, 1951; V.M. Hancher to State Board of Education, January 8, 1952, File 110Z, 1952–53, Virgil M. Hancher Papers, University of Iowa Archives.

77. Stephen B. L. Penrose to V. M. Hancher, October 30, 1951; V. M. Hancher to B. F. Wolverton, November 14, 1951, File 110Z, 1952–53, Virgil M. Hancher Papers, University of Iowa Archives.

78. H. H. Davis to Medical Faculty, June 1, 1951, December 18, 1951, File 110Z, 1952–53, Virgil M. Hancher Papers, University of Iowa Archives.

79. V. M. Hancher to H. H. Davis, February 4, 1952, File 110Z, 1952–53, Virgil M. Hancher Papers, University of Iowa Archives.

80. M. M. Weaver to V. M. Hancher, March 2, 1952, File 110Z, 1952–53, Virgil M. Hancher Papers, University of Iowa Archives.

81. Combined report of Committee on Medical Education and Hospitals and Special Committee of the House of Delegates, *Journal of the Iowa State Medical Society* 42 (July 1952), p. 345.

82. D. G. Anderson to V. M. Hancher, January 8, 1953, and February 2, 1953, File 110Z, 1952–53, Virgil M. Hancher Papers, University of Iowa Archives.

83. V. M. Hancher to D. G. Anderson, February 19, 1953, File 110Z, 1952–53, Virgil M. Hancher Papers, University of Iowa Archives.

84. See Stow Persons, *The University of Iowa in the Twentieth Century,* pp. 147–157.

85. Dewey Grantham, *Recent America: The United States Since 1945* (Arlington Heights, Ill.: Harlan Davidson, Inc., 1987), p. 183.

86. *Historical Statistics of the United States from Colonial Times to 1970* (Washington, D.C.: Department of Commerce, 1975), pp. 316–318.

CHAPTER 6

1. In Iowa, per capita expenditures for physicians' services tripled from 1965 to 1975 while hospital costs quadrupled. See U.S. Department of Health and Human Services, *Health: United States, 1982* (Washington, D.C.: HHS, 1982), p. 151.

2. *Annual Report, 1960–61,* p. 1.

3. *Ibid.*

4. *Annual Report, 1961–62,* p. 1.

5. *Annual Report, 1961–62, 1963–64,* Appendix II.

6. *Historical Statistics of the United States,* pp. 316–318.

7. *Annual Report, 1958–59,* p. 2.

8. For background to the passage of Medicare and Medicaid legislation, see Paul Starr, *The Social Transformation of American Medicine,* pp. 368–369; and Rosemary Stevens, *American Medicine and the Public Interest,* pp. 432–440.

9. *Health: United States, 1982,* p. 139.

10. Jonathan Bromberg, "Patient-Generated Medical School Income," *Journal of Medical Education* 49 (1974), pp. 202–203; "Medical Service Plan Income," *Journal of Medical Education*

45 (1970), p. 375; *Journal of the American Medical Association* 234 (December 29, 1975), p. 1346.

11. *Annual Report, 1965–66, 1966–67, 1967–68, 1974–75.*

12. John Eckstein, "Public Opinion: Effects on Medical Education and Research," *Journal of Laboratory and Clinical Medicine* 85 (January 1975), pp. 8–14.

13. *Annual Report, 1974–75*, p. 4

14. William B. Bean to Howard Bowen, February 2, 1967, File 65F, 1967–68, Howard Bowen Papers, University of Iowa Archives.

15. Robert H. Williams, "Departments of Medicine in 1970, I: Staff Policies," *Annals of Internal Medicine* 50 (May 1959), pp. 1252–1276.

16. *Annual Report, 1963–64*, p. 8.

17. James Clifton to Howard Bowen, April 4, 1968, File 65F, 1967–68, Howard Bowen Papers, University of Iowa Archives. On May 20, 1978, ten years after Elmer DeGowin's retirement, the Iowa Clinical Society of Internal Medicine and the Iowa Region of the American College of Physicians conducted a special symposium in hematology and endocrinology in his honor.

18. *Journal of the American Medical Association* 195 (November 15, 1965), p. 803; 214 (November 23, 1970), p. 1510; 234 (December 29, 1975), pp. 1334, 1336. In 1965, departments of internal medicine accounted for nearly 25 percent of all full-time clinical faculty, while in 1975, that percentage fell to just over 18.

19. Henry P. Jolly, *Participation of Women and Minorities on U.S. Medical School Faculties* (Washington, D.C.: Association of American Medical Colleges, 1977), p. 30.

20. College of Medicine, Executive Committee Minutes, December 2, 1968.

21. Jolly, *Participation of Women and Minorities on U.S. Medical School Faculties*, p. 30.

22. For general discussion, see Robert G. Petersdorf, "The Evolution of Departments of Medicine," *New England Journal of Medicine* 303 (1980), pp. 495–496.

23. Executive Committee Minutes, November 11, 1968, File 64, "Medical Affairs, Vice President for Medical Affairs, 1968–69," Howard Bowen Papers, University of Iowa Archives.

24. Rothstein, *American Medical Schools and the Practice of Medicine*, p. 234; John A. Cooper, "Undergraduate Medical Education," in John Z. Bowers and Elizabeth F. Purcell, eds., *Advances in American Medicine: Essays at the Bicentennial*, vol. 1, pp. 296–297.

25. "College of Medicine Report to the President," February 24, 1970, File 65, 1969–70, Willard Boyd Papers, University of Iowa Archives.

26. Howard R. Bowen, *The University of Iowa: The President's Report, September 1, 1965*, p. 60.

27. Ward Darley, "Medical School Financing and National and Institutional Planning," *Journal of Medical Education* 41 (February 1966), pp. 97–109; *Journal of the American Medical Association* 214 (November 23, 1970), p. 1520; *Journal of the American Medical Association* 234 (December 29, 1975), p. 1346.

28. *Annual Report, 1974–75*, pp. 2–3.

29. John Eckstein, "Public Opinion: Effects on Medical Education and Research," pp. 8–14.

30. *Journal of the American Medical Association* 234 (December 29, 1975), pp. 1334–1335.

31. Stow Persons, *The University of Iowa in the Twentieth Century*, p. 184.

32. Robert C. Hardin, Oral History Interview, September 11, 1976, University of Iowa Archives.

33. *Annual Report, 1973–74*, p. 18.

34. *Annual Report, 1962–63*, Appendix I.

35. *Annual Report, 1968–69*, p. 1; *Annual Report, 1967–68*, p. 1.

36. "Hospitals Most Frequently Cited as Place of Residency Training," *Journal of Medical Education* 36 (September 1961), pp. 1228–1229.

37. "Full-Time Faculty School of Graduation," *Journal of Medical Education* 36 (February 1961), pp. 178–179.

38. Medical Council Minutes, March 20, 1969, File 64, "Medical Affairs, Vice-President," 1968–69, Howard R. Bowen Papers, University of Iowa Archives.

39. Glen R. Shepherd, "History of Continuation Medical Education in the United States Since

1930," *Journal of Medical Education* 35 (August 1960), p. 741.

40. *Annual Report, 1962–63,* p. 9.

41. Ralph W. Yarborough, "Alleviating Fragmented Systems of Health Care: The Regional Medical Programs," *Journal of Medical Education* 45 (June 1970), pp. 411–414.

42. See, for example, Gordon K. MacLeod, "Linkage of a Teaching Medical Center to a Multispecialty Group Practice," *Journal of Medical Education* 45 (April 1970), pp. 225–231.

43. Iowa Regional Medical Program, *Annual Report, 1970.*

44. F. G. Ober, "President's Address," *Journal of the Iowa Medical Society* 56 (July 1966), p. 647. The so-called "AMA Amendment" in the original legislation specified that existing patterns of financing, hospital administration, and professional practice should not be disturbed.

45. *Muscatine Community Health Center: Operational Plan* (March 1973).

46. W. B. Bean to D. Stone, February 28, 1969, File 65, 1968–69, Howard R. Bowen Papers, University of Iowa Archives.

47. William B. Bean, *Walter Reed: A Biography* (Charlottesville, Va.: University of Virginia Press, 1982). See also Bean's Fielding H. Garrison Lecture to the American Assciation for the History of Medicine, "Walter Reed and the Ordeal of Human Experiments," *Bulletin of the History of Medicine* 51 (1977), pp. 75–92.

48. W. B. Bean to H. R. Bowen, April 23, 1969, File 65F, 1968–69, Howard R. Bowen Papers, University of Iowa Archives.

49. H. R. Bowen to D. Stone, April 23, 1969, File 65, 1968–69, Howard R. Bowen Papers, University of Iowa Archives.

50. N. S. Halmi to W. L. Boyd, January 8, 1970, File 65, 1969–70, Willard L. Boyd Papers, University of Iowa Archives.

51. W. O. Rieke to J. Clifton, February 2, 1970, File 65G, "Internal Medicine," 1969–70, Willard L. Boyd Papers, University of Iowa Archives.

52. R. C. Hardin to H. R. Bowen, August 29, 1967; Bowen to Hardin, September 1, 1967, File 65, 1967–68, Howard R. Bowen Papers, University of Iowa Archives.

53. William B. Bean, "Introduction," in Walter Bierring, *A History of the Department of Internal Medicine,* p. 10.

54. William B. Bean, "A Department of Internal Medicine," *Journal of Medical Education* 29 (June 1954), p. 17.

55. William B. Bean, "Opportunity for Research in General Practice," *Journal of the American Medical Association* 154 (February 20, 1954), pp. 639–642.

56. William B. Bean, "Criticism in Medicine," *Perspectives in Biology and Medicine* 1 (Winter 1958), p. 226.

57. William B. Bean, "Some Musings on Reviewing Medical Books," *Archives of Internal Medicine* 97 (April 1956), pp. 497–501.

58. William Bean, "Embryon Truths and Verities Yet in Their Chaos," *Archives of Internal Medicine* 102 (August 1958), pp. 179–188.

59. William B. Bean, "Recent Setbacks in Medicine," *Northwest Medicine* 55 (February 1956), pp. 157–160.

60. John M. Eisenberg, "Sculpture of a New Academic Discipline: Four Faces of Academic General Internal Medicine," *The American Journal of Medicine* 78 (February 1985), pp. 283–292.

61. See Earl P. Steinberg and Robert S. Lawrence, "Where Have All the Doctors Gone?" *Annals of Internal Medicine* 93 (1980), pp. 619–623.

62. *Annual Report, 1962–63,* Appendix I.

63. *Annual Report, 1963–64,* p. 3.

64. *Annual Report, 1967–68,* p. 2.

65. R. C. Hardin to Merritt Ludwig, February 2, 1968, File 65, 1967–68, Howard R. Bowen Papers, University of Iowa Archives.

66. David Schwartzman, *Innovation in the Pharmaceutical Industry* (Baltimore: Johns Hopkins University Press, 1976), pp. 158–159.

67. That emphasis reflected Walter Kirkendall's long-term interests. See, for example,

Kirkendall, "Indications for Treatment and Present Day Drug Therapy in Essential Hypertension," *Postgraduate Medicine* 33 (1963), pp. 540–544.

68. For discussion of the factors affecting subspecialty development, see Paul B. Beeson, "The Natural History of Medical Subspecialties," *Annals of Internal Medicine* 93 (1980), pp. 624–626.

69. *Annual Report, 1974–75*, p. 6.

70. Eugene Braunwald, "Can Medical Schools Remain the Optimal Site for the Conduct of Clinical Investigation?" *Journal of Clinical Investigation* 56 (July 1975), pp. i–vi.

71. Robert G. Petersdorf, "The Evolution of Departments of Medicine," *New England Journal of Medicine* 303 (1980), p. 494. See, also, Petersdorf, "Departments of Medicine—1973," *New England Journal of Medicine* 291 (1974), pp. 440–446.

72. Arnold S. Relman, "The New Medical-Industrial Complex," *New England Journal of Medicine* 303 (October 23, 1980), pp. 963–970.

73. E. Grey Dimond, "Lessons from the East," *The Pharos* 52 (Spring 1989), p. 26.

CHAPTER 7

1. Richard D. Wittrup, "The University Hospital: Teaching Hospital or Referral Center," *Journal of Medical Education* 41 (May 1966), pp. 451–456.

2. William Rothstein, *American Medical Schools and the Practice of Medicine*, pp. 10–14.

3. "Physician Supply and the Talent Pool: A National Problem," *Journal of Medical Education* 37 (June 1962), pp. 618–619; Edwin B. Hutchins and Helen Hofer Gee, "The Study of Applicants, 1959–60," *Journal of Medical Education* 36 (April 1961), pp. 289–304.

4. Davis G. Johnson, "The Study of Applicants, 1964–65," *Journal of Medical Education* 40 (November 1965), pp. 1017–1030; *Journal of the American Medical Association* 195 (November 15, 1965), p. 753.

5. *Journal of the American Medical Association* 214 (November 23, 1970), p. 1512; 234 (December 29, 1974), pp. 1336, 1338.

6. Edwin Hutchins and Helen Hofer Gee, "The Study of Applicants, 1960–61," *Journal of Medical Education* 37 (November 1962), pp. 1203–1216.

7. Howard R. Bowen, *The University of Iowa: The President's Report, September 1, 1965*, pp. 8–9.

8. *Journal of the American Medical Association* 214 (November 23, 1970), p. 1488; 234 (December 29, 1975), p. 1410.

9. J. Frank Whiting, Lee Powers, and Ward Darley, "The Financial Situation of the American Medical Student," *Journal of Medical Education* 36 (July 1961), pp. 745–775.

10. "Sources of Medical School Loan Assistance Monies," *Journal of Medical Education* 37 (August 1962), pp. 780–781.

11. File 60, 1974–75, Willard Boyd Papers, University of Iowa Archives.

12. *Journal of the American Medical Association* 195 (November 15, 1965), pp. 753, 809; Edwin Hutchins and Helen Hofer Gee, "The Study of Applicants, 1960–61," p. 1206; Howard R. Bowen, *The University of Iowa*, p. 17; *Journal of the American Medical Association* 234 (December 29, 1975), pp. 1336, 1338, 1410.

13. See Bernard W. Nelson, Richard A. Bird, Gilbert M. Rogers, "Expanding Educational Opportunities in Medicine for Blacks and Other Minority Students," *Journal of Medical Education* 45 (October 1970), pp. 731–736.

14. *Journal of the American Medical Association* 214 (November 23, 1970), p. 1517; 234 (December 29, 1975), p. 1339; Association of American Medical Colleges, *Minority Student Opportunities in United States Medical Schools, 1975–76* (Washington, D.C.: The Association, 1976), p. 54.

15. Howard R. Bowen, *The President's Report*, p. 17.

16. Howard R. Bowen to Robert C. Hardin, June 10, 1968, File 65, 1967–68, Howard R. Bowen Papers, University of Iowa Archives.

17. "Import of Medical Manpower," *Journal of Medical Education* 39 (November 1964), pp. 1056–1057; Kelly M. West, "Foreign Interns and Residents in the United States," *Journal of Medical Education* 40 (December 1965), pp. 1110–1129; *Journal of the American Medical Association* 177 (September 2, 1961), p. 628; *Journal of the American Medical Association* 195 (November 15, 1965), p. 773; *Journal of the American Medical Association* 234 (December 29, 1974), p. 1355.

18. John A. D. Cooper, Liaison Committee Report, File 65G, 1960–61, Virgil M. Hancher Papers, University of Iowa Archives.

19. *Annual Report, 1960–61,* p. 6; File 65 G, 1961–62, Virgil M. Hancher Papers, University of Iowa Archives.

20. *Annual Report, 1963–64,* p. 8.

21. *Annual Report, 1964–65,* p. 8.

22. Franz Reichsman, Francis Browning, and Raymond Hinshaw, "Observations of Undergraduate Clinical Teaching in Action," *Journal of Medical Education* 39 (February 1964), pp. 147–163.

23. *Annual Report, 1960–61,* Appendix I.

24. *Annual Report, 1968–69,* p. 8.

25. See Evans R. Collins, "Teaching and Learning in Medical Education," *Journal of Medical Education* 37 (July 1962), pp. 671–680.

26. For description and examples, see Bruce Joyce and Marsha Weil, *Models of Teaching* (Englewood Cliffs, N.J.: Prentice-Hall, Inc., 1980), pp. 9–10.

27. David P. Ausubel, "A Transfer of the Training Approach to Improving the Functional Retention of Medical Knowledge," *Journal of Medical Education* 37 (July 1962), pp. 647–655.

28. For an example of a comparative study of costs and outcomes, see Jerome S. Allender, Lionel M. Bernstein, and George E. Miller, "Differential Achievement and Differential Cost in Programmed Instruction and Conventional Instruction in Internal Medicine," *Journal of Medical Education* 40 (September 1965), pp. 825–831.

29. William Rothstein, *American Medical Schools and the Practice of Medicine,* pp. 310–311.

30. Lee Powers, Joseph Whiting, and K. C. Oppermann, "Trends in Medical School Faculties," *Journal of Medical Education* 37 (October 1962), pp. 1065–1091; *Journal of the American Medical Association* 177 (September 2, 1961), p. 632; *Journal of the American Medical Association* 195 (November 15, 1965), p. 768.

31. William Rothstein, *American Medical Schools and the Practice of Medicine,* pp. 315–317.

32. *Journal of the American Medical Association* 195 (November 15, 1965), pp. 765–766.

33. See, for example, "The Dilemma of the Internship," *Journal of Medical Education* 39 (May 1964), pp. 437–443; William Rothstein, *American Medical Schools and the Practice of Medicine,* pp. 302–303.

34. William Rothstein, *American Medical Schools and the Practice of Medicine,* pp. 318–319.

35. "Federal Grants for Undergraduate and Research Training, 1948–63," *Journal of Medical Education* 39 (December 1964), pp. 1132–1133.

36. For a survey, see John C. MacQueen, "A Study of Iowa Medical Practitioners," *Journal of the Iowa Medical Society* (November 1968), pp. 1129–1135.

37. See, for example, Lowell T. Coggeshall, *Planning for Medical Progress Through Education* (Washington, D.C.: Association of American Medical Colleges, 1965).

38. Robert C. Hardin, "Does Iowa Need Another Medical School," File 64, "Medical Affairs, Vice-President," 1968–69, Howard R. Bowen Papers, University of Iowa Archives.

39. *Journal of the American Medical Association* 234 (December 29, 1975), pp. 1357–1358.

40. John Eckstein, "Public Opinion: Effects on Medical Education and Research," pp. 8–14.

41. Lance R. Garlock to Howard Bowen, October 22, 1968, File 64, "Medical Affairs, Vice-President," 1968–69, Howard R. Bowen Papers, University of Iowa Archives.

42. The foregoing is taken chiefly from the Raymond Sheets Papers, "Diary, January 12, 1961–May 5, 1962"; Sheets Papers, Minutes and Other Documents Related to the Committee on Administrative Structure of the College of Medicine, 1961–63, University of Iowa Archives; and

"Medical Deanship," File 65, 1961–62, Virgil M. Hancher Papers, University of Iowa Archives.

43. File 65, 1961–62, Virgil M. Hancher Papers, University of Iowa Archives.

44. Robert C. Hardin, Oral History Interview, September 11, 1976, University of Iowa Archives.

45. Stow Persons, *The University of Iowa in the Twentieth Century*, p. 177.

46. Albert W. Snotke, "The Teaching Hospital," *Journal of Medical Education* 37 (April 1962), pp. 255–263.

47. Virgil M. Hancher to Medical Faculty, April 24, 1950, File 115 [Confidential], 1949–50, Virgil M. Hancher Papers, University of Iowa Archives.

48. Memo from Howard R. Bowen to Medical Faculty, July 6, 1966, University of Iowa Department of Internal Medicine Archives.

49. William B. Bean to Howard R. Bowen, June 28, 1968, File 65F, 1967–68, Howard R. Bowen Papers, University of Iowa Archives.

50. Manual of Procedure Draft, File 65, 1967–68, Howard R. Bowen Papers, University of Iowa Archives.

51. Raymond Sheets Papers, Minutes and Other Documents Related to the Ad Hoc Committee on Faculty Participation in the College of Medicine Affairs, 1967–68, University of Iowa Archives; Stow Persons, *The University of Iowa in the Twentieth Century*, pp. 236–241.

52. James Clifton to Raymond Sheets, January 26, 1968, Minutes and Other Documents Related to the Ad Hoc Committee on Faculty Participation in College of Medicine Affairs, 1967–68, Raymond Sheets Papers, University of Iowa Archives.

53. Daniel B. Stone to William O. Rieke, August 14, 1969, File 65, 1969–70, Willard Boyd Papers, University of Iowa Archives.

54. Minutes of the Deanship Selection Committee, May 26, 1969, File 65, 1968–69, Howard Bowen Papers, University of Iowa Archives.

55. William B. Bean to William O. Rieke, December 9, 1969, File 65; Walter M. Kirkendall to Rieke, December 11, 1969, File 65G, 1969–70, Willard L. Boyd Papers, University of Iowa Archives.

56. William O. Rieke to Search Committee Members, January 5, 1970, File 65, 1969–70, Willard L. Boyd Papers, University of Iowa Archives.

57. College of Medicine, Medical Council Minutes, January 17, 1991.

CHAPTER 8

1. *Iowa Alumni Review* 45 (January 1992), p. 37.

2. *Des Moines Register,* May 5, 1991.

3. *Des Moines Register,* November 24, 1991; April 2, 1992.

4. HSA's, Health Systems Agencies, are regional planning agencies whose function is to oversee the allocation of health care resources. PPS, the Prospective Payment System, implemented in the early 1980s, fixed hospital charges for patients falling into designated DRG's, or Diagnosis-Related Groups, a system adapted from research done at Yale University in the early 1970s. MVPS, the Medicare Volume Performance Standard, meant to encourage physicians to bill fewer services, specifies a declining fee schedule as the aggregate of service billings increases. RBRVS, the Resource-Based Relative Value System, is designed to adjust disparities in fee schedules between specialists and generalists and between rural and urban practitioners.

5. For examples of the literature, see Paul M. Ellwood, "Outcomes Management—A Technology of Patient Experience," *New England Journal of Medicine* 318 (June 9, 1988), pp. 1549–1556; Allan S. Detsky and I. Gary Naglie, "A Clinician's Guide to Cost-Effectiveness Analysis," *Annals of Internal Medicine* 113 (July 15, 1990), pp. 147–154; Lockhart B. McGuire, "A Long Run for a Short Jump: Understanding Clinical Guidelines," *Annals of Internal Medicine* 113 (November 1, 1990), pp. 705–708.

6. See Steven Estaugh, "Teaching the Principles of Cost-Effective Clinical Decision-Making

to Medical Students," *Inquiry* 18 (Spring 1981), pp. 28–36.

7. USPHS, *Women's Health: Report of the Public Health Service Task Force on Women's Health Issues* (Washington, D.C.: United States Department of Health and Human Services, 1985); AMA Council on Ethical and Judicial Affairs, "Gender Disparities in Clinical Decision Making," *Journal of the American Medical Association* 266 (July 24/31, 1991), pp. 559–562.

8. See, for example, Robert H. Fletcher and Suzanne W. Fletcher, "Clinical Research in General Medicine Journals," *New England Journal of Medicine* 301 (1979), pp. 180–183.

9. See Jody W. Zylke, "Investigation Results in Disciplinary Action Against Researchers, Retraction of Articles," *Journal of the American Medical Association* 262 (October 1989), 1910–1915; "New Requirements for Authors: Signed Statements of Authorship Responsibility and Financial Disclosure," *Ibid.,* pp. 2003–2005.

10. Charles D. May, "Selling Drugs by 'Educating' Physicians," *Journal of Medical Education* 36 (January 1961), p. 1.

11. See *Journal of the American Medical Association* 265 (January 1991), p. 501; "Physicians and the Pharmaceutical Industry," *Annals of Internal Medicine* 112 (April 15, 1990), pp. 624–626. See, also, "The Relationship Between Physicians and the Pharmaceutical Industry," *Journal of the Royal College of Physicians of London* 20 (October 1986), pp. 235–242.

12. David Rogers and Robert Blendon, "The Academic Medical Center: A Stressed American Institution," *New England Journal of Medicine* 298 (1978), pp. 940–950.

13. Eric Cassell, "The Changing Concept of the Ideal Physician," *Daedalus* 115 (Spring 1986), p. 197.

14. John W. Colloton, "Academic Medicine's Changing Covenant with Society," *Academic Medicine* 64 (1989), pp. 55–60.

15. See, for example, Robert H. Ebert, "Medical Education at the Peak of the Era of Experimental Medicine," *Daedalus* 115 (Spring 1986), p. 76.

16. Roy Porter, *The History of Medicine: Past, Present, and Future* (Uppsala: Institutionen for ide-och lardomshistoria, Uppsala Universitet, 1983), p. 15; Paul Starr, *The Social Transformation of American Medicine,* p. 7.

17. The following biographical sketch draws heavily upon a March 17, 1992, interview with François Abboud, notes from which are in the department's historical collections.

18. James Conway and K. Shirley Smith, "Aging of Arteries in Relation to Hypertension," *Circulation* 15 (June 1957), pp. 827–835.

19. François M. Abboud and J. H. Huston, "The Effects of Aging and Degenerative Vascular Disease on the Measurement of Arterial Rigidity in Man," *Journal of Clinical Investigation* 40 (June 1961), pp. 933–939; "Measurement of Arterial Aging in Hypertensive Patients," *Journal of Clinical Investigation* 40 (October 1961), pp. 1915–1921.

20. In keeping with that interdisciplinary trend, research space in the John Eckstein Building opened in the late 1980s was assigned to individual scientists rather than to departments, with priority to interdisciplinary group projects.

21. François Abboud, "Investing in Excellence," *Journal of Laboratory and Clinical Medicine* 100 (July 1987), pp. 3–12.

22. François Abboud, "Challenges and Values," *Circulation* 83 (June 1991), pp. 2128–2132.

23. *Colleague* 4 (Fall 1987), p. 2.

24. "Medical Education in the United States: Undergraduate Medical Education," *Journal of the American Medical Association* 262 (August 25, 1989), pp. 1011–1019.

25. Minutes of the Meeting of the Councils on Promotions, UIHC, VA, and COM, Department of Internal Medicine, December 1991.

26. American College of Physicians, "Promotion and Tenure of Women and Minorities on Medical School Faculties," *Annals of Internal Medicine* 114 (January 1, 1991), pp. 63–68.

27. *Iowa City Press Citizen,* September 28, 1992.

28. Department of Internal Medicine, Staff Meeting Minutes, March 23, 1989; January 31, 1991.

29. "Medical Education in the United States: U.S. Medical School Finances," *Journal of the*

American Medical Association 262 (August 25, 1989), pp. 1020–1028.

30. J. William Hollingsworth and Philip K. Bondy, "The Role of Veterans Affairs Hospitals in the Health Care System," *New England Journal of Medicine* 322 (June 28, 1990), pp. 1851–1857.

31. "Medical Education in the United States: Highlights of the 1989 Education Issue," *Journal of the American Medical Association* 262 (August 25, 1989), pp. 1001–1002.

32. "Sources of Construction Funds for Teaching Hospitals, 1977," *Journal of Medical Education* 54 (August 1979), pp. 669–671.

33. Department of Internal Medicine, *Annual Report, 1989–90,* pp. 142–143.

34. Medical Council Minutes, February 1, 1990.

35. CVC News Release, January 26, 1987.

36. After his death in 1989 at age 49, Melvin Marcus won the Distinguished Achievement Award of the American Heart Association's Council on Circulation, and the AHA named its Young Investigator Award in his honor. See Allyn L. Mark, "In Memoriam: Melvin L. Marcus, 1940–1989," *Circulation* 81 (June 1990), pp. 1981–1982.

37. François Abboud, *Colleague* 3 (Winter 1987), p. 11.

38. "In Case You Haven't Heard," August 1991, Dean's Office, The University of Iowa College of Medicine.

39. Paul Seebohm, "Learning to Interact with Colleagues—Statewide!" *Iowa Medicine* 78 (1988), pp. 161–163.

40. Bernard S. Bloom and Osler L. Peterson, "Physician Manpower Expansionism: A Policy Review," *Annals of Internal Medicine* 90 (February 1979), pp. 249–256.

41. "Medical Education in the United States: Undergraduate Medical Education," *Journal of the American Medical Association* 262 (August 25, 1989), pp. 1011–1019; 264 (August 15, 1990), pp. 801–809.

42. Michael C. Geokas and Barbara J. Branson, "Recruiting Students for Medicine," *Annals of Internal Medicine* 111 (September 1, 1989), pp. 433–436.

43. Robert G. Petersdorf, "In Defense of Medicine," *The Pharos* 54 (Summer 1991), pp. 2–7.

44. Anne E. Crowley, Sylvia I. Etzel, Edward S. Petersen, "Undergraduate Medical Education," *Journal of the American Medical Association* 254 (September 27, 1985), pp. 1568–1569.

45. "Medical Education in the United States: Undergraduate Medical Education," *Journal of the American Medical Association* 262 (August 25, 1989), pp. 1011–1019; 264 (August 15, 1990), pp. 801–809; Timothy Ready and Herbert W. Nickens, "Black Men in the Medical Education Pipeline: Past, Present, and Future," *Academic Medicine* 66 (April 1991), pp. 181–187.

46. *Colleague* 5 (Winter 1989), p. 30; Iowa City *Press Citizen,* September 23, 1988; *Daily Iowan,* February 13, 1989.

47. Admissions Committee Report, University of Iowa College of Medicine, June 15, 1991.

48. Christopher Lyttle, et al., "National Study of Internal Medicine Manpower: XVI. Subspecialty Fellowship Programs, 1988 Update," *Annals of Internal Medicine* 111 (October 1, 1989), pp. 604–611.

49. Alvin R. Tarlov and Mary Kay Schleiter, "National Study of Internal Medicine Manpower: VIII. Internal Medicine Residency and Fellowship Training, 1983 Update," *Annals of Internal Medicine* 99 (September 1983), pp. 380–387.

50. Michael W. Cox, et al., "National Study of Internal Medicine Manpower: XI. Internal Medicine Residency and Fellowship Training in the 1980s," *Annals of Internal Medicine* 106 (May 1987), pp. 734–740. The 48 percent rate at which women moved from residencies to fellowships in all medical specialties lagged considerably behind the 60 percent rate for men: Christopher Lyttle, et al., "National Study of Internal Medicine Manpower," pp. 604–611.

51. Alvin R. Tarlov, Peter A. Weil, Mary Kay Schleiter, "National Study of Internal Medicine Manpower: III. Subspecialty Fellowship Training, 1976–77," *Annals of Internal Medicine* 91 (September 1979), pp. 287–294.

52. Tarlov and Schleiter, "National Study of Internal Medicine Manpower"; "Medical Education in the United States: Graduate Medical Education," *Journal of the American Medical*

Association 262 (August 25, 1989), pp. 1029–1037.

53. Ronald M. Andersen, et al., "National Studies of Internal Medicine Manpower: XVII. Changes in the Characteristics of Internal Medicine Residents and Their Training Programs," *Annals of Internal Medicine* 113 (August 1, 1990), pp. 243–249.

54. Mark D. Schwartz, et al., "Medical Student Interest in Internal Medicine," *Annals of Internal Medicine* 114 (January 1, 1991), pp. 6–15. See, also, Richard J. Reitemeier, "The Leadership Crisis in Internal Medicine: What Can Be Done?" *Annals of Internal Medicine* 114 (January 1, 1991), pp. 69–75. The growth in internal medicine residency programs, then, reflected hospital administrators' desires to expand patient services rather than a need for more subspecialty practitioners or a surge of interest from qualified applicants; see Andersen, et al., "National Studies of Internal Medicine Manpower."

55. Ronald M. Andersen, et al., "National Study of Internal Medicine Manpower: XV. A Decade of Change in Residency Training in Internal Medicine," *Annals of Internal Medicine* 110 (June 1, 1989), pp. 922–929.

56. John J. Norcini, et al., "Trends in Medical Knowledge as Assessed by the Certifying Examination in Internal Medicine," *Journal of the American Medical Association* 262 (November 3, 1989), pp. 2402–2404.

57. Philip A. Tumulty, "What Is a Clinician and What Does He Do?" *New England Journal of Medicine* 283 (july 2, 1970), pp. 20–24.

58. Liaison Committee on Medical Education, "Functions and Structure of a Medical School," *Journal of the American Medical Association* 254 (September 27, 1985), pp. 1557–1564.

59. John M. Eisenberg, "Sculpture of a New Academic Discipline: Four Faces of Academic General Internal Medicine," *The American Journal of Medicine* 78 (February 1985), pp. 283–292.

60. Paul B. Beeson and Russell Maulitz, "The Inner History of Internal Medicine," in *Grand Rounds*, p. 48.

61. Robert H. Friedman and Janet T. Pozen, "The Academic Viability of General Internal Medicine: The Views of Department of Medicine Chairmen," *Annals of Internal Medicine* 103 (September 1985), pp. 439–444.

62. See Mack Lipkin, Jr., et al., "Primary Care Internal Medicine: A Challenging Career Choice for the 1990s," *Annals of Internal Medicine* 112 (March 1, 1990), pp. 371–378.

63. George L. Baker and Johanna Jones, "Largest Ever Graduating Class," *Journal of the Iowa State Medical Society* 67 (April 1977), p. 133; see, also, Paul Seebohm, "Manpower Situation," *Journal of the Iowa State Medical Society* 67 (April 1977), pp. 139–140.

64. College of Medicine Faculty Minutes, December 16, 1991.

65. *Des Moines Register,* April 3, 1989.

66. *Des Moines Register,* April 2, 1989.

67. Jack M. Colwill, "Where Have All the Primary Care Applicants Gone," *New England Journal of Medicine* 326 (February 6, 1992), p. 388.

68. See, for example, "Looking for U of I's Role in Caring for Iowa," *The Des Moines Sunday Register,* July 26, 1992.

69. "Final Report of the University Review Committee for the College of Medicine," April 15, 1991.

70. *Iowa City Press Citizen,* January 19, 1991. James Clifton, Eckstein's colleague in internal medicine, became interim dean.

EPILOGUE

1. J. H. Means, "Profession or Business?" *New England Journal of Medicine* 261 (October 1959), p. 791.

2. See Charles Rosenberg and Janet Golden, eds., *Framing Disease: Studies in Cultural History* (New Brunswick, N.J.: Rutgers University Press, 1992). See also George J. Annas, "Who's Afraid of the Human Genome," *Hastings Center Report* 19 (July/August 1989), pp. 19–21.

3. Bernardine P. Healy, "Beyond the College Walls," *Academic Medicine* 67 (March 1992), pp. 137–140.

4. See Joseph T. English, "The Changing Scene—II," *Journal of Medical Education* 45 (December 1970), pp. 968–973; Daniel Fox, "History and Health Policy," *Journal of Social History* 18 (Spring 1985), pp. 349–364.

5. David B. Smith and Arnold D. Kaluzny, *The White Labyrinth*, pp. 56.

6. Robert Ebert, "Medical Education at the Peak of the Era of Experimental Medicine," *Daedalus* 115 (Spring 1986), p. 76.

7. See Edmund D. Pellegrino, "The Ethics of Medicine: The Challenges of Reconstruction," *Transactions and Studies of the College of Physicians of Philadelphia*, ser. 5 9 (1987), pp. 180–181. For an extended discussion, see David J. Rothman, *Strangers at the Bedside: A History of How Law and Ethics Transformed Medical Decision Making* (New York: Basic Books, 1991).

8. Larry R. Churchill, "Reviving a Distinctive Medical Ethic," *Hastings Center Report* 19 (May/June 1989), pp. 28–34.

9. Roger Bulger, "The Modern Context for a Healing Profession," in Bulger, ed., *In Search of the Modern Hippocrates* (Iowa City, Iowa: The University of Iowa Press, 1987, p. 10.

10. Edmund Pellegrino, "The Ethics of Medicine," p. 188; Edmund Pellegrino, "Toward an Expanded Medical Ethics: The Hippocratic Ethic Revised," in *In Search of the Modern Hippocrates*, pp. 45–64; see, also, E. Langdon Burwell, "Are People Listening to Physicians Today?" *The Internist* 30 (April 1988), pp. 6–7, 14.

11. See, for example, Thomas W. Furlow, Jr., "Clinical Etiquette: A Critical Primer," *Journal of the American Medical Association* 260 (November 4, 1988), pp. 1558–1559; William B. Bean, "Medical Practice: Past, Present, and Future," *Journal of Medical Education* 51 (December 1976), pp. 979–985; Andrew C. Puckett, Jr., et al., "The Duke University Program for Integrating Ethics and Human Values into Medical Education," *Academic Medicine* 64 (May 1989), pp. 231–235.

12. See Edmund Pellegrino, "The Most Humane of the Sciences; the Most Scientific of the Humanities," in *Humanism and the Physician* (Knoxville, Tenn.: University of Tennessee Press, 1979), pp. 16–37.

13. Minutes of the Meeting of the Council on Promotions, UIHC, VA, COM, Department of Internal Medicine, December 19, 1991.

14. Robert G. Petersdorf, "The Imperative for Health Services Research," *Academic Medicine* 67 (April 1992), p. 244; see, also, the University of Iowa Department of Internal Medicine's *Colleague* 6 (May–August 1990), pp. 2–3.

15. Arnold Thackry, "History of Science in the 1980s," *Journal of Interdisciplinary History* 12 (Autumn 1981), pp. 299–314.

APPENDIX

Faculty of the Department of Internal Medicine, March 1996

EDITH KING PEARSON PROFESSOR OF CARDIOVASCULAR RESEARCH, PROFESSOR OF INTERNAL MEDICINE & DIRECTOR OF THE CARDIOVASCULAR RESEARCH CENTER
PROFESSOR OF PHYSIOLOGY & BIOPHYSICS

DIVISION OF ALLERGY-IMMUNOLOGY

CASALE, THOMAS B., M.D.	PROFESSOR & DIVISION DIRECTOR
BALLAS, ZUHAIR K., M.D.	PROFESSOR
RICHERSON, HAL B., M.D.	PROFESSOR
SEEBOHM, PAUL M., M.D.	PROFESSOR EMERITUS
WEILER, JOHN M., M.D.	PROFESSOR
SMITH, JEANNE M., M.D.	ASSOCIATE PROFESSOR EMERITUS
MULLER, BARBARA A., M.D.	ASSISTANT PROFESSOR/CLINICAL & DIRECTOR OF AMBULATORY CARE SERVICES

DIVISION OF CARDIOVASCULAR DISEASES

HEISTAD, DONALD D., M.D.	UI FOUNDATION DISTINGUISHED PROFESSOR & DIVISION DIRECTOR, CO-DIRECTOR OF AGING CENTER, & DEPUTY DIRECTOR of CARDIOVASCULAR RESEARCH CENTER PROFESSOR OF PHARMACOLOGY
KERBER, RICHARD E., M.D.	PROFESSOR & ASSOCIATE DIVISION DIRECTOR
BROWN, DONALD D., M.D.	PROFESSOR
ECKSTEIN, JOHN W., M.D.	PROFESSOR EMERITUS & DEAN EMERITUS
FELDER, ROBERT B., M.D.	PROFESSOR
JANUARY, LEWIS E., M.D., D.Sc.	PROFESSOR EMERITUS & SPECIAL ASSISTANT TO THE CHAIRMAN
KIRCHNER, PETER T., M.D.	PROFESSOR [RADIOLOGY]
MARK, ALLYN L., M.D.	ROY J. CARVER PROFESSOR OF MEDICINE & ASSOCIATE DEAN FOR RESEARCH DEVELOPMENT
MARTINS, JAMES B., M.D.	PROFESSOR
SCHMID, PHILLIP G., Jr., M.D.	PROFESSOR & ASSOCIATE CHIEF OF STAFF FOR RESEARCH & DEVELOPMENT, VAMC
SKORTON, DAVID J., M.D.	PROFESSOR & UI VICE PRESIDENT FOR RESEARCH PROFESSOR OF ELECTRICAL & COMPUTER ENGINEERING
SPECTOR, ARTHUR A., M.D.	PROFESSOR [BIOCHEMISTRY]
WINNIFORD, MICHAEL D., M.D.	PROFESSOR
DELLSPERGER, KEVIN C., M.D., Ph.D.	ASSOCIATE PROFESSOR
FARACI, FRANK M., Ph.D.	ASSOCIATE PROFESSOR ASSOCIATE PROFESSOR OF PHARMACOLOGY
FUNK, DAVID C., M.D.	ASSOCIATE PROFESSOR EMERITUS
GROVER-McKAY, MALEAH, M.D.	ASSOCIATE PROFESSOR ASSOCIATE PROFESSOR OF RADIOLOGY

[ ] Indicates primary department of faculty who hold a secondary appointment in Internal Medicine

FACULTY, 1996 (*continued*)

GUTTERMAN, DAVID D., M.D.	ASSOCIATE PROFESSOR
KALIL, DARRYL A., M.D.	ASSOCIATE PROFESSOR/CLINICAL
KIENZLE, MICHAEL G., M.D.	ASSOCIATE PROFESSOR & ASSOCIATE DEAN FOR CLINICAL AFFAIRS
LEE, HON-CHI, M.D., Ph.D.	ASSOCIATE PROFESSOR
McBRIDE, JOHN W., Jr., M.D.	ASSOCIATE PROFESSOR/CLINICAL
McKAY, CHARLES R., M.D.	ASSOCIATE PROFESSOR
ROSSEN, JAMES D., M.D.	ASSOCIATE PROFESSOR
VANDENBERG, BYRON F., M.D.	ASSOCIATE PROFESSOR
CHAPLEAU, MARK W., Ph.D.	ASSISTANT PROFESSOR
GORDON ELLEN E.I., M.D.	ASSISTANT PROFESSOR
HOPSON, JAMES R., M.D.	ASSISTANT PROFESSOR
LAMPING, KATHRYN G., Ph.D.	ASSISTANT PROFESSOR
MULHERN, KEVIN M., M.D.	ASSISTANT PROFESSOR/CLINICAL
OREN, RON M., M.D.	ASSISTANT PROFESSOR
OSKARSSON, HELGI J., M.D.	ASSISTANT PROFESSOR
SIGMUND, CURT D., Ph.D.	ASSISTANT PROFESSOR
	ASSISTANT PROFESSOR OF PHYSIOLOGY & BIOPHYSICS
SOMERS, VIREND K., M.D., D.Phil.	ASSISTANT PROFESSOR
WEISS, ROBERT M., M.D.	ASSISTANT PROFESSOR
MEDH, JHEEM D., Ph.D.	ADJUNCT ASSISTANT PROFESSOR & ASSISTANT RESEARCH SCIENTIST
PARDINI, BENET J., Ph.D.	ADJUNCT ASSISTANT PROFESSOR & ASSOCIATE RESEARCH SCIENTIST
HAYNES, WILLIAM G., M.D.	VISITING ASSOCIATE
MILLER, FRANCIS J., JR., M.D.	ASSOCIATE
WEINTRAUB, NEAL L., M.D.	ASSOCIATE

DIVISION OF CLINICAL PHARMACOLOGY

KNAPP, HOWARD R., M.D., Ph.D.	ASSOCIATE PROFESSOR & DIVISION DIRECTOR
	ASSOCIATE PROFESSOR OF PHARMACOLOGY

DIVISION OF ENDOCRINOLOGY-METABOLISM

BAR, ROBERT S., M.D.	PROFESSOR & DIVISION DIRECTOR, & DIRECTOR OF DIABETES & ENDOCRINOLOGY RESEARCH CENTER
SCHLECHTE, JANET A., M.D.	PROFESSOR & DIRECTOR FOR POSTGRADUATE PROGRAMS, & DIRECTOR OF CLINICAL RESEARCH CENTER
CHAPPELL, DAVID A., M.D.	ASSOCIATE PROFESSOR
MacINDOE, JOHN H., M.D.	ASSOCIATE PROFESSOR & DIRECTOR OF CONTINUING MEDICAL EDUCATION
SIVITZ, WILLIAM I., M.D.	ASSOCIATE PROFESSOR
SPANHEIMER, ROBERT G., M.D.	ASSOCIATE PROFESSOR
YOREK, MARK A., Ph.D.	ASSOCIATE PROFESSOR
SHARP, STEPHAN C., M.D.	ASSISTANT PROFESSOR/CLINICAL
THOMAS, MICHAEL J., M.D., Ph.D.	ASSISTANT PROFESSOR

DIVISION OF GASTROENTEROLOGY-HEPATOLOGY

WEINSTOCK, JOEL V., M.D.	PROFESSOR & DIVISION DIRECTOR
CHRISTENSEN, JAMES, M.D.	PROFESSOR
CLIFTON, JAMES A., M.D.	ROY J. CARVER PROFESSOR EMERITUS & INTERIM DEAN EMERITUS
FIELD, F. JEFFREY, M.D.	PROFESSOR & ASSOCIATE CHAIR FOR EDUCATIONAL PROGRAMS
HUBEL, KENNETH A., M.D.	PROFESSOR
LaBRECQUE, DOUGLAS R., M.D.	PROFESSOR
SCHEDL, HAROLD P., Ph.D., M.D.	PROFESSOR EMERITUS
SCHULZE, KONRAD S., M.D.	PROFESSOR
SUMMERS, ROBERT W., M.D.	PROFESSOR
CONKLIN, JEFFREY L., M.D.	ASSOCIATE PROFESSOR
JOHLIN, FREDERICK C., Jr., M.D.	ASSOCIATE PROFESSOR
ELLIOTT, DAVID E., M.D., Ph.D.	ASSISTANT PROFESSOR
MURRAY, JOSEPH A., M.D.	ASSISTANT PROFESSOR
RAO, SATISH S-C., M.D., Ph.D.	ASSISTANT PROFESSOR
SCHMIDT, WARREN N., Ph.D., M.D.	ASSISTANT PROFESSOR
TRUSZKOWSKI, JOSEPH A., M.D.	ASSISTANT PROFESSOR/CLINICAL
VOIGHT, MICHAEL J., M.D.	ASSISTANT PROFESSOR/CLINICAL
DONNER, CHARLES S., M.D.	ASSOCIATE
HILLEBRAND, DONALD J., M.D.	ASSOCIATE

DIVISION OF GENERAL MEDICINE, CLINICAL EPIDEMIOLOGY & HEALTH SERVICES RESEARCH

HELMS, CHARLES M., M.D., Ph.D.	PROFESSOR & ACTING DIVISION DIRECTOR
BELGUM, DAVID R., Ph.D.	PROFESSOR EMERITUS [RELIGION]
GALBRAITH, WILLIAM B., M.D.	PROFESSOR/CLINICAL & DIRECTOR OF PRIMARY CARE TRAINING
KATHOL, ROGER G., M.D.	PROFESSOR [PSYCHIATRY]

SMITH, IAN M., M.D.	PROFESSOR EMERITUS
TOBACMAN, LARRY S., M.D.	PROFESSOR
	PROFESSOR OF BIOCHEMISTRY
WALLACE, ROBERT B., M.D.	PROFESSOR [PREVENTIVE MEDICINE]
HEGEMAN, ROBERT J., M.D.	ASSOCIATE PROFESSOR/CLINICAL [SURGERY]
HERWALDT, LOREEN A., M.D.	ASSOCIATE PROFESSOR
SCHROTT, HELMUT G., M.D.	ASSOCIATE PROFESSOR [PREVENTIVE MEDICINE]
ZEITLER, RODNEY R., M.D.	ASSOCIATE PROFESSOR
DOEBBELING, BRADLEY N., M.D.	ASSISTANT PROFESSOR
FLANAGAN, JAMES R., Ph.D., M.D.	ASSISTANT PROFESSOR
GOERDT, CHRISTOPHER J., M.D.	ASSISTANT PROFESSOR/CLINICAL
KAUFMAN, LISA M., M.D.	ASSISTANT PROFESSOR/CLINICAL
MULHAUSEN, PAUL L. M.D.	ASSISTANT PROFESSOR
NISLY, NICOLE L., M.D.	ASSISTANT PROFESSOR/CLINICAL
TOBACMAN, JOANNE K., M.D.	ASSISTANT PROFESSOR
BERG, MARY ANNE, M.D.	ASSOCIATE
McFARLIN, BRET, D.O.	ASSOCIATE
YODER, KATHERINE E., M.D.	ASSOCIATE

ASSOCIATES (UI Select):

BOZEK, THOMAS T., M.D.	ASSOCIATE [UI Select]
NEAHRING, JENNIFER C., M.D.	ASSOCIATE [UI Select]

DIVISION OF
HEMATOLOGY-ONCOLOGY

BURNS, C. PATRICK, M.D.	PROFESSOR & DIVISION DIRECTOR
CLAMON, GERALD H., M.D.	PROFESSOR
DeGOWIN, RICHARD L., M.D.	PROFESSOR
GINGRICH, ROGER D., M.D., Ph.D.	PROFESSOR
MACFARLANE, DONALD E., M.D., Ph.D.	PROFESSOR
DREICER, ROBERT, M.D.	ASSOCIATE PROFESSOR & ASSOCIATE DIRECTOR FOR CLINICAL RESEARCH FOR UI CANCER CENTER
	ASSOCIATE PROFESSOR OF UROLOGY
HARMAN, GLENN S., M.D.	ASSOCIATE PROFESSOR/CLINICAL
RIGGS, CHARLES E., Jr., M.D.	ASSOCIATE PROFESSOR & MEDICAL DIRECTOR OF CLINICAL CANCER CENTER
WEINER, GEORGE J., M.D.	ASSOCIATE PROFESSOR & ASSOCIATE DIRECTOR OF EDUCATION FOR UI CANCER CENTER
BERG, DANIEL J., M.D.	ASSISTANT PROFESSOR
HOHL, RAYMOND J., M.D., Ph.D.	ASSISTANT PROFESSOR
	ASSISTANT PROFESSOR OF PHARMACOLOGY
KAMBHU, SUSAN A., M.D.	ASSISTANT PROFESSOR
KARWAL, MARK, M.D.	ASSISTANT PROFESSOR/CLINICAL
LEE, CHOON-KEE, M.D.	ASSISTANT PROFESSOR
LENTZ, STEVEN R., M.D., Ph.D.	ASSISTANT PROFESSOR
LINK, BRIAN K., M.D.	ASSISTANT PROFESSOR
CARLISLE, THOMAS L., M.D., Ph.D.	INSTRUCTOR

DIVISION OF INFECTIOUS DISEASES

BRITIGAN, BRADLEY E., M.D.	PROFESSOR & DIVISION DIRECTOR
DENSEN, PETER, M.D.	PROFESSOR & ASSOCIATE DEAN FOR MEDICAL EDUCATION
HELMS, CHARLES M., M.D., Ph.D.	PROFESSOR
NAUSEEF, WILLIAM M., M.D.	PROFESSOR
KIRCHHOFF, LOUIS V., M.D.	ASSOCIATE PROFESSOR
STAPLETON, JACK T., M.D.	ASSOCIATE PROFESSOR
WILSON, MARY E., M.D.	ASSOCIATE PROFESSOR
	ASSOCIATE PROFESSOR OF MICROBIOLOGY
KLION, AMY D., M.D.	ASSISTANT PROFESSOR
KOZAL, MICHAEL J., M.D.	ASSISTANT PROFESSOR
KUSNER, DAVID J., M.D., Ph.D.	ASSISTANT PROFESSOR
MEIER, JEFFERY L., M.D.	ASSISTANT PROFESSOR
SCHLESINGER, LARRY S., M.D.	ASSISTANT PROFESSOR
WINOKUR, PATRICIA L., M.D.	ASSISTANT PROFESSOR
DENNING, GERENE, Ph.D.	ADJUNCT ASSISTANT PROFESSOR & ASSISTANT RESEARCH SCIENTIST
GAYNOR, CECILIA D., M.D.	ASSOCIATE

DIVISION OF NEPHROLOGY

STOKES, JOHN B., III, M.D.	PROFESSOR & DIVISION DIRECTOR, & ASSOCIATE CHAIR FOR ACADEMIC PROGRAMS
DiBONA, GERALD F., M.D.	PROFESSOR & DEPARTMENT VICE CHAIRMAN, & CHIEF, MEDICAL SERVICES, VAMC

299

FACULTY, 1996 (*continued*)

HUNSICKER, LAWRENCE G., M.D.	PROFESSOR
LIM, VICTORIA S., M.D.	PROFESSOR
BERTOLATUS, JOHN A., M.D.	ASSOCIATE PROFESSOR
DIXON, BRADLEY S., M.D.	ASSOCIATE PROFESSOR
GORDON JOEL A., M.D.	ASSOCIATE PROFESSOR & ASSOCIATE DIRECTOR FOR POSTGRADUATE PROGRAMS
KARNISKI, LAWRENCE P., M.D.	ASSOCIATE PROFESSOR
LAWTON, WILLIAM J., M.D.	ASSOCIATE PROFESSOR
FLANIGAN, MICHAEL J., M.D.	ASSISTANT PROFESSOR
KOPP, ULLA C., Ph.D.	ASSISTANT PROFESSOR
THOMAS, CHRISTIE P., M.D.	ASSISTANT PROFESSOR
HEGEMAN, REBECCA L., M.D.	ASSOCIATE
HOCHSTETLER, LINDA A., M.D.	ASSOCIATE
LAPLACE, JOAN R., D.O.	ASSOCIATE
SIDRYS, DEBBEE S., M.D.	ASSOCIATE
SOMERS, DOUGLAS L., M.D.	ASSOCIATE

DIVISION OF PULMONARY DISEASES, CRITICAL CARE & OCCUPATIONAL MEDICINE

HUNNINGHAKE, GARY W., M.D.	PROFESSOR & DIVISION DIRECTOR
BEDELL. GEORGE N., M.D.	PROFESSOR EMERITUS
KASIK, JOHN E., M.D., Ph.D.	PROFESSOR & CHIEF OF STAFF - VAMC
MERCHANT, JAMES A., M.D., Dr.P.H.	PROFESSOR [PREVENTIVE MEDICINE]
SHASBY, D. MICHAEL, M.D.	PROFESSOR & DIRECTOR OF FISCAL PROGRAMS
WELSH, MICHAEL J., M.D.	PROFESSOR & INVESTIGATOR, HOWARD HUGHES MEDICAL INSTITUTE PROFESSOR OF PHYSIOLOGY & BIOPHYSICS
ZAVALA, DONALD C., M.D.	PROFESSOR EMERITUS
FIESELMANN, JOHN F., M.D.	ASSOCIATE PROFESSOR & DIRECTOR, JOINT OFFICE FOR CLINICAL OUTREACH SERVICES & CONTRACTING FOR PATIENT CARE
HEMPEL, STEPHEN L., M.D.	ASSOCIATE PROFESSOR
KERN, JEFFREY A., M.D.	ASSOCIATE PROFESSOR
McGOWAN, STEPHEN E., M.D.	ASSOCIATE PROFESSOR
McLENNAN, GEOFFREY, M.D.	ASSOCIATE PROFESSOR
PETERSON, MICHAEL W., M.D.	ASSOCIATE PROFESSOR
SCHWARTZ, DAVID A., M.D.	ASSOCIATE PROFESSOR ASSOCIATE PROFESSOR OF PREVENTIVE MEDICINE
SPRINCE, NANCY L., M.D.	ASSOCIATE PROFESSOR [PREVENTIVE MEDICINE]
ZWERLING, CRAIG S., M.D., Ph.D.	ASSOCIATE PROFESSOR [PREVENTIVE MEDICINE]
BERGER, HERBERT A., M.D.	ASSISTANT PROFESSOR
DAVIDSON, BEVERLY L., Ph.D.	ASSISTANT PROFESSOR
FUORTES, LAURENCE J., M.D.	ASSISTANT PROFESSOR [PREVENTIVE MEDICINE]
GEIST, LOIS J., M.D.	ASSISTANT PROFESSOR
GROSS, THOMAS J., M.D.	ASSISTANT PROFESSOR
HARTLEY, PATRICK G., M.D.	ASSISTANT PROFESSOR/CLINICAL
HORNICK, DOUGLAS B., M.D.	ASSISTANT PROFESSOR
KLINE, JOEL N., M.D.	ASSISTANT PROFESSOR
MALLAMPALLI, RAMA K., M.D.	ASSISTANT PROFESSOR
MOY, ALAN B., M.D.	ASSISTANT PROFESSOR
WILSON, JEFF S., M.D.	ASSISTANT PROFESSOR
HOPKINS, HARVEY A.J., M.D.	ASSOCIATE
JAGIELO, PAUL J., M.D.	ASSOCIATE
LEAVELL, KEITH J., M.D.	ASSOCIATE
MASTRONARDE, JOHN G., M.D.	ASSOCIATE

DIVISION OF RHEUMATOLOGY

ASHMAN, ROBERT F., M.D.	PROFESSOR & DIVISION DIRECTOR PROFESSOR OF MICROBIOLOGY
COWDERY, JOHN S., M.D.	PROFESSOR & ASSOCIATE CHAIR FOR CLINICAL PROGRAMS
GOEKEN, NANCY E., Ph.D. PROFESSOR OF PATHOLOGY	PROFESSOR
BISHOP, GAIL A., Ph.D.	ASSOCIATE PROFESSOR [MICROBIOLOGY]
FIELD, ELIZABETH H., M.D.	ASSOCIATE PROFESSOR
KORETZKY, GARY A., M.D., Ph.D.	KELTING ASSOCIATE PROFESSOR OF RHEUMATOLOGY ASSOCIATE PROFESSOR OF PHYSIOLOGY & BIOPHYSICS
KRIEG, ARTHUR M., M.D.	ASSOCIATE PROFESSOR
NAIDES, STANLEY J., M.D.	ASSOCIATE PROFESSOR
STROTTMANN, M. PAUL, M.D.	ASSOCIATE PROFESSOR ASSOCIATE PROFESSOR OF ORTHOPAEDIC SURGERY
LAWRY, GEORGE V., II, M.D.	ASSISTANT PROFESSOR
RACHOW, JOHN W., Ph.D., M.D.	ASSISTANT PROFESSOR
SAAG, KENNETH G., M.D.	ASSISTANT PROFESSOR
VOGELGESANG, SCOTT A., M.D.	ASSISTANT PROFESSOR/CLINICAL

COMMUNITY CLINICAL FACULTY*

BROOKS, MICHAEL S.	CLINICAL ASSISTANT PROFESSOR	CEDAR RAPIDS
EYANSON, STEVEN	CLINICAL ASSISTANT PROFESSOR	CEDAR RAPIDS
HARB, NIDAL H.	CLINICAL INSTRUCTOR	CLINTON
LARSON, ERLING	CLINICAL ASSOCIATE PROFESSOR	DAVENPORT
MOTTO, EDWIN A.	CLINICAL ASSOCIATE PROFESSOR	DAVENPORT
GILLILLAND, JAMES L.	CLINICAL ASSISTANT PROFESSOR	DAVENPORT
HABAK, PHILIP A.	CLINICAL ASSISTANT PROFESSOR	DAVENPORT
VICKSTROM, DOUGLAS	CLINICAL ASSISTANT PROFESSOR	DAVENPORT
CHANDRAN, PREM K.G.	CLINICAL ASSOCIATE PROFESSOR	DES MOINES-INT MED RESIDENCY PROG
CRAIG, STEVEN R.	CLINICAL ASSOCIATE PROFESSOR	DES MOINES-INT MED RESIDENCY PROG
GLYNN, RUSSELL D.	CLINICAL ASSOCIATE PROFESSOR	DES MOINES-INT MED RESIDENCY PROG (VA)
LOUNGANI, RAMESH R.	CLINICAL ASSOCIATE PROFESSOR	DES MOINES-INT MED RESIDENCY PROG (VA)
SHADUR, CRAIG A.	CLINICAL ASSOCIATE PROFESSOR	DES MOINES-INT MED RESIDENCY PROG
WILLIAMS, CHAD	CLINICAL ASSOCIATE PROFESSOR	DES MOINES-INT MED RESIDENCY PROG
YANS, JAVAD	CLINICAL ASSOCIATE PROFESSOR	DES MOINES-INT MED RESIDENCY PROG
ALEXANDER, SARAMMA J.	CLINICAL ASSISTANT PROFESSOR	DES MOINES-INT MED RESIDENCY PROG
ALLEN, DANIEL PAUL	CLINICAL ASSISTANT PROFESSOR	DES MOINES-INT MED RESIDENCY PROG
ANDRINGA, DALE J.	CLINICAL ASSISTANT PROFESSOR	DES MOINES-INT MED RESIDENCY PROG
BAKER, LYNDA A.	CLINICAL ASSISTANT PROFESSOR	DES MOINES-INT MED RESIDENCY PROG (VA)
BASSIRI, RAHIM M.	CLINICAL ASSISTANT PROFESSOR	DES MOINES-INT MED RESIDENCY PROG
CHANDRAN, VIMALA V.	CLINICAL ASSISTANT PROFESSOR	DES MOINES-INT MED RESIDENCY PROG (VA)
ESPELAND, SUSAN L.	CLINICAL ASSISTANT PROFESSOR	DES MOINES-INT MED RESIDENCY PROG
FLOOD, MICHAEL T.	CLINICAL ASSISTANT PROFESSOR	DES MOINES-INT MED RESIDENCY PROG
GERLEMAN, BRENT F.	CLINICAL ASSISTANT PROFESSOR	DES MOINES-INT MED RESIDENCY PROG (VA)
GHALI, MAGDI G.H.	CLINICAL ASSISTANT PROFESSOR	DES MOINES-INT MED RESIDENCY PROG
GIBSON, JON D.	CLINICAL ASSISTANT PROFESSOR	DES MOINES-INT MED RESIDENCY PROG
GLAZIER, ADAM J., JR.	CLINICAL ASSISTANT PROFESSOR	DES MOINES-INT MED RESIDENCY PROG
HADE, JOEL E.	CLINICAL ASSISTANT PROFESSOR	DES MOINES-INT MED RESIDENCY PROG
HANSON, RANDALL R.	CLINICAL ASSISTANT PROFESSOR	DES MOINES-INT MED RESIDENCY PROG
HICKLIN, GREGORY A.	CLINICAL ASSISTANT PROFESSOR	DES MOINES-INT MED RESIDENCY PROG
LARSON, CHARLES C.	CLINICAL ASSISTANT PROFESSOR	DES MOINES-INT MED RESIDENCY PROG
LEMON, DAVID K.	CLINICAL ASSISTANT PROFESSOR	DES MOINES-INT MED RESIDENCY PROG
NAYERSINA, HOOSHMAND	CLINICAL ASSISTANT PROFESSOR	DES MOINES-INT MED RESIDENCY PROG (VA)
PARK, HEE-CHULL	CLINICAL ASSISTANT PROFESSOR	DES MOINES-INT MED RESIDENCY PROG (VA)
PIROS, JAMES G.	CLINICAL ASSISTANT PROFESSOR	DES MOINES-INT MED RESIDENCY PROG
PURTLE, MARK W.	CLINICAL ASSISTANT PROFESSOR	DES MOINES-INT MED RESIDENCY PROG
QUESTAD, DEANNA L.	CLINICAL ASSISTANT PROFESSOR	DES MOINES-INT MED RESIDENCY PROG
STARK, CRAIG A.	CLINICAL ASSISTANT PROFESSOR	DES MOINES-INT MED RESIDENCY PROG
VEACH, LISA A.	CLINICAL ASSISTANT PROFESSOR	DES MOINES-INT MED RESIDENCY PROG
VERSTEEG, DIRK A.	CLINICAL ASSISTANT PROFESSOR	DES MOINES-INT MED RESIDENCY PROG
VITURAWONG, VICHIT	CLINICAL ASSISTANT PROFESSOR	DES MOINES-INT MED RESIDENCY PROG (VA)
BEAR, PHILIP A.	CLINICAL INSTRUCTOR	DES MOINES-INT MED RESIDENCY PROG
BUNGE. STEVEN M.	CLINICAL INSTRUCTOR	DES MOINES-INT MED RESIDENCY PROG
COVERT, CHRISTOPHER M.	CLINICAL INSTRUCTOR	DES MOINES-INT MED RESIDENCY PROG
DUNLAP, STEVEN K.	CLINICAL INSTRUCTOR	DES MOINES-INT MED RESIDENCY PROG
GHRIST, JOHN H.	CLINICAL INSTRUCTOR	DES MOINES-INT MED RESIDENCY PROG
GUEST, KATRINA A.	CLINICAL INSTRUCTOR	DES MOINES-INT MED RESIDENCY PROG
KARAZIJA, PAUL A.	CLINICAL INSTRUCTOR	DES MOINES-INT MED RESIDENCY PROG
LOVELL, JAMES P.	CLINICAL INSTRUCTOR	DES MOINES-INT MED RESIDENCY PROG
LOZIER, CHARLES O.	CLINICAL INSTRUCTOR	DES MOINES-INT MED RESIDENCY PROG
RADIA, MARY A.	CLINICAL INSTRUCTOR	DES MOINES-INT MED RESIDENCY PROG
RUZKOWSKI, CHARLES J.	CLINICAL INSTRUCTOR	DES MOINES-INT MED RESIDENCY PROG
ROSENBERGER, JAY A.	CLINICAL INSTRUCTOR	DES MOINES-INT MED RESIDENCY PROG
SENNEFF, MARTHA J.	CLINICAL INSTRUCTOR	DES MOINES-INT MED RESIDENCY PROG
WILKINSON, SUSAN M.	CLINICAL INSTRUCTOR	DES MOINES-INT MED RESIDENCY PROG
BROWN, THOMAS M., JR.	CLINICAL ASSISTANT PROFESSOR	DES MOINES-IOWA LUTHERAN
GORDON, DAVID F.	CLINICAL ASSISTANT PROFESSOR	DES MOINES-IOWA LUTHERAN
IANNONE, LIBERATO A.	CLINICAL ASSISTANT PROFESSOR	DES MOINES-IOWA LUTHERAN
RIVER, GEORGE L.	CLINICAL ASSISTANT PROFESSOR	DUBUQUE
RUNDE, MARK P.	CLINICAL INSTRUCTOR	DUBUQUE
CHAMPION, M. CRAIG	CLINICAL ASSOCIATE PROFESSOR	IOWA CITY-TOWNCREST
LARSEN, KARL	CLINICAL ASSOCIATE PROFESSOR	IOWA CITY-TOWNCREST
NICKNISH, THOMAS R.	CLINICAL ASSOCIATE PROFESSOR	IOWA CITY-TOWNCREST
FEELEY, JAMES E.	CLINICAL ASSISTANT PROFESSOR	IOWA CITY-TOWNCREST
LITTLE, MARTA M.	CLINICAL ASSISTANT PROFESSOR	IOWA CITY-TOWNCREST
SIRNA, SARA J.	CLINICAL ASSISTANT PROFESSOR	IOWA CITY-TOWNCREST
CAMPBELL, CAM F.	CLINICAL INSTRUCTOR	IOWA CITY-TOWNCREST

*Non-salaried faculty

301

FACULTY, 1996 (*continued*)

EWING, R. JOE	CLINICAL INSTRUCTOR	IOWA CITY-TOWNCREST
AUSTIN, MILTON F.	CLINICAL INSTRUCTOR	KEOKUK
DAVIS, WILSON L., JR.	CLINICAL INSTRUCTOR	KEOKUK
HAKES, THOMAS E.	CLINICAL INSTRUCTOR	KEOKUK
CAPLAN, ROBERT H.	CLINICAL ASSOCIATE PROFESSOR	LACROSSE, WI-GUNDERSEN CLINIC
DAHLBERG, PHILIP J.	CLINICAL ASSISTANT PROFESSOR	LACROSSE, WI-GUNDERSON CLINIC
WINGA, EDWARD R.	CLINICAL ASSISTANT PROFESSOR	LACROSSE, WI-GUNDERSON CLINIC
GLASSER, JAMES E.	CLINICAL INSTRUCTOR	LACROSSE, WI-GUNDERSEN CLINIC
KEIMOWITZ, RUDOLPH M.	CLINICAL INSTRUCTOR	LACROSSE, WI-GUNDERSEN CLINIC
LOCKHART, JACK M.	CLINICAL INSTRUCTOR	LACROSSE, WI-GUNDERSEN CLINIC
WILDE, JAMES G.	CLINICAL INSTRUCTOR	LACROSSE, WI-GUNDERSEN CLINIC
ZURBRIGGEN, THOMAS L.	CLINICAL INSTRUCTOR	LACROSSE, WI-GUNDERSEN CLINIC
TRIMBLE, RICHARD B.	CLINICAL ASSOCIATE PROFESSOR	MASON CITY
BATE, WALTER W.	CLINICAL ASSISTANT PROFESSOR	MASON CITY
BEASLEY, BYRON T.	CLINICAL ASSISTANT PROFESSOR	MASON CITY
THORESON, JOSEPH D.	CLINICAL ASSISTANT PROFESSOR	MASON CITY
CAUGHLAN, CHARLES R.	CLINICAL INSTRUCTOR	MASON CITY
SILBERSTEIN, PETER T.	CLINICAL INSTRUCTOR	MASON CITY
BENNETT, JOHN P.	CLINICAL ASSISTANT PROFESSOR	MT. PLEASANT
BALLER, JOHN T.	CLINICAL ASSISTANT PROFESSOR	SIOUX CITY
VANBRAMER, EDWARD L.	CLINICAL INSTRUCTOR	SIOUX CITY
RICHARDS, CARL J.	CLINICAL ASSOCIATE PROFESSOR	WATERLOO
JOSEPHSON, NATHAN	CLINICAL ASSOCIATE PROFESSOR	DM AREA CONSORTIUM

EMERITUS FACULTY

BEASLEY, OSCAR C.	CLIN ASSOC PROFESSOR EMERITUS	IOWA CITY-TOWNCREST
SCHROCK, CHRISTIAN E.	CLIN ASSOC PROFESSOR EMERITUS	IOWA CITY-TOWNCREST
SPELLMAN, GEORGE G., SR.	CLIN ASSOC PROFESSOR EMERITUS	SIOUX CITY
STAPLES, LAWRENCE F.	CLIN ASSOC PROFESSOR EMERITUS	DES MOINES-IOWA METHODIST

INDEX

Abboud, François M.
awards, 168
biography, an American success story, 214-219
Cardiovascular Research Center, 180
Central Society for Clinical Research, 168
as chair of Internal Medicine, 218
changing aspects of medical research, 217-219
editorial role, 219
as head of Cardiovascular Diseases Division, 217
health services research, 259
ICU and, 176
John Eckstein and, 216-217
photograph, 94, 156, 247
role in medical societies, 219
as president of the American Heart Association, 219
as president of the American Association of Physicians, 219
ABIM. *See* American Board of Internal Medicine
Academic medicine
from 1945-1960, 113-116
from 1960-1975, 157-159
from 1975-1990, 211-214
in 1990s, 257-260
beginnings of, 31
government and, 57, 77
pharmaceutical industry and, 213
politics and, 255, 256
public distrust of, 213
research *vs.* teaching, 185-186
revenue-raising activities in, 225
Accountability, in health care, 212
Accreditation, increase in standards for, 62-64

ACP. *See* American College of Physicians
Adjunct assistant professors, establishment of position, 222
Administration
from 1960-1975, 173-175, 186-187
Executive Committee, 144-149
faculty involvement in
from 1910-1928, 52-54
from 1960-1975, 201-207
growth of committee system, 149-151
Administrative Structure, Committee on, 203
Admissions
improving standards for, 21
restrictions, 61-62, 134
tests, 258
African Americans
as medical school faculty, 163
as medical students
from 1960-1975, 189
from 1975-1990, 234
Agency for Health Care Policy and Research, 259
Agriculture
Depression and, 58
opponents to funding for new university hospital, 44, 46
positive outlook in 1922, 47
1980s recession in, 211-212
AIDS Advisory Committee of the Health Resources and Services Administration, 230
AIDS Training and Education Center, Midwest, 230
Alcock, Nathaniel G.
characteristics, 104
on federal funding for medical education, 143-144
on postwar physician shortage, 136